Multi-Criteria Decision Analysis to Support Healthcare Decisions

AF716033

Kevin Marsh • Mireille Goetghebeur
Praveen Thokala • Rob Baltussen
Editors

Multi-Criteria Decision Analysis to Support Healthcare Decisions

Springer

Editors
Kevin Marsh
Evidera
London
United Kingdom

Praveen Thokala
University of Sheffield
Sheffield
United Kingdom

Mireille Goetghebeur
School of Public Health
University of Montreal
and LASER Analytica
Montréal
Québec
Canada

Rob Baltussen
Radboud University Medical Center
Nijmegen
The Netherlands

ISBN 978-3-319-83763-5 ISBN 978-3-319-47540-0 (eBook)
DOI 10.1007/978-3-319-47540-0

© Springer International Publishing AG 2017
Softcover reprint of the hardcover 1st edition 2017
This work is subject to copyright. All rights are reserved by the Publisher, whether the whole or part of the material is concerned, specifically the rights of translation, reprinting, reuse of illustrations, recitation, broadcasting, reproduction on microfilms or in any other physical way, and transmission or information storage and retrieval, electronic adaptation, computer software, or by similar or dissimilar methodology now known or hereafter developed.
The use of general descriptive names, registered names, trademarks, service marks, etc. in this publication does not imply, even in the absence of a specific statement, that such names are exempt from the relevant protective laws and regulations and therefore free for general use.
The publisher, the authors and the editors are safe to assume that the advice and information in this book are believed to be true and accurate at the date of publication. Neither the publisher nor the authors or the editors give a warranty, express or implied, with respect to the material contained herein or for any errors or omissions that may have been made. The publisher remains neutral with regard to jurisdictional claims in published maps and institutional affiliations.

Printed on acid-free paper

This Springer imprint is published by Springer Nature
The registered company is Springer International Publishing AG
The registered company address is: Gewerbestrasse 11, 6330 Cham, Switzerland

Contents

Chapter 1
Introduction

Kevin Marsh, Mireille Goetghebeur, Praveen Thokala, and Rob Baltussen

Abstract Multi-criteria decision analysis (MCDA) has the potential to support better healthcare decision making. But a number of challenges need to be overcome before it can achieve its potential. These are both technical – which weighting methods are most appropriate and how should uncertainty be dealt with – and political, the need to work with decision makers to get their support for such approaches. This collection is a first attempt to identify and address these challenges by bringing together MCDA practitioners from what has to date been a relatively fragmented research community. This introductory chapter describes the potential of MCDA in healthcare; provides an outline of the chapters in the collection, the process of developing the collection; and identifies key question, the answers to which will determine the future direction of MCDA in healthcare.

1.1 Introduction

Increased awareness of how multi-criteria decision analysis (MCDA) can support healthcare decision making has resulted in an increased interest in and application of MCDA in healthcare. As with any new technique, however, achieving the potential of MCDA in healthcare faces a number of challenges. To those unfamiliar with MCDA, the diversity of approaches and uses can often be a barrier to its use,

K. Marsh (✉)
Evidera, London, UK
e-mail: kevin.marsh@evidera.com

M. Goetghebeur, MEng PhD
School of Public Health, University of Montreal
and LASER Analytica, Montréal, Québec, Canada
e-mail: mm.goetghebeur@umontreal.ca

P. Thokala
University of Sheffield, Sheffield, UK
e-mail: p.thokala@sheffield.ac.uk

R. Baltussen
Radboud University Medical Center, Nijmegen, The Netherlands
e-mail: Rob.Baltussen@radboudumc.nl

© Springer International Publishing AG 2017
K. Marsh et al. (eds.), *Multi-Criteria Decision Analysis to Support Healthcare Decisions*, DOI 10.1007/978-3-319-47540-0_1

making it difficult to understand what it is and how it can best be used. This obstacle is compounded by the fragmented nature of the MCDA research community, with practitioners coming from different academic and policy backgrounds, recommending different approaches and there being no space for this community to meet, share ideas, learn from each other and develop a more coherent vision for the application of MCDA in healthcare. We envisioned this collection of papers as a first step in overcoming some of these obstacles.

MCDA is the collective heading for several analytical techniques used to support decision making in the context of multiple, conflicting criteria (Belton and Stewart 2002). These techniques support decision makers to agree which assessment criteria are relevant, the importance attached to each and how to use this information to assess alternatives. By doing so, they can help increase the consistency, transparency and legitimacy of decisions.

MCDA comprises a broad set of methodological approaches, originating from operations research, yet with a rich intellectual grounding in other disciplines (Kaksalan et al. 2011). They are widely used in both public- and private-sector decisions on transport, immigration, education, investment, environment, energy, defence, etc. (Dodgson et al. 2009). The healthcare sector has been relatively slow to apply MCDA. But as more researchers and practitioners have become aware of the techniques, there has been a sharp increase in its healthcare application (Diaby et al. 2013; Marsh et al. 2014).

The application of MCDA to healthcare should be seen as a natural extension of evidence-based medicine (EBM) and associated practices, such as health technology assessment. Over the past 40 years, the provision of healthcare has been revolutionised by the use of EBM – the systematic reviewing, appraisal and use of clinical research to aid the delivery of optimum clinical care to patients (see Belsey 2009). Whilst the achievements of EBM are not to be underestimated, it has to date only addressed part of the challenge facing healthcare decision making – the rigorous measurement of the performance of alternatives. This emphasis of EBM is continued by MCDA. But MCDA also provides a set of techniques for determining which elements of performance should be measured, how stakeholder preferences for changes performance should be elicited and how data on performance and preferences should be combined to assess alternatives. By doing so, MCDA allows the rigour which EBM has brought to the quantification of performance to be extended to the understanding of stakeholders preferences (Weernink et al. 2014).

Healthcare decisions are rarely simple, involving multiple factors, multiple options, imperfect information and diverse stakeholder preferences. EBM has established the importance of rigorous measurement of alternatives against multiple factors. Using this information can, however, still involve significant cognitive burden. Decision makers have difficulty processing and systematically evaluating relevant information, a process that involves trading off between multiple factors. In these circumstances, relying on informal processes or judgements can lead to suboptimal decisions (Baltussen and Niessen 2006). MCDA provides support and structure to the decision-making process to overcome such challenges.

A challenge for users of MCDA, however, is that there are many different MCDA methods available; the current field is fragmented, with methods being selected based on researchers' background and previous experience, rather than a systematic consideration of the 'best' approach; and there is little guidance on how to choose between the available approaches (Marsh et al. 2014). The objective of this collection is to support the use of MCDA in healthcare by, for the first time, bringing together researchers specialising in numerous approaches and healthcare decisions and giving the reader the benefit of this rich experience. To support the reader to select between MCDA techniques, we illustrate and critically appraise this diversity of MCDA approaches as applied to healthcare, summarise the ethical and theoretical foundations of MCDA and offer good practice guidelines when using MCDA in healthcare to help the reader select between MCDA techniques.

1.2 Process of Developing the Book

We were approached by Springer in April 2014 to produce a collection of papers on MCDA, specifically 'Healthcare Decisions Supported by Multi-Criteria Decision Analysis'. Our first steps were to put together an outline of the book (see below), develop a brief description of each chapter and identify authors who we would ideally want to lead the writing of each chapter. We were delighted at the response from our lead authors, who were all enthusiastic about contributing to the collection.

In what is quite unusual for most books, we were able to organise a face-to-face workshop to bring authors together to present and discuss their chapters. The workshop was held in Amsterdam late June 2015 and was made possible by funding from Radboud University Medical Center, through a personal VICI grant obtained by Rob Baltussen from the Netherlands Organisation for Scientific Research (NWO). There was a great turnout, with all but one of the chapters being represented by an author. All the chapters were presented, received comments from a nominated discussant (lead author from another chapter) and discussed by the attendees. This workshop provided everyone with a better idea of how the collection is structured, where their chapters fits in, and with comments to take on board as they finalised their chapters. We would like to thank Evelinn Mikkelsen for her support in organising this workshop.

1.3 Outline of the Book

This book is organised into different sections, each with a different emphasis. Before we get into the detail, it should be noted that most of the examples presented in the book are weighted-sum MCDA models (value measurement approaches). Whilst we acknowledge that there are other MCDA approaches (see Chapter 15 for an overview of these non-value measurement methods), most of the applications of MCDA in healthcare are value measurement methods, and thus, this has also been the focus of this book.

Section one presents the foundations of MCDA as it is applied to healthcare decisions, providing guidance on the ethical and theoretical underpinnings of MCDA, and how to select MCDA methods appropriate to different decision settings. Chapter 2 presents the theoretical foundations, and Chapter 3 presents the ethical aspects of MCDA in healthcare. Chapter 4 highlights the diversity of weighting/scoring methods in MCDA and addresses their relative merits and weaknesses. Chapter 5 considers alternative approaches for dealing with uncertainty in MCDA.

Section two comprises a collection of case studies spanning the decision continuum, including portfolio development, benefit-risk assessment, health technology assessment, priority setting, resource optimisation, clinical practice and shared decision making. Chapter 6 presents optimisation of a robotics research and development portfolio using MACBETH. Chapter 7 illustrates the use of MCDA for benefit-risk analysis of drugs. Chapter 8 presents the experiences of Health Technology Assessment (HTA) agencies with MCDA in Colombia, Italy and Belgium. Chapter 9 presents the experiences of using MCDA for priority setting in low- and middle-income countries. Chapter 10 presents a case study of the use of MCDA for resource allocation in South Yorkshire, UK. Chapter 11 presents the use of conjoint analysis and analytic hierarchy process for shared decision making in clinical settings. Chapter 12 highlights the similarities between health research priority setting and health intervention priority setting and presents suggestions for future methodological research. Chapter 13 presents applications of MCDA for clinical practice guidelines and clinical research prioritisation.

Section three explores future directions in the application of MCDA to healthcare. Chapter 14 highlights the issues and opportunities associated with the use of MCDA within HTA. Chapter 15 presents the non-value-based measurement methods and when conditions under which they would be appropriate. Finally, Chapter 16 presents the good practice general principles that need consideration during the design, conduct and analysis of MCDA in healthcare.

1.4 Future Direction

This collection presents the current state of reflection, knowledge and applications on MCDA for healthcare decision making worldwide. Future developments rest on providing clear answers to simple questions: Why do we need MCDA in healthcare? What can it bring? Is it worth it?

As healthcare users, providers and payers around the world are facing critical ethical dilemmas, current decision-making approaches are reaching their limits. EBM was developed to ensure best choices at a clinical level, health economics to ensure informed allocation of resources and HTA to ensure best choices and health system sustainability. However, the need to go beyond these approach is highlighted by the controversy on an 'acceptably cost-effective' treatment for hepatitis C, which is challenging the sustainability of healthcare systems worldwide (Neuman and Cohen 2015) and issues raised by the reimbursement of treatments for patients with rare diseases which require consideration of many aspects that are not formally contained in current HTA methods (Wagner et al. 2016). Our time calls for ways to define value of interventions based on the social values on which healthcare systems are founded to guide prioritisation and investment in interventions with highest value and disinvestment of those with low value. MCDA is poised to build on EBM and HTA to provide an integrative methodology to help tackle these current challenges and transition into healthcare of the twenty-first century.

As illustrated in the present collection, MCDA offers a structured approach to support reasonable and accountable decision making (Daniels and Sabin 1997). Doing this at either individual or collective levels, it can support many decisions to improve population outcomes and promote sustainability, including shared decision making, clinical research, clinical practice guidelines, portfolio development, health technology assessment, priority setting and resource optimisation.

Transitioning to a wider use of MCDA will require some adaptation to address healthcare specificities. Technical aspects of MCDA will have to be developed with the end of healthcare decision makers in mind. This will require answer to the following questions: Whose preference matter for different decisions? Which weighting methods are most appropriate for different decisions? How can uncertainty in MCDA be dealt with to support decision makers? How can opportunity cost be measured in a MCDA framework? Research and debates are required on best approaches to tackle these issues.

Beyond the technical questions, further work is required to manage decision makers' concerns about the function of MCDA. Specifically, decision makers may have the perception that MCDA is a way to replace reflection and to algorithmically make decisions. It is important to educate decision makers that MCDA is designed to support reflection to ensure balanced and accountable decision-making processes. Decision makers should also be engaged on the principles that inform decision making and how these relate to the assumptions underlying alternative MCDA approaches.

In conclusion, MCDA can help us develop a healthcare system focused on what truly matters to patients and populations, in a fair and sustainable manner. Given this potential, the time has come for MCDA developers and users to answer the above questions and demonstrate the value that these methods can bring. We hope this collection is a first step in the process, demonstrating where MCDA has been used in healthcare to date, drawing the lessons from this experience and identifying the research agenda required for MCDA to achieve its potential.

References

Baltussen R, Niessen L (2006) Priority setting of health interventions: the need for multi-criteria decision analysis. Cost Eff Resour Alloc 4:14

Belsey J (2009) What is evidence-based medicine? Hayward Medical Communications, London

Belton V, Stewart TJ (2002) Multiple criteria decision analysis: an integrated approach. Kluwer Academic Publishers, Boston

Daniels N, Sabin J (1997) Limits to health care: fair procedures, democratic deliberation, and the legitimacy problem for insurers. Philos Public Aff 26(4):303–350

Diaby V, Campbell K, Goeree R (2013) Multi-criteria decision analysis (MCDA) in health care: a bibliometric analysis. Oper Res Health Care 2(1–2):20–24

Dodgson J, Spackman M, Pearman A, Phillips L. (2009) Multi-criteria analysis: a manual. Department for Communities and Local Government. London. http://www.communities.gov.uk/documents/corporate/pdf/1132618.pdf

Kaksalan M, Wallenius J, Zionts S (2011) Multiple criteria decision making from early history to the 21st century. World Scientific, Singapore

Neuman P, Cohen J (2015) Measuring the value of prescription drugs. N Engl J Med 20:1–4

Marsh K, Lanitis T, Neasham D et al (2014) Assessing the value of health care interventions using multi-criteria decision analysis: a review of the literature. Pharmacoeconomics 32(4):345–65

Wagner M, Khoury H, Willet J, Rindress D, Goetghebeur M (2016) Can the EVIDEM framework tackle issues raised by evaluating treatments for rare diseases: analysis of issues and policies, and context-specific adaptation. Pharmacoeconomics 34(3):285–301

Weernink MGM, Janus SIM, van Til JA, Raisch DW, van Manen JG, Ijzerman MJ (2014) A systematic review to identify the use of preference elicitation method in healthcare decision making. Pharm Med 28:175–185

Part I
Foundations of MCDA in Healthcare

Chapter 2
Theoretical Foundations of MCDA

Dean A. Regier and Stuart Peacock

Abstract Decision-makers in the healthcare sector face a global challenge of developing robust, evidence-based methods for making decisions about whether to fund, cover, or reimburse medical technologies. Allocating scarce resources across technologies is difficult because a range of criteria are relevant to a healthcare decision, including the effectiveness, cost-effectiveness, and budget impact of the technology; the incidence, prevalence, and severity of the disease; the affected population group; the availability of alternative technologies; and the quality of the available evidence. When comparing healthcare technologies, decision-makers often need to make trade-offs between these criteria. Multi-criteria decision analysis (MCDA) is a tool that helps decision-makers summarize complex value trade-offs in a way that is consistent and transparent. It is comprised of a set of techniques that bring about an ordering of alternative decisions from most to least preferred, where each technology is ranked based on the extent to which it creates value through achieving a set of policy objectives. The purpose of this chapter was to provide a brief overview of the theoretical foundations of MCDA. We reviewed theories related to problem structuring and model building. We found problem structuring aimed to qualitatively determine policy objectives and the relevant criteria of value that affect decision-making. Model building theories sought to construct consistent representations of decision-makers' preferences and value trade-offs through value measurement models (multi-attribute value theory, multi-attribute utility theory, and the analytical hierarchy process), outranking (ELECTRE), and reference (weighted

D.A. Regier (✉)
Canadian Centre for Applied Research in Cancer Control (ARCC), Cancer Control Research, British Columbia Cancer Agency, Vancouver, BC, Canada

School of Population and Public Health, University of British Columbia, Vancouver, BC, Canada
e-mail: dregier@bccrc.ca

S. Peacock
Canadian Centre for Applied Research in Cancer Control (ARCC), Cancer Control Research, British Columbia Cancer Agency, Vancouver, BC, Canada

Faculty of Health Sciences, Simon Fraser University, Burnaby, BC, Canada

© Springer International Publishing AG 2017

K. Marsh et al. (eds.), *Multi-Criteria Decision Analysis to Support Healthcare Decisions*, DOI 10.1007/978-3-319-47540-0_2

and lexicographic goal programming) models. We conclude that MCDA theory has largely been developed in other fields, and there is a need to develop MCDA theory that is adapted to the healthcare context.

2.1 Introduction

Decision-makers in the healthcare sector face a global challenge of employing robust, evidence-based methods when making decisions about whether to fund, cover, or reimburse medical technologies. Historically, technology assessment agencies promoted cost-effectiveness analysis as the primary decision aid for appraising competing claims on limited healthcare budgets. The recommended metric to summarize cost-effectiveness, the incremental cost-effectiveness ratio (ICER), has the incremental costs of competing technologies in the numerator and quality-adjusted life years (QALY) gained in the denominator (Drummond 2005). Judgment surrounding value for money is determined against a cost-effectiveness threshold, which represents the opportunity cost to the healthcare sector of choosing one technology over another. While cost-effectiveness analysis is a necessary component when informing resource-constrained decisions, it is not a sufficient condition. This is because a range of criteria are relevant, including the incidence, prevalence, and severity of the disease; the population group affected; the availability of alternative technologies; the quality of the available evidence; and whether the technology contributes technological innovation (Devlin and Sussex 2011). Technology assessment agencies have gone as far as publishing the criteria they consider in their decision-making contexts, including how each criterion may be reflected in funding decisions (NICE 2008; Rawlins et al. 2010).

Publishing the criteria that decision-makers consider when setting priorities can provide clarity for stakeholders on how committees make decisions (Devlin and Sussex 2011). Making explicit the extent to which decision criteria influence program funding will enhance the legitimacy, transparency, and accountability of decisions and will encourage public trust in the decision-making process (Regier et al. 2014a; Rowe and Frewer 2000). Further, it will improve the consistency of decisions, can provide an opportunity for decision-makers to engage the public, and can serve to sharpen the signal to industry about what aspects of innovation are important and where research and development efforts should be directed (Devlin and Sussex 2011).

Multi-criteria decision analysis (MCDA) represents a set of methods that decision-makers can use when considering multiple criteria in priority-setting activities. It is a decision aid that helps stakeholders summarize complex value trade-offs in a way that is consistent and transparent, thus leading to fairer decision-making (Peacock et al. 2009). MCDA makes explicit the criteria applied and the relative importance of the criteria. As such, MCDA is a process that integrates objective measurement with value judgment while also attempting to manage subjectivity

(Belton and Stewart 2002). To enable these goals, the theories and methodologies supporting MCDA need to allow for both the technical and nontechnical aspects of decision-making; they need to include sophisticated quantitative algorithms while also providing structure to a decision-making process. All help to promote the replicability and transparency of policy decisions (Belton and Stewart 2002).

The purpose of this chapter is to provide an overview of the theoretical foundations of MCDA. Particular attention is given to two key parts of MCDA: problem structuring and model building. Problem structuring refers to determining policy objectives through methods that illuminate the policy-relevant criteria. Model building requires constructing consistent representations of decision-makers' values and value trade-offs. MCDA theory in healthcare is under-researched - for this reason, we draw on theories developed in other disciplines in the following sections.

2.2 Principles of MCDA and Decision-Making

MCDA begins with decision-makers encountering a choice between at least two alternative courses of action. A key principle of MCDA is that decision-makers consider several objectives when judging the desirability of a particular course of action (Keeney and Raiffa 1993). It is unlikely that any one program will satisfy all objectives or that one course of action dominates another. Each program will meet the policy objectives at different levels, and trade-offs will be inherent when making decisions (Belton and Stewart 2002). Policy objectives can be thought of as the criteria against which each program is judged. Choosing one program over another will entail opportunity cost. The decision is one where multiple objectives (criteria) need to be balanced and acceptable. The aim of decision-makers is to make the best choice between alternative courses of action that are characterized by multiple criteria (Belton and Stewart 2002). Doing so can help ensure that decisions are consistent with the policy objectives.

These key principles suggest several basic assumptions of MCDA. First, decisions are made under constrained resources – not all programs can be funded and choosing one program over another will entail opportunity cost. Second, decision-makers' objectives are within their personal discretion and are not normatively determined by theories from ethics or economics, such as utilitarianism or social justice (Peacock et al. 2009). Third, a program cannot be thought of as a homogenous "good." Instead, multiple levels of criteria can describe each alternative program and decision-makers weigh and value each criterion level (Lancaster 1966). Decision-makers can relate the criteria levels to the program alternatives, and incremental changes in criteria can cause a switch from one good with a specific bundle of characteristics to another good with a different combination that is more beneficial. A fourth assumption supporting MCDA value theories is that trade-offs and the relative importance of criteria can be established or that such scores can allow for a rank ordering of programs (Baltussen and Niessen 2006; Baltussen et al. 2006).

2.3 Problem Structuring

Problem structuring is the process of stakeholders identifying policy objectives and decision criteria that they determine are of value (Belton and Stewart 2002). Model building and the use of quantitative methods to determine value were the focus of early MCDA applications. The literature has increasingly acknowledged the importance of problem structuring (Phillips 1984; Schoner et al. 1999). This is due to the recognition that failing to adequately frame and structure the policy problem increases the likelihood of committing a type III error, that is, getting the right answer to the wrong question (Kimball 1957). The theory behind problem structuring begins with understanding the nature of MCDA. Definitionally, MCDA is an aid to decision-making that relates alternative courses of action to conflicting multiple criteria requiring value trade-offs. The decision criteria are determined in relation to decision-makers' objectives. It follows that decision-makers can have differing values with varying sets of objectives and preferences. Decision-makers can dispute which objectives are "right" when choosing between healthcare programs, whether it be to maximize health status, to solve a political problem, or to balance trade-offs between health status and equity. Equally, the solution to any objective is debateable because decision-makers' weightings of criterion will not be homogeneous, possibly leading to different solutions to the problem. Using Ackoff's (1979a, b) lexicon of defining types of decision problems, Belton and Stewart (2010) argue that the MCDA problem can be termed "messy" because both the definition and solution to the problem are arguable. Contributing to the messy categorization is that MCDA criteria can be based on evidence from the hard or soft sciences (objectives are quantitative versus qualitatively assessed) (Goetghebeur et al. 2008). Hester and Adams (2014) defined messy problems as the intersection between hard and soft sciences (Fig. 2.1).

A key component to addressing messy-type problems is the use of facilitation to identify values and frame the multi-criteria problem (Keeney and Mcdaniels 1992). Following Keeney (1992), decision-makers' core values determine strategic objectives, criteria, and decisions. While decision-makers are likely to know their latent values, their values can change as new information becomes available (Schoner et al. 1999). The goal of facilitation is to translate latent values to make statements regarding the objectives and the set of criteria, the set of alternatives from which to make decisions, and the methods that will be used characterize criteria weights (Belton and Stewart 2002).

Diverging perspectives between decision-makers coupled with system-wide implications suggest that decision-makers may elect to include input from multiple stakeholders. Stakeholders can be identified by focusing on the nature of the health system (Checkland 1981). In soft systems methodology, one framework proposed the following checklist to understand the system and stakeholders under the acronym CATWOE: *Customers* are individuals who are directly affected by the system; *Actors* are individuals carrying out the system activities; *Transformation* is the purpose of the system; *World View* includes the societal purposes of the system; *Owners* are

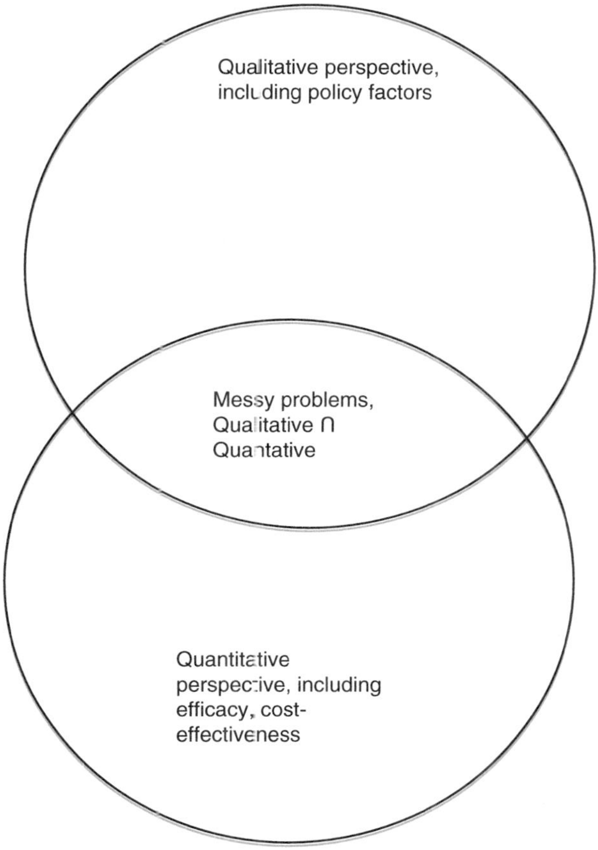

Fig. 2.1 An illustration of messes

those who control system activities; and *Environment* includes the demands and constraints external to the system. Stakeholders can include representatives from government, key decision-makers at institutions, clinicians, healthcare professionals, patients, the lay public, or drug developers. It is emphasized that the inclusion of stakeholders and the extent that stakeholders' views are included in the facilitation process is under the discretion of decision-makers (Belton and Stewart 2002).

Consideration should be given to the idea that stakeholders can exert varying degrees of power to over- or under-influence a particular decision, or to be included as a token participant with little input into the discourse (Arnstein 1969). To mitigate the potential for power structures, facilitation can focus on using deliberative theories that adhere to a process of respectful engagement, where stakeholders' positions are justified and challenged by others, and conclusions represent group efforts to find common ground (O'Doherty et al. 2012; MacLean and Burgess 2010). The facilitator can strive to understand what is going on in the group and should attend to relationships between participants while being aware that they need to intervene to forward the work of the group (Phillips and Phillips 1993).

Whether or not stakeholders with different backgrounds are included in problem structuring, varying frames will emerge during facilitation (Roy 1996). A frame is a cognitive bias that exists when individuals react differently to a criterion depending on how the information is represented (e.g., number of years gained versus number of years lost) (Belton and Stewart 2010). Through facilitation, decision-makers need to acknowledge frames such that stakeholders can similarly understand the criterion. To do this, Belton and Stewart (2002) identified the following set of general properties to consider, which include domains related to value relevance, measurability, nonredundancy, judgmental independence, completeness, and operationality.

- *Relevance*: Can decision-makers link conceptual objectives to criteria, which will frame their preferences? For example, a criterion may include the cost-effectiveness of a competing program, and an associated objective would be to pursue programs that provide value for money.
- *Measurability*: MCDA implies a degree of measuring the desirability of an alternative against criteria. Consideration should be given regarding the ability to measure or characterize the value of the specified criteria in a consistent manner by allowing for criteria to be decomposed to a number of criteria attribute levels.
- *Nonredundancy*: The criteria should be mutually exclusive with a view to avoid double counting and to allow for parsimony. When eliciting objectives and defining criteria, decision-makers may identify the same concept but under different headings. If both are included, there is a possibility the criteria will be attributed greater importance by virtue of overlap. If persistent disagreement regarding double counting exists in the facilitation process, double counting can be avoided through differentiating between process objectives (how an end is achieved) and fundamental objectives, ensuring that only the latter are incorporated (Keeney and Mcdaniels 1992).
- *Judgmental independence*: This refers to preferences and trade-offs between criteria being independent of one another. This category should be taken in light of preference value functions.
- *Completeness and operationality*: Refers to all important aspects of the problem are being captured in a way that is exhaustive but parsimonious. This is balanced against operationality, which aims to model the decision in a way that does not place excessive demands on decision-makers.

There is a broad literature based on psychology and behavioral economics outlining how judgment and decision-making depart from "rational" normative assumptions (Kahneman 2003). For a comprehensive review of techniques directed at improving judgment, interested readers are referred to Montibeller and von Winterfeldt (2015).

2.4 Model Building

Model building refers to constructing a behavioral model that can quantitatively represent decision-makers' preferences or value judgments. MCDA models originate from different theoretical traditions, but most have in common two components: (1) preferences are first expressed for each individual criterion; and (2) an aggregation model allows for comparison between criteria with a view to combine preference estimates across criteria (Belton and Stewart 2002). The aggregation model establishes a preference ordering across program alternatives. A bird's-eye view of the decision objective(s) is represented through a hierarchical value tree, where there are m criteria at the lowest level of the hierarchy (Fig. 2.2). The broadest objective is at the top. As decision-makers move down the hierarchy, more specific criteria are defined. This continues until the lowest-level criteria are defined in such a way that a clear ordering of value can be determined for each alternative (Belton and Stewart 2002). Generally, aggregation can be applied across the tree or in terms of the parent criteria located at higher levels of the hierarchy.

The following section highlights several underlying theories used in MCDA that support model building through value measurement models, including multi-attribute value theory, multi-attribute utility theory, and the analytical hierarchy process; outranking, focusing on ELECTRE; and reference models using weighted goal and lexicographic goal programming. While the theories described are not comprehensive, we have chosen methods that represent the major theoretical approaches supporting MCDA.

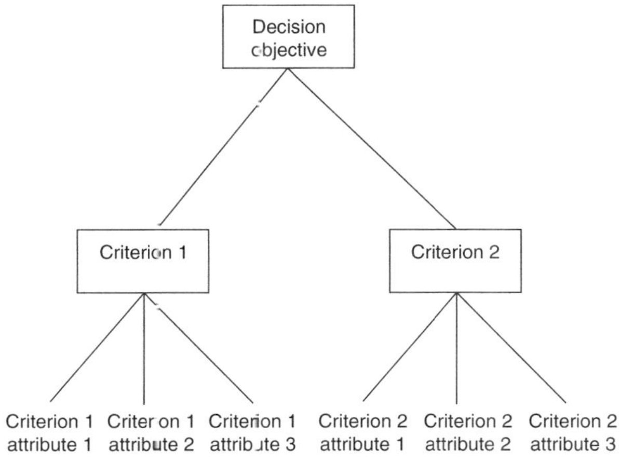

Fig. 2.2 Hierarchical value tree

2.4.1 Value Measurement

Value measurement models aggregate preferences across criterion to allow decision-makers to characterize the degree to which one alternative program is preferred to another (Belton and Stewart 2002). The challenge is to associate decision-makers' preferences to a quantitative real number such that each program alternative can be compared in a consistent and meaningful way. Value measurement approaches have been cited as the most applied methods in MCDA in the healthcare context (Dolan 2010).

2.4.1.1 Multi-attribute Value Theory

The principle that decision-makers want to make consistent decisions is the key building block for multi-attribute value theory. The notion of consistency is formalized through two preference-based assumptions: (i) completeness – any two alternatives can be compared such that alternative a is preferred to alternative b, or b is preferred to c, or they are equally preferred – and (ii) transitivity, if a is preferred to b and b is preferred to c, then a is preferred to c. These assumptions – called axioms in economic utility theory (Mas-Colell et al. 1995) – provide the necessary building blocks for a mathematical proof of the existence of a real-valued function that can represent preferences. That is, these assumptions allow for statements regarding the ability of quantitative values for a program alternative, denoted as $V(a)$ for alternative program a, to represent preferences such that $V(a) \geq V(b)$ if and only if $a \gtrsim b$, where $\gtrsim$ is a binary preference relation meaning "at least as good as"; or $V(a) = V(b)$ if and only if $a \sim b$, where $\sim$ denotes indifference between the value of a good. Depending on the context and complexity of the decision problem, the assumptions of completeness and transitivity can be violated in real-world contexts (Camerer 1995; Rabin 1998). In value measurement theory, these axioms provide a guide for coherent decisions but are not applied literally (Belton and Stewart 2002). That is, the axioms are not dogma.

The next set of definitions outline the value score of the criteria. A partial value function, denoted a $v_i(a)$ for program a, is needed such that $v_i(a) > v_i(b)$ when criteria i for program a are preferred to b after consideration of the opportunity costs (also called "trade-offs," i.e., a sacrifice of one aspect of a good that must be made to achieve the benefit of another aspect of the good). When a performance level of criterion i is defined as attribute $z_i(a)$ for alternative a (i.e., $z_1(a)$, $z_2(a)\ldots$ $z_m(a)$) and if the value of a criterion is independent of the other z_i criteria and is increasing in preference, it is denoted as $v_i(z_i)$ (Keeney and Raiffa 1993). Of note, the value of a given configuration that is consistent with these properties is equivalent to $v_i(a) = v_i(z_i(a))$; as such, $z_i(a)$ is called a partial or marginal preference function (Belton and Stewart 2002).

A widely applied aggregation of decision-makers' preferences is the additive or weighted sum approach (Belton and Stewart 2002):

$$V(a) = \sum_{i=1}^{m} w_i v_i(a) \tag{2.1}$$

where $V(a)$ is the overall value of alternative a, w_i is the relative importance of criterion i, and $v_i(a)$ is the score of a program alternative on the ith criterion (Belton and Stewart 2002; Thokala and Duenas 2012). The partial value functions, v_i, are bound between 0 (worst outcome) and a best outcome (e.g., 1). They can be valued using a variety of techniques, including using a direct rating scale (Keeney 1992). The importance of criteria i is represented through swing weights, where the weight, w_i, represents the scale and relative importance of the ith criterion (Diaby and Goeree 2014; Goodwin and Wright 2010; Belton and Stewart 2002).

The aggregate form of the value function is the simplest application, but relies on several assumptions to justify additive aggregation. The first assumption is first-order preference independence, which states that decisions can be made on a subset of criteria irrespective of the other criteria (Keeney and Raiffa 1993). Suppose there are two alternatives under consideration, and they are different on $r<m$ criteria. Define D to be the set of criteria on which the alternatives differ. Assume the criteria that are not in set D are held constant (i.e., they are identical between the alternatives). By definition, the partial value functions are equal for the criteria not in set D. As such program a is preferred to program b if and only if

$$\sum_{i \in D} w_i v_i(a) > \sum_{i \in D} w_i v_i(b) \tag{2.2}$$

This implies that decision-makers can have meaningful preference orderings on a set of criteria without considering the levels of performance on other criteria, provided that the other criteria remain fixed.

The second assumption is that the partial value function is on an interval scale. The interval scale assumption dictates that equal increments on a partial value function represent equal quantitative distances within the criterion (e.g., on a scale between 1 and 10, the value of the difference between 1 and 2 is the same as the difference between 8 and 9). In this way, interval scales provide information about order and possess equal trade-offs across equal intervals within the scale.

The final assumption is the trade-off condition, which satisfies the notion that the weights are scaling constants that render the value scales commensurate (Keeney and Raiffa 1993; Belton and Stewart 2002). This condition is achieved through swing weights, which represent the gain in value by going from the worst value to the best value in each criterion. For example, suppose two partial value functions for two criteria are constructed. Next, suppose that program alternatives a and b differ in terms of two criteria, r and s, which are equally preferred. As such $V(a) = V(b)$. This implies that $w_r v_r(a) + w_s v_s(a) = w_r v_r(b) + w_s v_s(b)$. For this equality to hold, simple algebra demonstrates that the weights are required such that $w_r/w_s = v_s(a) - v_s(b)/v_s(a) - v_s(b)$.

2.4.1.2 Multi-Attribute Utility Theory (MAUT)

MAUT is an extension of von Neumann-Morgenstern (VNM) expected utility theory (Von Neumann and Morgenstern 1953) because it incorporates multi-attribute alternatives (Keeney and Raiffa 1993). The theoretical underpinnings of VNM are similar to value measurement, but MAUT crucially allows for preference relations that involve uncertain outcomes of a particular course of action, which involves risk typically represented through lotteries. To accommodate the idea of risky choices, preferences between lotteries are incorporated directly into to the assumptions of preference relations. The first VNM axiom is preferences exist and are transitive, i.e., risky alternatives can be compared such that either *a* is preferred to *b*, or *b* is preferred to *c*, or they are equally preferred; and if *a* is preferred to *b* and *b* is preferred to *c*, then *a* is preferred to *c*. The second axiom is independence, which states that the preference ordering between two risky goods is independent of the inclusion of a third risky good. To illustrate, suppose in the first stage there are three risky goods (*a*, *b*, *c*), where risky good *a* is associated with probability p_1 and risky good *b* with probability $(1-p_1)$. The independence axioms suggest that if $a \geq b$, then $p_1a+(1-p_1)c \geq p_1b+(1-p_1)c$. The axiom assumes that if a decision-maker is comparing good *a* to good *b*, their preference should be independent of probability p_1 and good *c*. This is also called the independence of irrelevant alternatives assumption because if risky good *c* is substituted for part of *a* and part of *b*, it should not change the rankings. The third axiom, continuity, is a mathematical assumption that preferences are continuous. It states that if there are three outcomes such that outcome z_i is preferred to z_j and z_j is preferred to z_k, there is a probability p_1 at which the individual is indifferent between outcome z_j with certainty or receiving the risky prospect made of outcome z_i with probability p_1 and outcome z_k with probability $1-p_1$.

These axioms guarantee the existence of a real-valued utility function such that *a* is preferred to *b* if and only if the expected utility of *a* is greater than the expected utility of *b* (Mas-Colell et al. 1995). The axiom of continuity provides the guide to making decisions: choose the course of action associated with the greatest sum of probability-weighted utilities. This is the expected utility rule. To apply this rule, the probability and utility associated with possible consequence of each course of an action needs to be assessed, and the probability and utility are multiplied together for each consequence (Fig. 2.3). The products are then added together to obtain the expected utility, $U(z_i)$, of an alternative course action. The process is repeated for each course of action, and the program with the largest expected utility is chosen.

The characterization of VNM utility into a multi-criteria problem depends on utility functions for multiple criteria, $u_i(z_i)$, for $i=1\ldots m$ being aggregated into a multi-attribute utility function, $U(z_i)$, that is consistent with lotteries over the criteria. The most common form of the multi-attribute utility function is additive:

$$U(z)=\sum_{i=1}^{m}k_i u_i(z_i) \tag{2.3}$$

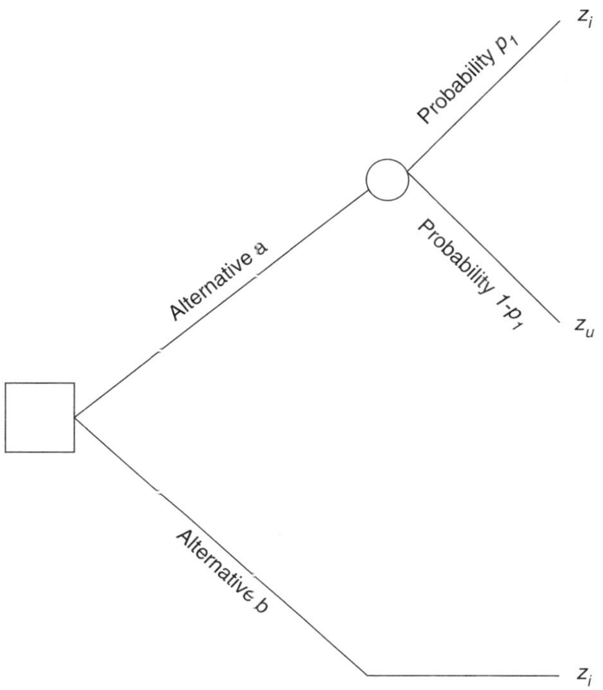

Fig. 2.3 Expected utility theory using the standard gamble method

where k_i is a scaling constant such that $\sum_{i=2}^{m} k_i = 1$ (Drummond 2005). There are two additional assumptions that are needed to guarantee the existence of an additive utility function: utility independence and additive independence. Utility independence among criteria occurs when there is no interaction between preferences over lotteries among one criterion and the fixed levels for the other criterion; that is, the relative scaling of levels for a given criterion level is constant within each criterion. Additive independence is stronger and suggests that there is no interaction for preference among attributes at all. As such, preference depends on the criterion levels and do not depend on the manner in which the levels of different attributes are combined. The restrictive assumption regarding additive independence can be eased, leading to multiplicative or multi-linear forms of the multi-attribute utility function (Keeney and Raiffa 1993; Drummond 2005).

2.4.1.3 Analytic Hierarchy Process

The analytic hierarchy process (AHP) is a theory of measurement based on mathematics and psychology (Mirkin and Fishburn 1979; Saaty 1980, 1994). It has three principles: (i) decomposition, where a decision problem is structured into a cluster of hierarchies; (ii) comparative judgments, where judgments of preference are made between criterion attribute levels in each cluster; and (iii) synthesis of priorities, which is the aggregation model. Described below are the four axioms that support AHP: the reciprocal property, homogeneity within criterion, the synthesis axiom, and the expectation axioms (Saaty 1986). The AHP axioms allow for the derivation of ratio scales of absolute numbers through decision-makers' responses to pairwise comparisons.

The reciprocal axiom requires that a paired comparison between criterion attribute levels, x_1 and x_2 and denoted as $P(x_1, x_2)$, exhibits a property such that if criterion level x_1 is preferred to x_2 and S represents the strength of preference, then the comparison of x_2 with x_1 is $P_c(x_2, x_1) = 1/S$ (Belton and Stewart 2002; Saaty 1980). That is, if x_1 is preferred twice as much as x_2, then x_2 is preferred one-half as much as x_1. The homogeneity axiom requires that preferences for attribute criterion levels should not differ too much in terms of strength of preference. For example, questions of a general form such as "How important is criteria level x_1 relative to x_2?" are asked (Fig. 2.4). The numerical value of importance is captured from categories that describe strength of preference and are within an order of magnitude from equally important (index 1) to extremely more important (index of 9). The synthesis axiom requires that preferences regarding criterion in a higher-level hierarchy are independent on lower-level elements in the hierarchy (Saaty 1986). Finally, the expectation axiom states that the outcome of the AHP exercise is one such that decision-makers' preferences or expectations are adequately represented by the outcomes of the exercise (Saaty 1986).

How important is x_1 relative to x_2 ?	Preference index assigned	Description
Equally preferred	1	Two criterion levels contribute equally
Moderately preferred	3	Experience and judgment moderately favour one level over another
Strongly preferred	5	Experience and judgment strongly favour one level over another
Very strongly preferred	7	A criterion level is strongly favoured and its dominance demonstrated in practice
Absolutely preferred	9	The evidence favouring one criterion level over another is of the highest possible order of affirmation
Intermediate values are assigned between adjacent categories	2,4,6,8	When compromise is needed

Fig. 2.4 Analytic hierarchy process preference index based on Saaty (1980)

The analysis of AHP paired comparisons judgment data includes the utilization of a comparison matrix. Elements on the principal diagonal of the matrix are equal to 1 because each criterion is at least as good as itself. The off-diagonal elements of the matrix are not symmetric and represent the numerical scale of preference strength expressed as a ratio (as required by the first axiom). The formal analysis requires that the set of value estimates, $v_i(a)$, be consistent with the relative values expressed in the comparison matrix. While there is complete consistency in the reciprocal judgments for any pair, consistency of judgments between alternatives is not guaranteed (Belton and Stewart 2002). The task is to search for the v_i that will provide a fit to the observations recorded in the comparison matrix. This is accomplished through the eigenvector corresponding with the maximum eigenvalue for the matrix. An alternative approach is to calculate the geometric mean of each row of the comparison matrix; each row corresponds to the weight for a specific criterion (Dijkstra 2011).

In the aggregation model for AHP, the importance weight, w_i, of the parent criterion in the hierarchy needs to be calculated. To do this, the above process of pairwise comparisons is applied, where the comparison is between the parent criteria in the hierarchy level. The final aggregation model that allows decision-makers to rank alternatives is similar to the value measurement approach because an additive aggregation is used:

$$P(a) = \sum_{i=1}^{m} w_i v_i(a) \tag{2.4}$$

where $P(a)$ is the priority of alternative i, $v_i(a)$ is the partial value function of a criterion level, and w_i is the overall weight of criterion.

2.4.2 *Outranking*

Outranking utilizes the concept of dominance between partial preference functions of the alternatives (Belton and Stewart 2002). In MCDA, dominance is defined as $z_i(a) \geq z_i(b)$ for all criteria i, where there is strict inequality on at least one criterion j, i.e., $z_j(a) \geq z_j(b)$ (Belton and Stewart 2002). Dominance rarely occurs in real-world decision-making. Outranking generalizes the definition of dominance by defining an outranking relation that represents a binary condition on a set of alternatives, denoted by A, such that program *a* will outrank *b* if there is evidence suggesting that "program *a* is at least as good as program *b*." The outranking relation is represented by *aSb* for $(a, b) \in$ A (Ehrgott et al. 2010). Of note, outranking investigates the hypothesis that *aSb* by focusing on whether there is compelling evidence for the hypothesis (i.e., "strong enough"), rather than focusing on strength of preference using compensatory preference structures (Belton and Stewart 2002). As a result, in addition to the possibility of dominance or indifference, there may be a lack of compelling evidence to conclude dominance or indifference (Belton and Stewart 2002).

The outranking relation is constructed using concordance and discordance indices. These indices characterize the sufficiency of evidence for or against one alternative outranking another. The concepts of concordance and discordance can be stated as follows:

- *Concordance*: For an outranking *aSb* to be true, there must be a sufficient majority of criterion to favor the assertion.
- *Non-discordance*: When concordance holds, none of the criteria in the minority should oppose too strongly the assertion that *aSb*; alternatively, *discordance* is where *b* is very strongly preferred to *a* on one or more of the minority of criteria which call into question the hypothesis that *aSb* (Figueira et al. 2005).

The process of characterizing concordance and discordance starts with evaluating the performance of each alternative on the criterion using a decision matrix summarizing the partial preference functions. The matrix is structured such that each row summarizes the partial preference function for the individual criterion which is located in each of the *m* columns. Outranking recognizes that partial preference functions are not precise (Belton and Stewart 2002). Indifference thresholds, defined as $p_i[z]$ and $q_i[z]$, are used to acknowledge a distinction between weak and strict preference, where alternative *a* is weakly preferred to alternative *b* for criterion *i* if $z_i(a) > z_i(b) + q_i[z_i(b)]$; it follows that $z_i(a) - z_i(b) > q_i[z_i(b)]$. Alternative *a* is strictly preferred to alternative *b* for criterion *i* if $z_i(a) > z_i(b) + p_i[z_i(b)]$ and $z_i(a) - z_i(b) > p_i[z_i(b)]$. In this notation, it would be necessary for $q_i[z_i(b)] > p_i[z_i(b)]$ to distinguish between weak and strict thresholds (Belton and Stewart 2002). Indifference between *a* and *b* can happen when there is not strict inequality between the partial preference function. While the decision matrix demonstrates if alternative *a* outperforms alternative *b* in each of the criterion, it does not account for the relative importance of the criteria. This is achieved through criterion weights (w_i). The weights measure the influence that each criterion should have in building the case for one alternative or another.

There are several approaches to estimating concordance or discordance, including the ELECTRE methods (Roy 1991), PROMETHEE (Brans and Vincke 1985), and GAIA (Brans and Mareschal 1994). We present ELECTRE1 below. The concordance index, *C(a,b)*, characterizes the strength of support for the hypothesis that program *a* is at least as good as program *b*. The discordance index, *D(a,b)*, measures the strength of evidence against *aSb*. In ELECTRE1, the concordance index is:

$$C(a,b) = \frac{\sum_{j \in Q(a,b)} w_j}{\sum_{i=1}^{m} w_i} \tag{2.5}$$

where *Q(a,b)* is the set of criterion for which *a* is equal or preferred to *b* as determined by the decision matrix. Note that the concordance index is bound between 0 and 1, and as *C(a,b)* approaches 1, there is stronger evidence in support of the claim that *a* is preferred to *b*. A value of 1 indicates that program *a* dominates *b* on all criterion.

The discordance index will differ depending on if the decision matrix values are cardinal or if the weights are on a scale that is comparable across criteria (Belton and Stewart 2002). When these conditions hold, the discordance index is:

$$D(a,b) = \frac{max_{i \in R(a,b)}[w_i(z_i(b) - z_i(a)]}{max_{i=1}^{m} max_{c,d \in A}[w_i \mid (z_i(c) - z_i(d) \mid]} \tag{2.6}$$

where *R*(*a*,*b*) is the set of criteria for which *b* is strictly preferred to *a* in the set of A alternatives. The index is calculated as the maximum weighted estimate for which program *b* is better than program *a* divided by the maximum weighted difference between any two alternatives on any criterion. Note that in the two alternative cases, an instance of *b* outperforming *a* would result in a value of 1. When the partial preference scores are not cardinal (e.g., they are qualitative relations) or when the criteria importance weights are not on a scale that is comparable across criteria, the discordance criterion is based on a veto threshold. That is, for each criterion i, there is a veto threshold defined as t_i such that program *a* cannot outrank *b* if the score for *b* on any criterion exceeds the score for *a* on that criterion. The discordance index is:

$$D(a,b) = \begin{cases} 1 \text{ if } z_i(b) - z_i(a) > t_i \text{ for any } i \\ 0 \text{ otherwise} \end{cases} \tag{2.7}$$

The concordance and discordance indices are evaluated against thresholds, denoted as *C** and *D**, to determine the relationship between program *a* and *b* according to the following: if *C*(*a*,*b*)>*C** and *D*(*a*,*b*)<*D** then *aSb*, otherwise *a* does not outrank *b*; program *bSa* if *C*(*b*,*a*)>*C** and *D*(*b*,*a*)<*D**, otherwise *b* does not outrank *a*. There is indifference between program *a* and *b* when *aSb* and *bSa*. The two are incomparable if neither program outranks the other, i.e., not *aSb* and not *bSa*. A summary of these outranking relations, adapted from Belton and Steward (2002), is in Fig. 2.5.

2.4.3 Goal Programming

Goal programming attempts to model complex multi-criteria problems using concepts linked to a decision heuristic called "satisficing" (Belton and Stewart 2002). Introduced by Simon (1976), satisficing is a cognitive heuristic where a decision-maker examines the characteristics of multiple alternatives until an acceptability threshold is achieved. This is in contrast to a compensatory

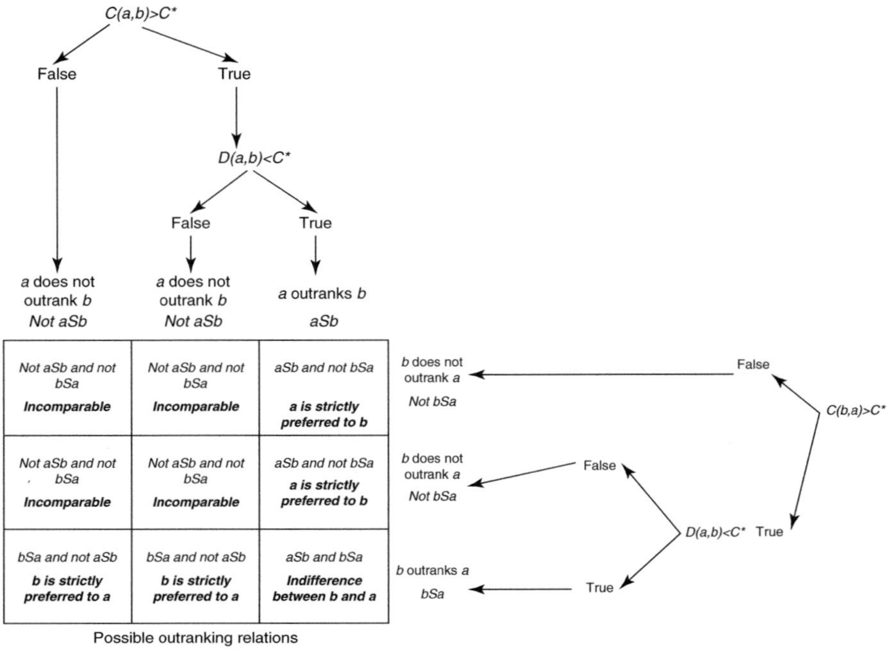

Fig. 2.5 Outranking relations from a pairwise comparison

framework, which assumes decision-makers have unlimited cognitive processing abilities and carefully consider all information(Regier et al. 2014b; Kahneman 2003; Simon 2010). Because of complexity, decision-makers seek a choice that is "good enough," i.e., a choice that is satisfactory rather than optimal.

Goal programming operationalizes satisficing by assuming decision-makers seek to achieve a satisfactory level of each criterion (Tamiz et al. 1995). Attention is shifted to other criteria when a desired threshold is achieved. Goal programming methods encapsulate the following two assumptions. First, each criterion is associated with an attribute that is measurable and represented on a cardinal scale. Thus, the methods utilize partial preference functions, denoted by $z_i(a)$, where $i = 1 \ldots m$ criteria for alternative a. Second, decision-makers express judgment in terms of goals or "aspiration levels" for the m criterion, which are understood in terms of desirable levels of performance (e.g., ICER is below a threshold of \$50,000 per QALY). In goal programming notation, goals are denoted by g_i where $i = 1, \ldots, m$. With the goals defined, an algorithm is used identify the alternatives which satisfy the goals in an order of priority (Thokala and Duenas 2012; Ignizo 1978).

Decision-makers' preferences for goals will differ depending on the context or frame of each criterion. That is, the direction of preference as reflected in each goal will differ depending if the attribute criterion, $z_i(a)$, is defined in the context of: maximization, with the goal representing a minimum level of satisfactory performance; or minimization of $z_i(a)$, with the goal of representing the maximum level of tolerance; or whether the goal is to reach a desirable level of performance for $z_i(a)$ (Belton and Stewart 2002). The difference between $z_i(a)$ and g_i is denoted by δ_i^- or δ_i^+, which respectively represents the quantitative amount the partial preference function is under- or overachieved.

The solution to the decision-makers problem of satisficing is investigated through mathematical optimization techniques (e.g., linear programming) that aim to achieve the best outcome given an objective that is subject to constraints (e.g., minimize the deviation of attribute values subject to a value function). Goal programming models can be categorized either through a weighted goal programming or one that focuses on lexicographic preferences. In weighted goal programming, deviations from goals are minimized after importance weights are assigned to each of the $z_i(a)$. This can be achieved through following algebraic formulation (Tamiz et al. 1998; Rifai 1996; Kwak and Schniederjans 1982):

$$\min Z = \sum_{i=1}^{m} \left(w_i^- \delta_i^- + w_i^+ \delta_i^+ \right)$$

$$\text{subject to } f_i\left(x\right) + \delta_i^- - \delta_i^+ = g_i \text{ for } i = 1, \ldots, m \tag{2.8}$$

where x is a vector of the decision variables that can be varied such that a criterion achieves a specified goal (e.g., the price of a drug), $f_i(x)$ is a linear objective function equivalent to the realization of the partial preference value $z_i(a)$ for an x vector, g_i is the target value for each $z_i(a)$. δ_i^- and δ_i^+ are the negative and positive deviation from the target values, and w_i^-, w_i^+ are the importance weights. Of note, the importance weights need to conform to a trade-off condition when the weighted sum approach is used (e.g., through swing weights).

In lexicographic goal programming, deviational variables are assigned into priority levels and minimized in a lexicographic order (Belton and Stewart 2002). A lexicographic ordering is one where a decision-maker prefers any amount of one criterion to any amount of the other criteria. Only when there is a tie does the decision-maker consider the next most preferred criterion. In goal programming, a sequential lexicographic minimization of each priority criterion is conducted while maintaining the minimal values reached by all higher priority level minimizations (Ijiri 1965):

$$\text{Lex} \min O = \left(g_1\left(\delta^+, \delta^-\right), g_2\left(\delta^+, \delta^-\right), \ldots, g_m\left(\delta^+, \delta^-\right) \right) \tag{2.9}$$

$$\text{subject to } f_i\left(x\right) + \delta_i^- - \delta_i^+ = g_i \text{ for } i = 1, \ldots, m$$

where all definitions above save O, which is an ordered vector of priorities (Tamiz et al. 1995). From a practical perspective, priority classes on each criterion are defined, and minimization of the weighted sum is conducted in relation to the goal.

Once the solution is obtained for the higher-order priority, the second priority class is minimized subject to the constraint that the weighted sum from goals in the first priority class does not exceed what was determined in the first step. The process is continued through each priority class in term.

2.5 Concluding Remarks

This chapter introduced the theoretical foundations and methods that support MCDA. MCDA provides decision-makers with a set of tools that can aid stakeholders in making consistent and transparent decisions. MCDA methods draw on theories that account for both the qualitative and quantitative aspects of decision-making. This is achieved through a process that includes a comprehensive approach to problem structuring and model building. We conclude by noting that there is a paucity of MCDA theory-related research in healthcare. We encourage future research that explores which MCDA methods best address stakeholders' needs in the context of the unique challenges we face in improving health and healthcare.

Acknowledgments The Canadian Centre for Applied Research in Cancer Control (ARCC) is funded by the Canadian Cancer Society Research Institute (ARCC is funded by the Canadian Cancer Society Research Institute grant #2015-703549). Dr. Stuart Peacock is supported by the Leslie Diamond Chair in Cancer Survivorship, Faculty of Health Sciences, Simon Fraser University.

References

Ackoff RL (1979a) Future of operational-research is past. J Oper Res Soc 30(2):93–104. doi:10.2307/3009290

Ackoff RL (1979b) Resurrecting the future of operational-research. J Oper Res Soc 30(3): 189–199. doi:10.2307/3009600

Arnstein SR (1969) Ladder of citizen participation. J Am Inst Plann 35(4):216–224. doi:10.1080/01944366908977225

Baltussen R, Niessen L (2006) Priority setting of health interventions: the need for multi-criteria decision analysis. Cost Effectiveness and Resource Allocation : C/E 4:14. doi:10.1186/1478-7547-4-14

Baltussen R, Stolk E, Chisholm D, Aikins M (2006) Towards a multi-criteria approach for priority setting: an application to Ghana. Health Econ 15(7):689–696. doi:10.1002/hec.1092

Belton V, Stewart T (2010) Problem structuring and multiple criteria decision analysis. In: Trends in multiple criteria decision analysis, vol 142, International series in operations research & management science. Springer, New York, p xvi, 412 p

Belton V, Stewart TJ (2002) Multiple criteria decision analysis: an integrated approach. Kluwer Academic Publishers, Boston

Brans JP, Mareschal B (1994) The Promcalc and Gaia decision-support system for multicriteria decision aid. Decis Support Syst 12(4–5):297–310. doi:10.1016/0167-9236(94)90048-5

Brans JP, Vincke PH (1985) A preference ranking organization method – (the Promethee method for multiple criteria decision-making). Manag Sci 31(6):647–656. doi:10.1287/mnsc.31.6.647

Camerer C (1995) Individual decision making. In: Kagel J, Roth A (ed) The Handbook of Experimental Economics. Princeton University Press, NJ
Checkland P (1981) Systems thinking, systems practice. J. Wiley, Chichester/New York
Devlin N, Sussex J (2011) Incorporating multiple criteria in HTA: methods and processes. Office of Health Economics, London
Diaby V, Goeree R (2014) How to use multi-criteria decision analysis methods for reimbursement decision-making in healthcare: a step-by-step guide. Expert Rev Pharmacoecon Outcomes Res 14(1):81–99. doi:10.1586/14737167.2014.859525
Dijkstra T (2011) On the extraction of weight from pairwise comparison matrices. CEJOR 21(1):103–123
Dolan JG (2010) Multi-criteria clinical decision support: a primer on the use of multiple criteria decision making methods to promote evidence-based, patient-centered healthcare. Patient 3(4):229–248. doi:10.2165/11539470-000000000-00000
Drummond M (2005) Methods for the economic evaluation of health care programmes, 3rd edn, Oxford medical publications. Oxford University Press, Oxford England/New York
Ehrgott M, Figueira J, Greco S (2010) Trends in multiple criteria decision analysis, vol 142, International series in operations research & management science. Springer, New York
Figueira J, Greco S, Ehrgott M (2005) Multiple criteria decision analysis : state of the art surveys. Springer, New York
Goetghebeur MM, Wagner M, Khoury H, Levitt RJ, Erickson LJ, Rindress D (2008) Evidence and value: impact on DEcisionMaking--the EVIDEM framework and potential applications. BMC Health Serv Res 8:270. doi:10.1186/1472-6963-8-270
Goodwin P, Wright G (2010) Decision analysis for management judgment, 4th edn. Wiley, Hoboken
Hester PT, Adams KM (2014) Problems and messes. 26:23–34. doi:10.1007/978-3-319-07629-4_2
Ignizo J (1978) A review of goal programming: a tool for multiobjective analysis. J Oper Res Soc 29:1109–1119
Ijiri Y (1965) Management goals and accounting for control. Studies in mathematical and managerial economics, vol 3. North Holland Pub. Co., Amsterdam
Kahneman D (2003) A perspective on judgment and choice – mapping bounded rationality. Am Psychol 58(9):697–720. doi:10.1037/0003-066X.58.9.697
Keeney RL (1992) Value-focused thinking: a path to creative decision making. Harvard University Press, Cambridge
Keeney RL, Mcdaniels TL (1992) Value-focused thinking about strategic decisions at Bc Hydro. Interfaces 22(6):94–109. doi:10.1287/Inte.22.6.94
Keeney RL, Raiffa H (1993) Decisions with multiple objectives : preferences and value tradeoffs. Cambridge University Press, Cambridge/New York
Kimball AW (1957) Errors of the 3rd kind in statistical consulting. J Am Stat Assoc 52(278): 133–142. doi:10.2307/2280840
Kwak NK, Schniederjans MJ (1982) An alternative method for solving goal programming-problems – a reply. J Oper Res Soc 33(9):859–860
Lancaster KJ (1966) New approach to consumer theory. J Polit Econ 74(2):132–157. doi:10.1086/259131
MacLean S, Burgess MM (2010) In the public interest: assessing expert and stakeholder influence in public deliberation about biobanks. Public Underst Sci 19(4):486–496. doi:10.1177/0963662509335410
Mas-Colell A, Whinston MD, Green JR (1995) Microeconomic theory. Oxford University Press, New York
Mirkin BG, Fishburn PC (1979) Group choice. Scripta series in mathematics. V. H. Winston; distributed by Halsted Press, Washington, D.C.
Montibeller G, von Winterfeldt D (2015) Cognitive and motivational biases in decision and risk analysis. Risk Anal 35(7):1230–1251. doi:10.1111/risa.12360

NICE (2008) Guide to the Methods of Technology Appraisals. National Institute of Clinical Excellence, London, England

O'Doherty KC, Hawkins AK, Burgess MM (2012) Involving citizens in the ethics of biobank research: informing institutional policy through structured public deliberation. Soc Sci Med 75(9):1604–1611. doi:10.1016/j.socscimed.2012.06.026

Peacock S, Mitton C, Bate A, McCoy B, Donaldson C (2009) Overcoming barriers to priority setting using interdisciplinary methods. Health Policy 92(2–3):124–132. doi:10.1016/j.healthpol.2009.02.006

Phillips LD (1984) A theory of requisite decision-models. Acta Psychol 56(1–3):29–48. doi:10.1016/0001-6918(84)90005-2

Phillips LD, Phillips MC (1993) Facilitated work groups – theory and practice. J Oper Res Soc 44(6):533–549. doi:10.1057/Jors.1993.96

Rabin M (1998) Psychology and economics. J Econ Lit 36(1):11–46

Rawlins M, Barnett D, Stevens A (2010) Pharmacoeconomics: NICE's approach to decision-making. Br J Clin Pharmacol 70(3):346–349. doi:10.1111/j.1365-2125.2009.03589.x

Regier DA, Bentley C, Mitton C, Bryan S, Burgess MM, Chesney E, Coldman A, Gibson J, Hoch J, Rahman S, Sabharwal M, Sawka C, Schuckel V, Peacock SJ (2014a) Public engagement in priority-setting: results from a pan-Canadian survey of decision-makers in cancer control. Soc Sci Med 122:130–139. doi:10.1016/j.socscimed.2014.10.038

Regier DA, Watson V, Burnett H, Ungar WJ (2014b) Task complexity and response certainty in discrete choice experiments: an application to drug treatments for juvenile idiopathic arthritis. J Behav Exp Econ 50:40–49. doi:10.1016/j.socec.2014.02.009

Rifai AK (1996) A note on the structure of the goal-programming model: assessment and evaluation. Int J Oper Prod Manag 16(1):40. doi:10.1108/01443579610106355

Rowe G, Frewer LJ (2000) Public participation methods: a framework for evaluation. Sci Technol Hum Values 25(1):3–29

Roy B (1991) The outranking approach and the foundations of electre methods. Theor Decis 31(1):49–73. doi:10.1007/Bf00134132

Roy B (1996) Multicriteria methodology for decision aiding, vol 12, Nonconvex optimization and its applications. Kluwer Academic Publishers, Dordrecht/Boston

Saaty TL (1980) The analytic hierarchy process : planning, priority setting, resource allocation. McGraw-Hill International Book Co, New York/London

Saaty TL (1986) Axiomatic foundation of the analytic hierarchy process. Manag Sci 32(7): 841–855. doi:10.1287/mnsc.32.7.841

Saaty TL (1994) Fundamentals of decision making and priority theory with the analytic hierarchy process, vol 6, 1st edn, Analytic hierarchy process series. RWS Publications, Pittsburgh

Schoner B, Choo E, Wedley W (1999) Comment on 'Rethinking value elicitation for personal consequential decision' by G wright and P goodwin. J Multi-Criteria Decis Anal 8:24–26

Simon HA (1976) Administrative behavior: a study of decision-making processes in administrative organization, 3dth edn. Free Press, New York

Simon HA (2010) A behavioral model of rational choice. Compet Policy Int 6(1):241–258

Tamiz M, Jones D, Romero C (1998) Goal programming for decision making: an overview of the current state-of-the-art. Eur J Oper Res 111(3):569–581. doi:10.1016/S0377-2217(97)00317-2

Tamiz M, Jones DE, Eldarzi E (1995) A review of goal programming and its applications. Ann Oper Res 58:39–53. doi:10.1007/Bf02032309

Thokala P, Duenas A (2012) Multiple criteria decision analysis for health technology assessment. Value Health : J Int Soc Pharmacoeconomics Outcomes Res 15(8):1172–1181. doi:10.1016/j.jval.2012.06.015

Von Neumann J, Morgenstern O (1953) Theory of games and economic behavior, 3dth edn. Princeton University Press, Princeton

Chapter 3
Identifying Value(s): A Reflection on the Ethical Aspects of MCDA in Healthcare Decisionmaking

Mireille Goetghebeur and Monika Wagner

Abstract *Background*: A number of ethical theories have been developed over many centuries, such as deontology, consequentialism (including utilitarianism), virtue ethics, and, more recently, for example, Rawls' *Theory of Justice* and Habermas' *Ethics of Discussion*, which have been investigated further in healthcare. These major ethical positions and procedural theories integrate many ethical aspects with which decisionmakers, in particular at policy level, are struggling to deliver the best treatments to patients, protect population health, and build sustainable healthcare systems (triple aim). While ethical dilemmas, rooted in this triple aim, are becoming more critical and the demand for accountable processes is rising, multi-criteria decision analysis (MCDA) offers an opportunity to integrate ethical aspects in an innovative manner to enhance accountability for reasonableness (A4R).

Objectives: This chapter is a first attempt to explore how MCDA may integrate ethical aspects inherent to healthcare decisionmaking. The reflection proposed here is primarily rooted in the real-life constraints of decisionmaking at the HTA/Ministry of Health (MoH) level, rather than in specific ethical positions.

Method: This chapter explores the ethical aspects of each MCDA development step, following the eight-step outline of the ISPOR Task Force on MCDA, as well as the legitimacy of decisions from the HTA/MoH perspective, using the triple aim as the goal to illustrate this exploration. For each step, we discuss the substantive and procedural elements of major ethical positions and procedural theories that such method can integrate.

M. Goetghebeur, MEng PhD (✉)
School of Public Health, University of Montreal
and LASER Analytica, Montréal, Québec, Canada
e-mail: mm.goetghebeur@umontreal.ca

M. Wagner
LASER Analytica, Montreal, Quebec, Canada

© Springer International Publishing AG 2017

K. Marsh et al. (eds.), *Multi-Criteria Decision Analysis to Support Healthcare Decisions*, DOI 10.1007/978-3-319-47540-0_3

Results: Legitimacy of decisions on healthcare interventions requires inclusion of representative stakeholders for both the design and operationalization of the MCDA to ensure that criteria included and their consideration are in agreement with the mission and values of the institution. Consideration of the triple aim as the goal of the MCDA (step 1) results in the definition of a broad range of criteria (step 2) derived from ethical aspects, such as the "imperative to help" at the patient level, the "prioritization of those who are worst off," and the aim to achieve the "greatest good for the greatest number" to best serve the population, as well as maintain the sustainability of the healthcare system. The first two MCDA steps foster reflection, collaboration, and communication across stakeholders to define common ground upon which to establish what constitutes the holistic value of interventions, i.e., integrating all ethical aspects of the triple aim. Synthesis of evidence to consider these criteria (step 4) requires elements of practical wisdom to provide clear, transparent, and systematic evidence. Other aspects of MCDA, such as weighting (step 3), scoring (step 5), aggregating of weights and scores (step 6), and managing uncertainty (step 7), include ethical elements of practical wisdom as well as additional procedural values, such as transparency of values, consistency, participation, accountability, and deliberation. The criteria and their consideration through the MCDA process can result in an accountable and reasonable measure of "holistic value" of interventions contributing the most to the triple aim.

Conclusion: This reflection suggests that MCDA can be designed to integrate numerous ethical aspects inherent to healthcare decisionmaking. By enhancing their operationalization, MCDA can support accountable and reasonable decision processes rooted in a holistic consideration of value of healthcare interventions. Reflection on the ethical aspects of MCDA in healthcare is in its infancy, and further research on each aspect presented here is warranted.

3.1 Introduction

A number of ethical theories have been developed over the centuries, such as deontology, consequentialism (including utilitarianism) (Cleret de Langavant 2001), virtue ethics, and, more recently, for example, Rawls' *Theory of Justice* and Habermas' *Ethics of Discussion*, which have been investigated further in healthcare. These positions integrate many ethical aspects with which decisionmakers, in particular at policy level (HTA, Ministry of Health (MoH)), are struggling to ensure quality of care and delivery of the best treatments to patients, to serve population health, and to maintain sustainability of the healthcare system (triple aim: care, health, costs (Berwick et al. 2008)). Ethical dilemmas, rooted in the difficulty to achieve the triple aim, are becoming more critical, and the demand for accountable processes is rising.

This chapter does not attempt to summarize the reflection of some of the greatest thinkers of humankind but to shed some light on the ethical elements that are evoked by the triple aim and A4R considerations by HTA/MoH; a high-level overview is provided to introduce basic concepts. Virtue ethics is the oldest concept in occidental ethics, set forth by Plato and Aristotle. It holds that an act is morally good if it corresponds to what a virtuous person would do. It emphasizes the character of the virtuous person, who applies practical wisdom and goodness to motivate and guide his/her decisions (Hursthouse 2013). In this context, the virtuous person is the norm, rather than duty (as in deontology) or pragmatism (as in consequentialism). Deontology, derived from the Greek deon ("duty"), is an ethical position that holds those actions to be morally right that conform to established rules or duties. Kant (1724–1804) held that the moral value of an action is not related to its consequences but to the moral duty to which it responds, which manifests as an imperative to act. The "imperative to help" in medicine was outlined by Hippocrates (460–370 BCE) in the Hippocratic Oath: "I will prescribe for the good of my patients according to my ability and my judgment and never do harm to anyone," underscoring the moral obligations of beneficence and non-maleficence, which, according to the oath, requires medical practitioners to use their "ability and judgment" or, in other terms, their expertise and knowledge of the consequences of the medical act. Consequentialism (including utilitarianism) holds that an action is good if its consequences are good. According to utilitarianism, developed by Bentham (1748–1832) and Mill (1806–1873), an action must be guided by its utility; thus, societies should pursue the "greatest good for the greatest number" (maximize utility), a theory that had a strong influence on public policies (Driver 2014).

Contemporary ethical approaches include, among others, the *Theory of Justice* set forth by Rawls, (Rawls 1971) which holds that "priority should be given to those who are worst off." Although there are various models of distributive justice (e.g., libertarian, communitarian, egalitarian, and utilitarian), solidarity, i.e., giving priority to those most in need, is a key concept rooted in an egalitarian justice model and upheld as a principle in many healthcare systems (Kieslich 2012; Hoedemaekers and Dekkers 2003). Daniels' model of distributive justice aims for fair distribution of life opportunities (Daniels 2001).

Procedural theories have also been set forth, such as Habermas' *Ethics of Discussion* (Habermas 1984) and, more recently, deliberative practices (Danis et al. 2010). In their seminal work on accountability for reasonableness (A4R), Daniels and Sabin proposed four conditions to ensure that a decisionmaking process is legitimate (Daniels and Sabin 1997; Daniels 1999): publicity (decisions and rationales accessible publicly), revision and appeals (opportunity for challenge and revision), enforcement (regulations to ensure that the other A4R conditions are met), and relevant reasons. The latter refers to the rationales upon which decisions are based and which should be rooted in principles that are accepted as relevant by "fair-minded" people.

Principlism, developed by Beauchamp and Childress, proposes four moral principles to guide decisionmaking in medicine: beneficence ("do good to others"), non-maleficence ("avoid harming others"), respect for autonomy ("treat others as free agents"), and justice ("fair distribution of benefits and burdens") (Beauchamp and Childress 2001).

These major ethical positions and procedural theories, considered to some extent conflicting, are at play in healthcare policy decisionmaking, and the pursuit to integrate them in pragmatic approaches is ongoing. Policy decisionmaking inevitably involves value judgments (Littlejohns et al. 2012) rooted in individual and social values that can be classified into substantive values (relevant reasons or criteria on which decisions are made, e.g., effectiveness, costs) and procedural values (values the process itself reflects and which are critical to legitimize the decision). (Clark and Weale 2012) While evidence-based medicine and health technology assessment emerged in the twentieth century to improve understanding of the consequences of healthcare interventions (or in other terms their true value) for better decisions at the clinical and policy levels (Battista and Hodge 2009; Jenicek 2006), there is a need for pragmatic and accountable processes to support the operationalization of social values, the integration of ethical aspects inherent to healthcare decisions, and the tackling of ethical dilemmas.

MCDA offers an opportunity to integrate ethical aspects in an innovative manner to enhance accountability for reasonableness (Daniels and Sabin 1997; Daniels 1999). Although MCDA has been used extensively in many fields for several decades (e.g., engineering), its exploration for application in healthcare is fairly recent. This chapter is a first attempt to explore how MCDA might integrate some of the ethical aspects inherent to healthcare decisionmaking. The reflection proposed here is primarily rooted in the real-life constraints of decisionmaking at the HTA/MoH level, rather than in specific ethical positions.

This chapter explores the ethical aspects of each MCDA development step, following the eight-step outline of the MCDA ISPOR task force, as well as the legitimacy of decisions, from the HTA/MoH perspective where ethical dilemmas are most challenging, to illustrate this exploration. It is acknowledged that MCDA can also serve more specific functions (e.g., benefit-risk assessment in its traditional sense), but for the sake of exploring MCDA and ethics from a broad perspective, we constructed this chapter to reflect on the development of an MCDA model that aims at identifying interventions that best achieve the triple aim. For each step of the MCDA, we discuss the substantive and procedural aspects of major ethical positions and procedural theories that such methods can integrate.

3.2 Who Should Decide? Legitimacy of Decisions and Representativeness of MCDA Users

Legitimacy of decisions on healthcare interventions requires inclusion of representative stakeholders in the deliberations that are supported by the MCDA framework, as well as in its design, to ensure that criteria included and the way they are considered are in agreement with the mission and values of the institution. Decisionmaking committees are meant to represent the society/population they are serving, and legitimacy rests on inclusion of the diversity of perspectives that stakeholders may have. According to Daniels' and Sabin's seminal A4R framework

(Daniels and Sabin 1997; Daniels 1999), the relevance condition for legitimacy requires that rationales for decisions rest on evidence, reasons, and principles that fair-minded people can agree are relevant for the decision. Martin et al. (2002) have explored who these fair-minded people should be and stated that the following constituencies be included in a representative decisionmaking committee: committee chair, administrator, medical specialist, medical generalist, public representative, and patient representative. More recently, according to Rosenberg-Yunger et al. (2012), decisionmaking committees should include multiple stakeholders including healthcare professionals, academics, managers/administrators, patients, and/or public representatives, while industry representatives should be involved on other aspects of the process but not in the decisionmaking committee. Garrido et al. (2016) suggested that HTA committee members "may include representatives of patients, providers, payers, government or manufacturers, as well as clinical and methodological experts." Procedural values of MCDA are illustrated in Fig. 3.1. MCDA allows capturing the perspectives of all participants in a structured manner,

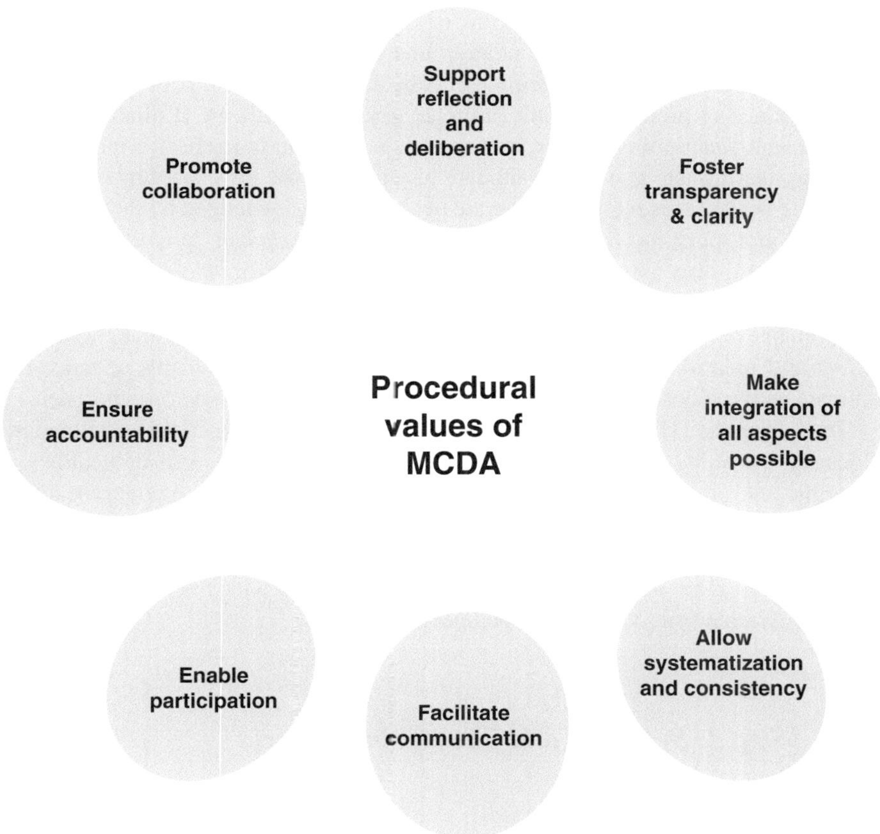

Fig. 3.1 Procedural values embedded in the development and application of MCDA

thus clarifying the individual and group reasoning and supporting deliberation among all committee members, which is hard to achieve without an appropriate method. By the same token, MCDA can be used to consult large groups of individuals. When designed to support reflection, MCDA provides a pragmatic means to enhance the legitimacy of decisions and their acceptability.

3.3 How to Decide?

3.3.1 Step 1: Defining the Decision Problem

In their seminal work on the triple aim of healthcare (care, health, and cost), Berwick et al. (2008), Centers for Medicare and Medicaid Services (2015) proposed that high-value healthcare will be achieved only if stakeholders pursue a broad system of linked goals related to patient health, population health, and healthcare system resource management.

Compassion is the ethical foundation and fundamental impetus of healthcare (Lown 2015), which aims at prevention of ill health, cure, relief of pain and suffering, and avoidance of premature death (ultimate goals of healthcare (Callahan 1999)). While a well-functioning healthcare system is not an end in itself, it is inextricably linked to the ultimate goals of healthcare because it is the only instrument through which the healthcare sector can generate health. As acknowledged by developers of the triple aim, pursuing this broad system of linked goals can "provide enormous gains" but are also associated with "potential disruption in the status quo" and require broad reflection across stakeholders. Integration of the triple aim into a comprehensive (or holistic) MCDA could provide a road map for all stakeholders to *reflect* and identify what constitutes high-value healthcare and thus advance the ultimate goals of healthcare through a *collaborative* and *participatory* approach.

Thus, from the HTA/MoH perspective, the decision problem could be defined as: "Identify the value of interventions with regard to the triple aim of healthcare, ensuring that all underlying ethical aspects are included." Regarding procedural values, the development of MCDA approaches to achieve the triple aim stimulates *reflection* and *collaboration,* while promoting exchange and *communication* across stakeholders. Thus it provides common ground upon which to establish what constitutes value from a triple aim perspective.

3.3.2 Step 2: Selecting and Structuring Criteria

Setting the triple aim as the goal (step 1) of the MCDA framework results in the selection of a broad range of criteria (step 2) to include ethical elements such as the "imperative to help" at the patient level; the "prioritization of those who are worst off," while aiming at the "greatest good for the greatest number" at the population level; as well as the "sustainability" of the healthcare system. Balancing these, often competing, ethical demands require practical wisdom to motivate and guide the decision, as illustrated in Fig. 3.2 (Hursthouse 2013). The resolution of these ethical dilemmas is ultimately driven by universal and specific values related to the ethical and legal traditions of each society which the decision committee at HTA or MoH levels represents (Schlander et al. 2014).

It is postulated that these ethical elements can be translated into objectives and operationalized into decision criteria (quantitatively or qualitatively, or a mix of

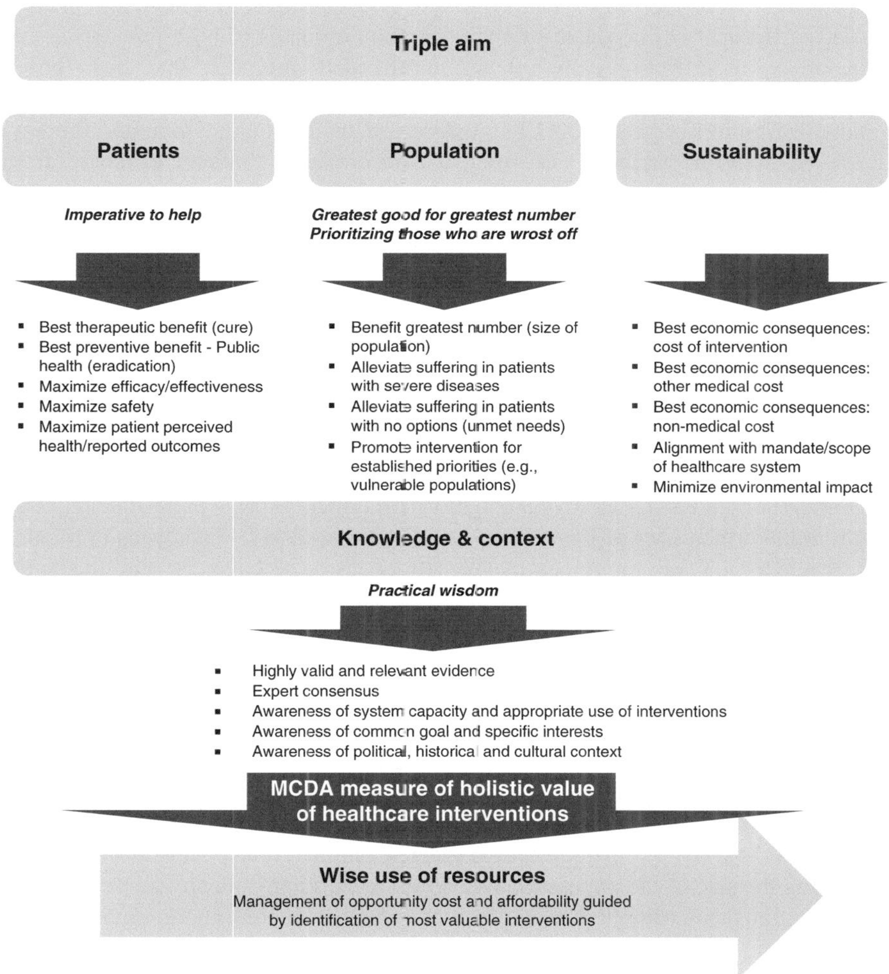

Fig. 3.2 Triple aim, underlying ethical aspects and transformation into criteria for an MCDA measure of holistic value of interventions to guide wise use of resources and management of opportunity costs

both) to design an MCDA framework that allows identifying interventions that contribute most to the triple aim of healthcare (i.e., the most beneficial or most valuable interventions). Of note, we acknowledge that the classification of Fig. 3.2, proposed as a starting point to advance reflection on these matters, is subject to debate.

3.3.2.1 Patient

Among the most evident criteria that contribute to the value of a healthcare intervention at the patient level is the type of health benefit it can provide. This is directly related to the fundamental impetus of compassion to relieve and prevent suffering. Ethical commitment of societies and clinicians to both prevention and alleviation of suffering calls for an evenhanded approach that does not a priori value therapeutic benefits above preventive benefits. The concept of quality-adjusted life years (QALYs) accommodates both prevention and therapy; however, being an artificial construct, it also creates a "mental distance" from natural notions, such as disease eradication, cure, or symptom relief, which relate closer to the way decisionmakers think. MCDA can integrate the type of preventive service and type of alleviating/therapeutic service as separate criteria to retain these natural notions in the deliberation while ensuring that all types of health benefit are part of the value measurement.

When exploring further the ethical impetus of beneficence, aiming at preventing and alleviating suffering to the greatest extent (i.e., toward the greatest improvement of the current situation) can be translated into criteria that reflect the extent of benefit from a clinical standpoint (effectiveness) as well as from a patient perspective ("patient-perceived health"). Also related to the patient perspective are the principles of respect for patient autonomy and dignity, two critical aspects of healthcare, as set forth in the principlism of Beauchamp and Childress (2001). Finally, as implied in the Hippocratic Oath, the imperative to help needs to be balanced with the safety and tolerability of the intervention, "never do harm" or non-maleficence. Both the immediate and the long-term unfavorable effects must be considered to address this ethical imperative.

3.3.2.2 Population

At the population level, prevention and alleviation of suffering in as many individuals as possible, that is, "doing good for the greatest number," can be operationalized by including the size of the population potentially benefiting from an intervention as a criterion, thus assigning higher value to interventions benefiting larger numbers of individuals.

"First helping those who are worst off," also often referred to as fairness in real-life situations, can be translated into the criterion disease severity. Thus, interventions targeting (i.e., preventing, curing, or alleviating) severe diseases will have higher value than those targeting less severe diseases. Ranking of diseases according to severity is not a simple task, although some work has been done in this direction (Shah 2009; Ottersen 2013; Lindemark et al. 2014). Individual judgment on what constitutes "severe" will vary based on personal experience, perspective, and perception of suffering. Unmet medical needs (e.g., orphan diseases or absence of effective intervention) also relate to the notion of prioritizing those who are worst off and can translate into a criterion of "unmet needs," which is a way to address inequalities across therapeutic areas.

National policy makers may further operationalize fairness by defining priorities based on those who are worst off in a given society (e.g., vulnerable populations, rare diseases, remote populations). Inclusion of a criterion that assesses to what extent an intervention is aligned with defined priorities ensures that interventions targeting established priorities are more valued than those not aligned with these priorities.

3.3.2.3 Healthcare Systems

To ensure sustainability, consideration of the economic consequences of an intervention in an MCDA model implies that interventions that reduce treatment costs or free up other medical and nonmedical resources (i.e., use and preserve medical, societal, and individual resources wisely from a broad perspective) have greater value than those that increase treatment costs or deplete medical and nonmedical resources. Including these criteria in an MCDA model stimulates development and promotion of healthcare interventions and programs that possess these intrinsic values, e.g., reducing treatment costs or freeing up other medical and nonmedical resources. Conversely, not including economic aspects in the MCDA framework may fail to discriminate between interventions that do or do not contribute to the triple aim. Daniels et al. (2015) recently pointed out the pharmacological treatment of chronic hepatitis C as an example of a potentially unsustainable intervention that poses difficult ethical issues if, due to high cost, coverage can be provided only for some and not for others (see also comment below on opportunity costs).

When integrating economic aspects in an MCDA framework, a distinction is often made by decisionmakers between costs consequences that will occur with less uncertainty (i.e., cost of the intervention per se and its implementation) and those that will occur with higher uncertainty, that is, the impact of the intervention on other medical as well as nonmedical costs, which are often modeled rather than based on real-life data. MCDA can be designed to provide clarity on this aspect by dealing with these costs through separate criteria.

Certain interventions present a challenge as they may be deemed by some to fall outside the mandate and scope of the healthcare system (e.g., growth hormone for height, assisted reproduction, lifestyle drugs). To address this, a criterion can be introduced in the MCDA to consider the ethical implications of covering these interventions by the healthcare system.

Finally, at the societal level, consideration of the environmental impact of healthcare interventions is becoming more and more an element of value (Tanios et al. 2013). Including a criterion on the impact of the intervention on the environment implies giving more value to interventions that cause minimal environmental damage and can create an impetus to develop and promote interventions that are environmentally sustainable for the benefit of all.

3.3.2.4 Knowledge and Context

Practical wisdom is a combination of explicit knowledge rooted in formal evidence, knowledge rooted in experience, knowledge of the context, common sense, and implicit judgments. Knowledge, based on understanding of the clinical and economic consequences of interventions, is a key element of practical wisdom and requires long-term real-life data. The ethical implications of data availability and quality are evident as claims about an intervention may or may not be substantiated in real life, implying a risk of selecting interventions that may contribute little to the triple aim. Knowledge comes from evidence generated through studies, which may be of variable relevance and quality, from direct experience of clinicians, which is to some extent captured in clinical practice guidelines, and from patients. If solid knowledge is considered an element of value, two criteria, quality of evidence and expert consensus, may be added. This design will ensure that interventions with solid knowledge will be valued higher than those with limited knowledge.

Since evidence generation comes at a cost, formal data collection tends to focus on new, complex interventions and products, while data for programs and simple interventions is often lacking, which creates a strong bias toward the former. To respond to this dilemma, one may consider that knowledge generation is a social responsibility and also that, in some cases, common sense is a reasonably acceptable source of knowledge. Including an MCDA criterion that measures the strength of evidence can create an impetus for broader research on what constitutes solid and meaningful evidence and perhaps a more formal integration of common sense to demonstrate value of all types of interventions.

The healthcare system's capacity to implement and ensure appropriate use of an intervention is a common consideration by HTA and MoH. This can be seen as an aspect of practical wisdom, which requires knowledge of the system's infrastructure, legislation, organization, barriers, and skills. Introducing an appropriate criterion into the MCDA (most likely qualitatively) gives structure to these considerations and implies that interventions that are easy to implement and have low inherent risks of inappropriate use are more valuable.

Awareness of the context in which the intervention is to be implemented is related to practical wisdom. Being aware of stakeholder pressures and barriers helps ensure that decisions are fair-minded and driven by the triple aim and not unduly influenced by special interests. Being aware of the political, historical, and cultural context is important for assessing the feasibility of implementing the intervention. For example, precedence of decisions on similar interventions or the impact of the intervention on research and innovation (as new treatments often provide new scientific knowledge) may have an impact on the overall value at the time of decisionmaking.

Beyond defining criteria by their underlying ethical positions, an MCDA model should also follow MCDA methodological requirements, briefly summarized below, as described in detail in the chapter by Dean et al. (UK Department for Communities and Local Government 2009):

- Nonredundancy *(avoid double counting criteria)*
- Mutual independence *(criteria can be assessed independently)*
- Operationalizability *(appropriate measurement scales and data are available)*
- Completeness *(all criteria important for decisionmaking are included)*
- Clustering *(criteria structured in a conceptually meaningful manner)*

Values related to the process of identifying and selecting criteria are critical as this process stimulates *reflection* on how to translate ethical positions into pragmatic tools across the decision continuum from developers to regulators, policymakers, clinicians, and patients. In addition, the process of selecting criteria to develop an MCDA model rooted in the triple aim fosters *systematization* and *consistency*, *participation*, and *collaboration* to assess and identify what constitutes value.

Regarding the type of MCDA and the MCDA process, implementation of an MCDA approach might be, in a first instance, a qualitative operationalization of criteria to support *deliberation* and *communication* across stakeholders. Quantitative operationalization of these criteria involves some additional ethical aspects and procedural values, which are outlined below.

3.3.3 Step 3 of MCDA: Weighting Criteria

Ethical aspects of weighting decision criteria include the wisdom that comes from becoming aware of the ethical trade-offs within which each of us operates (our individual value system), its variability across stakeholders and how it relates to the triple aim (and its underlying ethical aspects). Indeed, although weighting of criteria is inherent to any decisionmaking, it is often made implicitly.

Key procedural values related to criteria weighting include *participation* and *reflection* embedded in the process by which each stakeholder can reflect on trade-offs between criteria and clarify their positions with regard to how they tackle ethical dilemmas, which ethical aspect predominates in their reasoning and other aspects of the deliberation. In a committee, the diversity of perspectives thus revealed can be integrated into the evaluation using a weighting technique most suitable to the group. The selection process for standing committees or panelists applying MCDA has also ethical implications, for example, inclusion of patients or patient representatives may impact on the perceived legitimacy of decisions in an era of patient-centered care.

Many weight elicitation techniques are available and should be selected according to needs and preferences (Dolan 2010) (see Chapter 4). The weighting process itself promotes *transparency* of the values considered and enables consultation of large groups of stakeholders and citizens via surveys (*participation*), as was performed by the Ministry of Health in Colombia (see Chapter 8 by Castro et al.).

3.3.4 Step 4 of MCDA: Providing Evidence to Measure Performance

Consideration of criteria requires evidence for these criteria, including scientific and colloquial evidence and common sense. The type of data selected and provided to decisionmakers has ethical implications and involves numerous value judgments (Hofmann et al. 2014a, b). Efficient, understandable, and meaningful communication of evidence, including standardized presentation (e.g., absolute vs relative data, range of variations across studies), is essential to ensure informed decisionmaking. The process of distilling information is not trivial and must be done to provide sufficient and necessary data for decisionmakers to form their judgments and proceed toward a decision. Providing decisionmakers with unbiased and pragmatic support is crucial for measuring the true value of an intervention, which, although it remains uncertain, can be approached by exploring it from various perspectives, which MCDA facilitates. Thus, MCDA processes stimulate *transparency* and clarity of the evidence (scientific and colloquial) at the criteria level and *systematization* of the evidence distillation process.

In addition, at the group level (e.g., decisionmaking committee), MCDA provides a structured process to share insights and colloquial evidence among members of the group, which can significantly enriches reflection and promotes a *participatory* evaluation and deliberation process.

3.3.5 Step 5: Scoring the Criteria to Evaluate Performance of the Intervention

As recently highlighted, value judgments are involved in every aspect of assessing a healthcare intervention as well as in appraisal and decisionmaking (Hofmann et al. 2014a).

As with weighting, scoring fosters *participation*, *reflection*, and *systematization*. The choice of scoring method has strong implications for the level of *transparency* and *accountability* of the process. Constructed scoring scales capture a judgment of the evidence, thus making transparent how the available evidence was interpreted. (For example, for the criterion "comparative safety," the scale could be defined to range from "much better safety than comparator" to "much worse safety than comparator.") The alternative, defining the high and low end of the scale based on a mathematical transformation of data, for example, frequency of adverse events, can create a mental distance between the scores and the interpretation of data. Since decisionmakers ultimately have to make a judgment on the evidence, the extent to which the scoring process supports their judgment must be considered in designing an MCDA approach that ensures *accountability*.

3.3.6 Step 6: Aggregating Data for Ranking, Investing, and Disinvesting

A quantitative MCDA model requires combining weights and scores to measure value (value model), which allows ranking interventions based on a measure of value defined by the criteria included in the model.

However, comprehensive understanding of the value of an intervention often includes aspects that cannot easily be measured. Indeed, certain criteria identified through analysis of ethical underpinnings in the previous section (e.g., cultural context) may not be amenable to quantitative consideration because scoring scales cannot be defined systematically. Nevertheless, consideration of these criteria might impact the value of the intervention, highlighting the need for nuance that can be met by a comprehensive MCDA that includes both quantitative and qualitative criteria. Such an MCDA can thus provide guidance on investing in the most valuable interventions and disinvesting in less valuable interventions, rooted in a definition of value that integrates conflicting ethical positions related to the triple aim that are operationalized in the criteria.

3.3.7 Step 7: Dealing with Uncertainty

Acknowledging uncertainty and providing means to explore it support the legitimacy of the MCDA process.

A fundamental uncertainty is whether the criteria included actually capture all the concepts that reflect what one aims to measure. This requires a thorough iterative validation process of the concepts underlying the criteria, bearing in mind the principles of MCDA and the objectives that the framework is meant to achieve. Exploration of the face validity of results obtained with the MCDA exercise is a prerequisite to avoid major misrepresentations of participant views.

Weighting explores trade-offs, which are expected to vary across stakeholders representing different views of the society. Uncertainty here is more a question of the representativeness of the committee members for a system-level decision than of mathematical calculations. Mathematics, however, are helpful to capture the diversity and transform the participatory process into a value measurement with an estimation of variability using appropriate statistics.

Uncertainty related to scoring includes uncertainty on the evidence, which is a fact in decisionmaking, and uncertainty on the interpretation of the meaning of the evidence, which can be captured, for example, by allowing users to provide ranges of scores.

A number of technical aspects, such as developing value functions for each criterion, the uncertainty related to the assumptions that have to be made to develop these, and the aggregation model (linear vs more complex) are described in more detail in the chapter by Oudshorn et al. From the procedural value standpoint, simplicity is important to limit the mental distance between the MCDA framework and the natural reflection and deliberation that takes place in decisionmaking.

3.3.8 Step 8: Reporting Results, Deliberation, Decision, Communication, and Implementation

Results of the MCDA-supported reflection, be they quantitative, semiquantitative, or qualitative, must be reported with clarity to those who apply the framework to ensure that face validity can be ascertained. Reporting of results is not trivial and quite critical for legitimacy. It should be done ideally during the deliberation, as a key procedural value of MCDA is its ability to clarify and support the deliberation process (Baltussen et al. 2016; Jansen et al. 2016). MCDA helps also communicating the reasoning that takes place during the committee's deliberation. *Clarity* on this reasoning facilitates acceptability by stakeholders. In this way, MCDA can be viewed as a method to operationalize accountability for reasonableness (A4R).

Once value related to the triple aim (holistic value) has been measured through the MCDA, implementation requires a financial exercise to invest in those healthcare interventions with high value and disinvest in those with low value. Such holistic value measurement provides a solid basis for ranking interventions and guides wise use of resources, which is characterized by opportunity cost and feasibility considerations (Fig. 3.2). Indeed, opportunity costs, in the sense of resources forgone due to the implementation of a new intervention, are at the root of ethical management of collectively funded healthcare systems (Claxton et al. 2015). Management of opportunity costs and affordability requires a financial exercise to estimate the total economic impact of interventions on a given system (Peacock et al. 2007). MCDA can thus help build sustainable healthcare systems.

3.4 Conclusion

This reflection suggests that MCDA can operationalize numerous ethical aspects and enhance the A4R framework set forth by Daniels and Sabin almost two decades ago (Daniels and Sabin 1997). Healthcare decisionmakers at all levels increasingly face ethical dilemmas in accommodating various mandates and constraints including those of patients, clinicians, policymakers, payers, and developers. MCDA might provide an opportunity, a road map, to open the path to a collective reflection on accountable and socially responsible identification of interventions that contribute the most to the triple aim of healthcare. Indeed, building on the principles of the A4R framework, MCDA can be designed to make explicit the values, competing ethical dilemmas, and uncertainty inherent to healthcare decisionmaking while furthering participatory and transparent processes (Baeroe and Baltussen 2014; Baltussen and Niessen 2006).

When making a decision in the name of the population they serve, decisionmakers struggle to achieve a balance between the imperative to help individual patients, to serve the population as a whole in a fair manner, and to maintain health system sustainability. While the MCDA method does not resolve ethical dilemmas, its strength lies in its ability to explicitly identify, make, and communicate trade-offs among competing ethical claims. It does so by clearly defining the relevant criteria that reflect the values and principles of a given institution or society it represents and by helping stakeholders identifying trade-offs. This makes reasoning more powerful and more transparent, which can facilitate understanding and acceptance of the coverage decision. It can also foster development of healthcare interventions with best value regarding the triple aim.

Thus, selecting criteria for an MCDA for an HTA/MoH application has strong ethical implications. For example, if the criterion *disease severity* is included and considered under the assumption that an intervention for a severe disease has a higher value than for a disease that is not severe (this assumption is translated into the scoring scale: high end of the scale = severe disease; low end of the scale = very mild condition), the resulting MCDA value measurement of the healthcare intervention embeds, by design, the ethical aspect that those who are worst off (with a severe disease) should be prioritized, an aspect of fairness. They are prioritized in the sense that the intervention is given more value because it is for a severe disease relative to an intervention for a mild condition. By applying this reasoning to all the criteria of an MCDA rooted in the triple aim, the apparently conflicting goals, and their underlying ethical aspects:

- Serving the individual patient (imperative to help with best type of benefit, best efficacy, safety, and PRO – aspects of deontology)
- Serving the population (benefit large number of individuals [greatest benefit to greatest number – an aspect of utilitarianism]; prioritize those who are worst off and with severe diseases and unmet needs – an aspect of distributive justice)
- Ensuring sustainability (reduce cost of intervention and other costs – an aspect of utilitarianism) can be balanced based on knowledge (relevant and valid evidence, expert knowledge, contextual knowledge – an aspect of practical wisdom) and insights from committee members to make a decision that fair-minded people would find reasonable. Of note, this approach is at the root of the development of the open source, EVIDEM framework (Goetghebeur et al. 2008; Collaboration

2015; EVIDEM 2015), which was designed and is continuously developed with input from stakeholders from around the world over the past 10 years to put ethics in action.

This chapter is meant to initiate the discussion on the ethical aspects of MCDA. Because this field is in its infancy, further research on each aspect presented here is warranted.

Acknowledgment We wish to acknowledge Bjorn Hofmann (Institute of Health and Society, Center for Medical Ethics, Oslo, Norway) and Ken Bond (CADTH, Ottawa, Ontario, Canada) for their contribution to the development of this chapter, as well as Rob Baltussen (Radboud University, Nijmegen, Netherlands), Ghislaine Cléret de Langavant and Isabelle Ganache (Commissioner for Health and Welfare of the Government of Québec, Montreal, Québec, Canada), Payam Abrishami (ZIN, Netherlands), and Norman Daniels (Harvard School of Public Health, Cambridge, MA, USA) for their insightful advice and review.

References

Baeroe K, Baltussen R (2014) Legitimate healthcare limit setting in a real-world setting: integrating accountability for reasonableness and multi-criteria decision analysis. Publ Health Ethics 7(2):98–111

Baltussen R, Niessen L (2006) Priority setting of health interventions: the need for multi-criteria decision analysis. Cost Eff Resour Alloc 4:14

Baltussen R, Jansen MP, Mikkelsen E, Tromp N, Hontelez J, Bijlmakers L et al (2016) Priority setting for universal health coverage: we need evidence-informed deliberative processes, not just more evidence on cost-effectiveness. Int J Health Policy Manag 5:615–618

Battista RN, Hodge MJ (2009) The "natural history" of health technology assessment. Int J Technol Assess Health Care 25(Suppl 1):281–284

Beauchamp TL, Childress JF (2001) Principles of biomedical ethics. Oxford University Press, New York

Berwick DM, Nolan TW, Whittington J (2008) The triple aim: care, health, and cost. Health Aff (Millwood) 27(3):759–769

Callahan D (1999) Remembering the goals of medicine. J Eval Clin Pract 5(2):103–106

Centers for Medicare & Medicaid Services (2015) CMS partnership for patients. http://www.ihi.org/topics/cmspartnershipforpatients/Pages/default.aspx. Accessed 26 Nov 2015

Clark S, Weale A (2012) Social values in health priority setting: a conceptual framework. J Health Organ Manag 26(3):293–316

Claxton K, Sculpher M, Palmer S, Culyer AJ (2015) Causes for concern: is NICE failing to uphold its responsibilities to all NHS patients? Health Econ 24(1):1–7

Cleret de Langavant G (2001) La bioéthique Bioéthique: méthode et complexité. Presses de l'Université du Québec, pp 21–52

Daniels N (1999) Decisions about access to health care and accountability for reasonableness. J Urban Health 76(2):176–191

Daniels N (2001) Justice, health, and healthcare. Am J Bioeth 1(2):2–16

Daniels N, Sabin J (1997) Limits to health care: fair procedures, democratic deliberation, and the legitimacy problem for insurers. Philos Public Aff 26(4):303–350

Daniels N, Porteny T, Urritia J (2015) Expanded HTA:enhancing fairness and legitimacy. Int J Health Policy Manag 5(1):1–3

Danis M, Ginsburg M, Goold S (2010) Experience in the United States with public deliberation about health insurance benefits using the small group decision exercise, CHAT. J Ambul Care Manage 33(3):205–214

Dolan JG (2010) Multi-criteria clinical decision support. A primer on the use of multiple-criteria decision-making methods to promote evidence-based, patient-centered healthcare. Patient 3(4):229–248

Driver J (2014 Winter) The history of utilitarianism. In: Zalta EN (ed) The stanford encyclopedia of philosophy. Ed 2014. http://plato.stanford.edu/archives/fall2013/entries/ethics-virtue/

EVIDEM Collaboration (2015) Decision criteria – Conceptual background, definitions, design & instructions. https://www.evidem.org/components-decision.php. Accessed 29 Jul 2015

EVIDEM Collaboration (2015) Evidence and value: impact on DecisionMaking. https://www.evidem.org/. Accessed 17 Sep 2015

Goetghebeur MM, Wagner M, Khoury H, Levitt RJ, Erickson LJ, Rindress D (2008) Evidence and value: impact on DEcisionMaking–the EVIDEM framework and potential applications. BMC Health Serv Res 8:270

Habermas J (1984) The theory of communicative action. Beacon, Boston

Hoedemaekers R, Dekkers W (2003) Justice and solidarity in priority setting in health care. Health Care Anal 11(4):325–343

Hofmann B, Cleemput I, Bond K, Krones T, Droste S, Sacchini D et al (2014a) Revealing and acknowledging value judgments in health technology assessment. Int J Technol Assess Health Care 30(6):579–586

Hofmann B, Droste S, Oortwijn W, Cleemput I, Sacchini D (2014b) Harmonization of ethics in health technology assessment: a revision of the Socratic approach. Int J Technol Assess Health Care 30(1):3–9

Hursthouse R (2013 Fall) Virtue ethics. In: Zalta EN (ed) The stanford encyclopedia of philosophy. Ed 2012. ed.), URL http://plato.stanford.edu/archives/fall2013/entries/ethics-virtue/

Jansen MP, Helderman JK, Boer B, Baltussen R (2016) Fair processes for priority setting: putting theory into practice. Comment on "expanded HTA: enhancing fairness and legitimacy". Int J Health Policy Manag 5:1–3

Jenicek M (2006) Evidence-based medicine: fifteen years later. Golem the good, the bad, and the ugly in need of a review? Med Sci Monit 12(11):RA241–RA251

Kieslich K (2012) Social values and health priority setting in Germany. J Health Organ Manag 26(3):374–383

Lindemark F, Norheim OF, Johansson KA (2014) Making use of equity sensitive QALYs: a case study on identifying the worse off across diseases. Cost Eff Resour Alloc 12:16

Littlejohns P, Weale A, Chalkidou K, Faden R, Teerawattananon Y (2012) Social values and health policy: a new international research programme. J Health Organ Manag 26(3):285–292

Lown BA (2015) Compassion is a necessity and an individual and collective responsibility comment on "why and how is compassion necessary to provide good quality healthcare?". Int J Health Policy Manag 4(9):613–614

Martin DK, Abelson J, Singer PA (2002) Participation in health care priority-setting through the eyes of the participants. J Health Serv Res Policy 7(4):222–229

Ottersen T (2013) Lifetime QALY prioritarianism in priority setting. J Med Ethics 39(3): 175–180

Peacock SJ, Richardson JR, Carter R, Edwards D (2007) Priority setting in health care using multi-attribute utility theory and programme budgeting and marginal analysis (PBMA). Soc Sci Med 64(4):897–910

Rawls J (1971) A theory of justice. Belknap, Cambridge

Rosenberg-Yunger ZR, Thorsteinsdottir H, Daar AS, Martin DK (2012) Stakeholder involvement in expensive drug recommendation decisions: an international perspective. Health Policy 105(2–3):226–235

Schlander M, Garattini S, Holm S, Kolominsky-Rabas P, Nord E, Persson U et al (2014) Incremental cost per quality-adjusted life year gained? The need for alternative methods to evaluate medical interventions for ultra-rare disorders. J Comp Eff Res 3(4):399–422

Shah KK (2009) Severity of illness and priority setting in healthcare: a review of the literature. Health Policy 93(2–3):77–84

Tanios N, Wagner M, Tony M, Baltussen R, van TJ, Rindress D et al (2013) Which criteria are considered in healthcare decisions? Insights from an international survey of policy and clinical decision makers. Int J Technol Assess Health Care 29(4):456–465

UK Department for Communities and Local Government (2009) Multi-criteria analysis: a manual. London. https://www.gov.uk/government/uploads/system/uploads/attachment_data/file/7612/1132618.pdf

Velasco Garrido M, Børlum Kristensen F, Palmhøj Nielsen C, Busse R (2008) Health technology assessment and health policy-making in Europe. Current status, challenges and potential. http://apps.who.int/medicinedocs/en/d/ (Accessed 3 Feb 2016)

Chapter 4
Incorporating Preferences and Priorities into MCDA: Selecting an Appropriate Scoring and Weighting Technique

Kevin Marsh, Praveen Thokala, Axel Mühlbacher, and Tereza Lanitis

Abstract A key component of many multi-criteria decision analyses (MCDAs) is the elicitation of stakeholder preferences in the form or scores and weights. A challenge to the MCDA practitioner is that there is little guidance about how to choose between the many scoring and weighting techniques. This chapter describes and illustrates the four commonly used methods – direct rating (specifically an instance of the use of the Evidence and Value: Impact on Decision Making (EVIDEM) framework), Keeney-Raiffa MCDA, the analytical hierarchy process and discrete choice experiment – and identifies key differences between these techniques in order to support researchers to determine the most appropriate technique in different circumstances. It is concluded that there is no 'best' MCDA method, with the pertinence of methods depending on the objective of the analysis.

4.1 Introduction

Multi-criteria decision analysis (MCDA) has been widely applied outside of healthcare (Communities and Local Government (CLG) 2009), but its value to healthcare decision makers has only recently been realised. As they become more familiar with MCDA, healthcare decision makers and researchers are acknowledging its potential to improve decision making (Baltussen and Niessen 2006; Devlin and Sussex 2011; Marsh et al. 2014; Thokala and Duenas 2012). As a consequence, there has recently been an increase in the number of publications on MCDA in

K. Marsh (✉) • T. Lanitis
Evidera, London, UK
e-mail: Kevin.marsh@evidera.com

P. Thokala
University of Sheffield, Sheffield, UK
e-mail: p.thokala@sheffield.ac.uk

A. Mühlbacher
Hochschule Neubrandenburg, Neubrandenburg, Germany

© Springer International Publishing AG 2017

K. Marsh et al. (eds.), *Multi-Criteria Decision Analysis to Support Healthcare Decisions*, DOI 10.1007/978-3-319-47540-0_4

healthcare (Diaby et al. 2013), including a number of publications reporting MCDA applied to evaluate healthcare interventions and support decision making (Marsh et al. 2014); and this interest is not confined to methodological curiosity. Decision makers themselves are piloting and implementing MCDA. In Germany, the Institute for Quality and Efficiency in Health Care (IQWiG) has piloted the use of two types of MCDA – conjoint analysis and the analytical hierarchy process – to weigh clinical endpoints and generate efficiency frontiers based on aggregated outcomes (Mühlbacher et al. 2013; Hummel et al. 2013). The Lombardi region of Italy has adopted an MCDA framework for Health Technology Assessment (HTA) (Radaelli et al. 2014), and the use of MCDA is not just restricted to HTA. The European Medicines Agency (EMA) reviewed methodologies for quantitative benefit risk assessment (BRA), concluding that MCDA would be useful for difficult or contentious cases where the benefit-risk balance is marginal (European Medicines Agency (EMA) 2012); and MCDA has been successfully tested as a tool for supporting shared decision making (SDM) between clinicians and patients (Dolan 2008).

This interest in MCDA reflects its potential, if done well, to support transparent, consistency and rigorous decision making in healthcare. Healthcare decisions invariably require the assessment of interventions that differ on multiple dimensions, by stakeholders who disagree on the relative value of these dimensions, and under conditions of uncertainty. MCDA provides a framework and a range of analytical techniques to help support decision makers identify and agree the criteria against which interventions should be assessed, measure the performance of interventions against these criteria, explicitly state the weights they give to the criteria, aggregate performance and priority data into an overall assessment of interventions and explore the implications of uncertainty on this assessment (Communities and Local Government (CLG) 2009). Decision makers who have participated in MCDAs are generally positive about the support it provides, observing that it facilitates knowledge transfer, improves transparency and improves the quality of discussions (Marsh et al. 2014).

MCDA is an umbrella term for several analytical techniques. First, three broad methodologies are often distinguished – value measurement, goal programming and outranking methods (Thokala and Duenas 2012). This chapter is concerned with value measurement techniques, as these are by far the most prevalent in the healthcare literature (Marsh et al. 2014). Second, although value measurement techniques share several common steps, multiple techniques are adopted to implement these steps. This chapter is concerned with two of these steps – scoring and weighting. Multiple methods exist for eliciting scores and weights, such as direct rating, swing weighting, the analytic hierarchy process (AHP) and discrete choice experiments (DCEs) (Marsh et al. 2014).

The healthcare literature, however, provides little guidance on the selection of appropriate scoring and weighting methods, and MCDAs in healthcare rarely justify their selection of scoring and weighting techniques (Marsh et al. 2014). With this in mind, the objectives of this chapter are twofold: first, to describe and illustrate the different scoring and weighting approaches used in MCDA in healthcare to date and, second, to identify the key differences between these techniques in order to support researchers to determine the most appropriate techniques in different circumstances.

4.2 Overview of Weighting and Scoring Techniques

The objective of the weighting and scoring steps of the MCDA is to capture stakeholders' priorities and preferences for criteria, which can then be combined with data on performance to assess the relative overall value of options. Weights capture priorities or preferences between criteria, for instance, how important is criterion 1 compared with criterion 2. Scores capture priorities or preferences within a criterion – for instance, how important is a change from A to B compared with a change from C to D on criterion 1 – and sometimes an evaluation of performance on the criteria. Combining these two pieces of data, we are able to assess the relative importance of any change in performance within any of the criteria.

We use the phrase 'priorities or preferences' to reflect the fact that different concepts are used to characterise weights and scores. A distinction that is often drawn in the literature is between MCDA methods that correspond with the axioms of utility theory – transitivity, completeness and independence – and those that don't (Guitouni and Martel 1998; De Montis et al. 2005). We might use the term 'preferences' to describe weights and scores that are consistent with the requirements of utility theory and 'priorities' for those that are not.

We can usefully characterise weighting and scoring methods in other ways. First, methods used different elicitation modes. That is, scores and weights can be described using different types of scales, including categorical, ordinal, interval and ratio scales. Second, elicitation techniques can be described as ranking, direct rating, pairwise, choice based or matching (Weernink et al. 2014). Direct methods require stakeholders to provide data that directly address the scores and weights for individual criteria. Pairwise methods elicit data on the relative importance of two criteria, with multiple pairwise comparisons being used to derived weights and/or scores. Choice experiments require stakeholders to choose between hypothetical options, each described using multiple criteria, with responses to multiple choice sets being used to derive weights and scores. Matching methods require respondents to provide number(s) that will make them indifferent to a particular outcome described using multiple criteria.

This section illustrates weighting and scoring methods by describing four different scoring and weighting techniques: direct scoring and weighting (specifically, an example of the implementation of the Evidence and Value: Impact on Decision Making (EVIDEM) framework), Keeney-Raiffa MCDA (swing weighting with partial value functions), the AHP and DCE. These techniques were chosen as they are particularly prevalent in the healthcare literature (Marsh et al. 2014) and are representative of the diversity of approaches employed, though it is important to note that many other methods are available (Guitouni and Martel 1998). Table 4.1 indicates how each of these methods can be described using the categories described above.

Table 4.1 Overview of the scoring and weighting methods used in the illustrations described below

Example	Scoring	Weighting
Direct rating	Direct elicitation Ordinal scale	Direct elicitation Ordinal scale
Keeney-Raiffa MCDA	Bisection method Interval scales	Swing weighting Interval scale
AHP	Pairwise comparison Ordinal scale	Pairwise comparison Ordinal scale
DCE	Choice experiment Interval scale	

4.2.1 Direct Rating

An application of the EVIDEM framework is used to illustrate direct rating. The EVIDEM framework is used to inform HTA (Radaelli et al. 2014; Goetghebeur et al. 2008; Goetghebeur et al. 2010, 2012; Tony et al. 2011; Miot et al. 2012) and clinical decision making (Deal et al. 2013). The framework is collaboratively developed as a support tool for decision making and priority setting. The current version includes 13 quantifiable criteria (see Table 4.2) and 7 qualitative criteria, defined based on analyses of the literature and consultations with stakeholders (Tanios et al. 2013).

While EVIDEM can be applied using different weighting approaches (6 weighting methods are available with EVIDEM (van Til et al. 2014)), its specificity lies in the scoring of interventions against criteria (see Table 4.2). One particular implementation of the EVIDEM framework (a 5-point rating weighting method in combination with the EVIDEM scoring system) is an example of direct scoring and weighting.

The simplicity of the direct rating method means that it is frequently applied in healthcare decision making (Marsh et al. 2014). However the method is subject to a number of shortcomings. First, the use of categorical scales for scoring potentially results in a loss of information. That is, if the relationship between criteria measurements and scores is continuous, differences in between the anchors included on the categorical scale are not captured by the model. Second, criteria weights are elicited independently of the performance being evaluated.

4.2.2 Keeney-Raiffa MCDA

The literature contains a number of examples of swing weighting being combined with partial value functions (European Medicines Agency (EMA) 2011), which we are referring to as Keeney-Raiffa MCDA after the authors of the seminal text in which the approach is described. This is illustrated here using the hypothetical example of treatments with the following performance: risks of minor safety events of between 10 and 20 % and a risk of experiencing malignancy between 5 and 10 %.

Both swing weighting and partial value functions can be constructed using a local scale or a global scale. A local scale contains the range of values of a criterion

Table 4.2 Example of scoring scales used in EVIDEM v3.0

Domain/criteria		Scoring scale and anchors
Need	Disease severity	5 = very severe; 0 = not severe
	Size of affected population	5 = common disease; 0 = very rare disease
	Unmet needs	5 = many and serious unmet needs; 0 = no unmet needs
Comparative outcomes	Effectiveness	5 = much better than comparator; −5 = much worse than comparator
	Safety/tolerability	5 = much better than comparator; −5 = much worse than comparator
	Patient-perceived health	5 = much better than comparator; −5 = much worse than comparator
Type of benefit	Type of preventive benefit	5 = elimination of disease; 0 = no reduction in risk of disease
	Type of therapeutic benefit	5 = cure/lifesaving; 0 = no therapeutic benefit
Economic consequences	Cost of intervention	5 = substantial savings; −5 = substantial additional expenditures
	Other medical costs	5 = substantial savings; −5 = substantial additional expenditures
	Nonmedical costs	5 = substantial savings; −5 = substantial additional expenditures
Knowledge about the intervention	Quality of evidence	5 = highly relevant and valid; 0 = not relevant and/or invalid
	Expert consensus/clinical practice guidelines	5 = strong recommendation vs other alternatives; 0 = not recommended

Source: https://www.evidem.org/docs/2015/EVIDEM-v3-0-Decision-criteria-conceptual-background-definitions-and-instructions-June-2015.pdf

within the alternatives examined, while a global scale contains the full range of plausible values. In the example used here, local scales would cover the range performed noted above, while global scales would extend beyond these, up to and including 0–100 % should this range be considered feasible. The decision between local and global scaling should not make a difference to the ranking of options, but may impact the ability of the analytical framework to evaluate other treatments (Communities and Local Government (CLG) 2009).

4.2.2.1 Construction of Partial Value Functions

When the ranges of each criterion have been identified, partial value functions are developed to specify the relationship between changes along these ranges of performance and the score that will be input into the MCDA, often defined on a scale of 0–100. If a linear function defines this relationship, the specification of the partial value function is straightforward. If this function is non-linear, there are a number of methods that can support the elicitation of these functions from stakeholders (Belton and Stewart 2002; Keeney and Raiffa 1976). For example, a partial value function for the above 5–10 % range of risk of experiencing malignancy could be developed using the bisection method, by answering the following question: 'What aesthetic level is halfway between a 5 % risk (i.e. the most desirable value with 100 in the local function) and 10 % risk (i.e. worst value with 0 in the local function)?' (Suedel et al. 2009). This process can be iterated between several points in the scale to understand the shape of the value function.

4.2.2.2 Swing Weighting

The first step in the swing weighting exercise is to identify and assign 100 points to the criterion with the swing (range of performance) that matters most. This is followed by a pairwise comparison between this criterion and each of the others to determine the relative importance of criterion, and correspondingly allocate them points between 0 and 100. For example if the risk of experiencing malignancy with a treatment was assigned a weight of 100, we might ask stakeholders: 'If an improvement in the risk of experiencing malignancy of 10–5 % is given a weight of 100, on a scale of 0–100, how important is an improvement in the risk of minor safety events from 20 to 10 %?'. This process is then repeated for all remaining criteria to obtain the relative ratio scale of each criterion.

While swing weighting and constructing partial value functions are more cognitively demanding and time consuming than the simple direct rating approaches (e.g. as adopted by the EVIDEM approach), they have a number of advantages. First, a key benefit of swing weighting is that the weight on a criterion reflects the range of performance of the alternatives being evaluated (Communities and Local Government (CLG) 2009). Second, the use of continuous scales to define partial value functions allows more granularity in the construction of priorities.

4.2.3 Pairwise Comparison Using Ordinal Scales (Analytic Hierarchy Process)

The AHP was developed by Saaty in the 1970s (Saaty 1977, 1980) and was introduced to healthcare by Dolan in 1989 (Dolan 1989; Dolan et al. 1989). The application of AHP in health contexts has increased over recent years (Liberatore and Nydick 2008) (see Chapter 11). Within the last 5 years, around 200 studies have been listed in PubMed. Thereby there are several indication-specific analyses, for example, in the field of cardiovascular diseases (Lee et al. 2015), infectious diseases (Tu et al. 2013) or renal cancer (Suner et al. 2012).

A key feature of AHP is its use of hierarchies of criteria to divide complex decision problems into smaller pieces. However, in this paper we are interested in the pairwise comparisons undertaken within these hierarchies to determine the scores and weights given to criteria.

As an example, imagine we are interested in the priorities of patients that suffer from type 2 diabetes mellitus (T2DM). The decision problem can be divided into the primary decision criteria, which would be finding the optimal T2DM treatment (1. hierarchy). This can be subdivided into the relevant dimensions of a possible treatment, which would be the 'outcome effects' and 'possible side effects' (2. hierarchy). Each of these dimensions can be further subdivided. This means being described at a lower level. Outcome effects are 'control of blood glucose level', 'delay of insulin therapy' and 'reduction hypoglycaemic events'. Possible side effects are 'possible weight change', 'urinary tract infection', 'genital infections' and 'gastrointestinal problems' (3. hierarchy).

In order to determine the weights of criteria, patients are posed pairwise comparisons of criteria, indicating the relative importance of the criteria on a 9-point scale (see Fig. 4.1) The data obtained from these pairwise comparisons are used to estimate weights using the eigenvector calculation (Saaty 1980, 1990). Eigenvalues and eigenvectors are used to solve ordinary differential equations. To check if answers are consistent, Saaty proposed what is called consistency ratio. Before calculating the preference statements, a consistency check is performed, meaning that the answers have to fulfil the transitive property. If answers are transitive, this approach assumes consistency. According to Saaty an evaluation matrix is sufficiently consistent if the consistency ratio is smaller than 0.1 (Saaty 1980). Other authors are of the opinion that in complex hierarchies, a consistency ratio of 0.2 would be acceptable (Dolan 2008; IJzerman et al. 2008; van Til et al. 2008). If the consistency measure exceeds the given benchmark, the hierarchy elements should be assessed again, or the hierarchy should be fully reviewed (Saaty 1977, 1980).

The AHP has the potential to support decisions by structuring the expectations and opinions of the patients, insurants, experts and other stakeholders. Dolan (1995) concluded that using the AHP method, patients become able to analyse and structure complex clinical problems (Dolan 1995). Within the application of AHP, it is important to note that the axiom of transitivity is a necessary but not an excluding

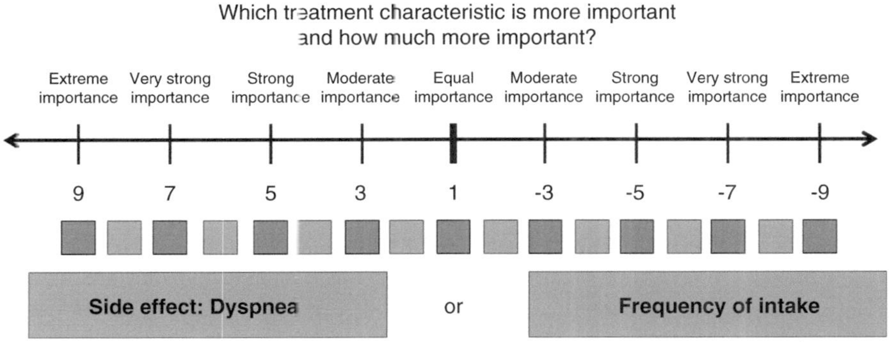

Fig. 4.1 Example of a pairwise comparison undertaken to determine criteria weights in AHP

condition (Scholl et al. 2005). This implies that inconsistent preference judgments are accepted to a certain degree (Haedrich et al. 1986). Furthermore, the lack of theoretical foundation and the lack of stability of the results are central points of criticism that should be considered before the application of AHP for preference measurement. The limited feasibility of interpretation as a result of the scale used in AHP as well as the not very realistic way of the pairwise comparisons of single elements should also be taken into consideration before the application of AHP (Manthey 2007; Dyer and Wendell 1985).

The AHP assumes that decision criteria are independent of one another. When this assumption is not appropriate, the analytic network process (ANP) can be used (Saaty and Vargas 2006). Rather than arranging decision criteria in a hierarchy, the ANP structures criteria in a network, allowing the identification and consideration of interrelationship between criteria. Furthermore, the ANP allows the traits of the alternatives under evaluation to impact weights. For instance, if all the alternatives were performed similarly on a criterion, the importance of that criterion would be reduced. Like the AHP, the ANP uses pairwise comparisons to elicit the weight of criteria. Although the ANP technique removes the deficiencies inherent in the AHP approach, the ANP is less prominent in the healthcare literature (Marsh et al. 2014).

4.2.4 Discrete Choice Experiment

DCE is a choice-based version of the conjoint analysis, which was made possible by the theoretical work of Lancaster (1966) and McFadden (1974). Instead of ranking or rating different therapeutic features (as in traditional importance elicitation formats and in conjoint analysis), DCE asks the participants to choose (decide) between hypothetical alternatives that are differently configured according to the criteria included in the MCDA (Ben-Akiva and Lerman 1985). By doing so, it forces respondents to make trade-offs between attributes, respective of their levels. Regression analysis is applied to data obtained from such choice-based surveys to determine the contribution of changes in criteria to the likelihood that respondents would prefer an intervention.

DCEs are increasingly used in the health economics and health services research. The research group of de Bekker-Grob published a paper in 2012 showing a strong increase of studies (de Bekker-Grob et al. 2012). This trend continued as demonstrated by the review of Whitty and colleagues that identified more than 1,100 preference studies in healthcare setting (Whitty et al. 2014).

As an example, imagine we are interested in the preferences of patients who have suffered a myocardial infarction and need long-term follow-up medication. Five characteristics of possible treatment options could be identified that are patient relevant during the decision-making process. These are ‘reduction of mortality

Characteristics	Treatment A	Treatment B
Frequency of intake To be taken ...	Three times a day	Once a day
Heart attack risk ... patients suffer from a new heart attack.	Low 5 of 100 Persons (5%)	Moderate 6 of 100 Persons (6%)
Bleedings 5% of the patients suffer from ...	Mild bleedings	Moderate bleedings
Shortness of breath Patients suffer (short-term) from ...	Severe Dyspnea	No Dyspnea
Risk of death ... patients die.	Low 4 of 100 Persons (4%)	High 6 of 100 Persons (6%)
	○	○

Fig. 4.2 Example of choice set in discrete choice experiment

risk'; the treatment causing side effects like 'shortness of breath', 'bleeding' and 'risk of a new myocardial infarction'; and the frequency of intake of the tablets (Mühlbacher and Bethge 2015). Within the DCE these characteristics are presented as treatment options. The patient is asked to indicate which treatment he/she would choose (see Fig. 4.2).

Each participant or patient is faced with a sequence of these decision tasks. By the estimation of several hundred of these trade-off decisions, enough data is generated for regression modelling techniques to be applied to determine participants' preferences for changes within and between criteria.

This method offers practical advantages, such as closeness to reality, as trade-off decisions are part of everybody's everyday life. The implementation of pairwise comparisons of a hypothetical alternative considerably reduces the degree of complexity of the tasks for the participants (Ryan et al. 2008). Nevertheless, there are several fields that need further addressing in research. For example, questions relating to the optimal experimental design, the identification of attributes and their related levels, the field of assumption for the regression models and further more. Several checklists and guidelines are available to help researchers address these issues when designing DCEs (Bridges et al. 2011; Lancsar and Louviere 2008; Johnson et al. 2013).

4.3 Which Scoring and Weighting Techniques Are Most Appropriate?

Studies that have addressed the relative merits of MCDA approaches have tended to do so at the level of methods, rather than specifically comparing scoring and weighting techniques. For instance, they often compare AHP with multi-attribute utility theory (MAUT) (see, for instance, Guitouni and Martel 1998; De Montis et al. 2005; Velasquezl and Hester 2013; De Montis et al. 2000; Getzner et al. 2005; Ivlev et al. 2014; Dolan 2010). However, given that scoring and weighting methods are perhaps the element of MCDA methods that distinguish them most, this literature still holds some interest for our purpose in this chapter.

Nevertheless, a comparison at the level of methods is of only limited use to those wanting to implement MCDA in healthcare. First, there are a number of specific techniques that are consistent with the principles of MAUT. Consequently, such an approach unnecessarily obscures the method choices available to researchers. We contend that it is more productive to compare specific scoring and weighting techniques, rather than MCDA methods. Second, this literature does not address the specific objectives and challenges posed by healthcare decision making. For instance, rather than simply selecting between a discrete number of options, it is often the objective of healthcare decision makers to undertake a detailed comparison of the relative value of options and/or criteria.

Consequently, this section draws on the insights from this literature, but presents the comparison at the level of scoring and weighting techniques, rather than methods. Furthermore, we put more emphasis on the 'validity' of the results generated by different approaches. We think this is necessary given the objective of some healthcare decision makers to understand the relative 'value' of interventions.

The healthcare literature contains empirical work comparing the results of weighting methods (van Til et al. 2014). But we are only aware of two manuscripts that attempt to assess the relative merits of different methods from a healthcare decision-making perspective (Ivlev et al. 2014; Dolan 2010). These put a lot of emphasis on practical factors, such as user-friendliness and resources required. These are important when determining the relevance of a method, but we believe a greater emphasis should be placed on the validity of the results obtained.

The remainder of this section is organised around the following factors that distinguish MCDA techniques:

1. The level of 'validity' required in the analysis
2. The cognitive burden that methods place on stakeholders
3. Interpreting and communicating the results of MCDA
4. Practical constraints

The relevance of these factors is illustrated using the four examples of scoring and weighting methods included in the previous section.

4.3.1 *'Validity' of Scores and Weights*

A method is valid if it measures what it claims to measure (Kelley 1927). In the context of MCDA, we interpret this as meaning that scoring and weighting methods are valid if they accurately capture priorities or preferences in a manner consistent with the requirements of the analytical model being employed.

It almost goes without saying that we would want an MCDA to produce valid results. As with any methodology, however, different ways to implement an MCDA can be placed on a scale reflecting an effort-validity trade-off. The importance of validity in the results of an MCDA will depend on the objective of the analysis. Validity is paramount if the objective is to produce a precise estimate of the value of an option to allow a complete ranking of the potential options, for instance, when informing pricing decisions or when designing a HTA methodology that can be repeatedly applied to multiple future assessments. When the objective is to rank options – for instance, when prioritising a predetermined list of options – it is possible to imagine a lower level of validity being acceptable. The demands on the method are less arduous, only requiring the determination of whether the value of one option is greater than another, rather than providing a precise measure of the value of each option. Though, even when ranking, the importance of validity increases as options become less easy to distinguish, which will be a function of the number of, among other things, options being ranked.

To understand what validity means in the context of MCDA, it is useful to consider the requirements of the analytical framework that underlies the approach adopted by most MCDAs undertaken in healthcare – the simple weighted sum approach. This is illustrated in the equation below:

$$V_j = \sum_{0}^{i} s_{ij}.w_i$$

where s_{ij} is the score for intervention j on criterion i and w_i is the weight attached to criterion i.

For the simple weighted sum approach to be applied, a number of principles must be adhered to. Criteria are assumed to be compensatory – an improvement in one criterion can offset a worsening of another. Several more requirements follow from this compensatory principle. First, weights must be scaling constants or value trade-offs, reflecting the rate at which changes in criteria compensate one another. Second, scores must have interval scale properties – equal increments on a scoring scale should represent equal increments of value, so, for instance, a change from 10 to 20 is of equal value as a change from 40 to 50.

4.3.1.1 Do Scores Display Interval Properties?

Interval properties are displayed by interval variables and ratio variables. For instance, of the examples above, the partial value functions, point allocation methods and the coefficients generated by the DCE display interval properties.

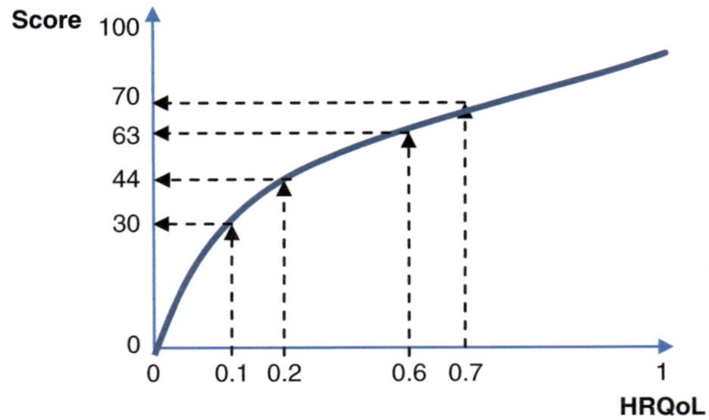

Fig. 4.3 Illustration of a non-linear partial value function

The ordinal scales illustrated above do not necessarily display interval properties. In the example of the application of the EVIDEM framework in the previous section, two ordinal scales are employed – a scale of 1–5 for weighting, where 1 denotes the lowest weight and 5 denotes the highest, and scale of 0–3 for scoring where 0 denotes the least valuable score and 3 the most valuable score. In neither of these instances can we say for sure that a change from 1 to 2 is necessarily worth the same value as a change from 2 to 3. The same point can be made about the ordinal scales employed by AHP. It is not possible to say that moving from a score of 2 (weakly preferred) to a score of 4 (moderate plus) has the same value as moving from a score of 5 (strong importance) to a score of 7 (very strong or demonstrated importance).

This can be illustrated by considering the task of eliciting the values attached to unit gains in health-related quality of life (HRQoL). It is generally thought that the value attached to a unit gain in HRQoL is greater than the lower baseline level of HRQoL. Figure 4.3 illustrates how this might manifest itself in a hypothetical partial value function used to translate HRQoL into a score. In this case, a 0.1 improvement in HRQoL on a scale of 0–1 is valued twice as much from a baseline of 0.1 (change in score of 14 points on a scale of 0–100) than the same change from a baseline of 0.6 (change in score of 7 points).

Both the ordinal scales illustrated above (EVIDEM's direct rating and AHP's pairwise comparison) can, in principle, reflect such non-linearities. However, a barrier to using such scales to accurately reflect such non-linearities is that they do not necessarily display interval properties.

As partial value functions and choice experiments generate scales with interval properties, they are better suited to capturing non-linearities. Whether choice experiments accurately reflect non-linearities depends on the functional form of the regression model applied by the research team. For instance, if only two levels are specified in the survey for a particular attribute (or criteria), it is equivalent to assuming that the partial value function for that attribute is linear. Alternatively, a complex DCE design could be adopted, comprising multiple levels on each attribute, allowing non-linearities to be explored, but at the cost of requiring an increased research budget. However, it is not entirely clear how the validity of such a design can be determined a priori, without actually eliciting the partial value function from stakeholders.

4.3.1.2 Do Weights Reflect Scaling Constant or Trade-Offs?

The hypothetical swing weighting exercise described in the previous section might produce the following result: a reduction in the risk of experiencing malignancy from 10 to 5 % is deemed the most important swing on a criterion and is assigned a weight of 100. Another criterion of swing – for instance, a reduction in the risk of experiencing minor safety events from 20 to 10 % – is allocated 50 points. The MCDA model will interpret these weights as trade-offs, implying that stakeholders would be left no worse off if they experienced an increase in the risk of minor safety events of 10–20 % and a reduction in the risk of malignancy from 10 to 7.5 %. It is not immediately obvious that stakeholders responding to the swing weighting exercise will be precisely aware of this implication. Rather, it is necessary that swing weighting exercises are carefully explained to participants, and results validated to ensure that scaling constants are being elicited.

Another obstacle to the elicitation of scaling constants during weighting exercises is the fact that some methods elicit assessment of importance, independent of a range of performance or consequence (Keeney 2002). Swing weighting is an example of a method that elicits weights for a particular range (the swing). The EVIDEM and AHP examples, however, elicit stakeholders' assessment of the importance of criteria independent of a range of performance. For instance, the EVIDEM example asks stakeholders how important an improvement in efficacy is on a scale of 1–5. It does not provide stakeholders the range of levels of improvement in efficacy being evaluated; without which it is difficult to envisage that the results of the weighting exercise will be scaling constants.

DCE requests that respondents make trade-offs. By posing stakeholders with choices between hypothetical options, each described with multiple criteria, it requires stakeholders to make trade-offs between changes in performance on these criteria. The responses will be scaling constants if respondents think rationally about the criteria – that is, in a manner that reflects the axioms of expected utility theory – and they do not fall back on heuristics to simplify the choice problem.

4.3.2 Cognitive Burden on Stakeholders

Scoring and weighting methods vary in the level of cognitive challenge they pose participants. This can in turn be divided into three dimensions. First, techniques vary in the elicitation modes they adopt. For instance, making a choice (as required by DCE) is something participants are used to doing and is thus more intuitive than providing a valuation (as is the case to varying extents with many other techniques). Related to this, the ordinal data collected in a DCE is easier for participants to provide than the cardinal data required by, for instance, point allocation techniques, which in turn is easier for participants to provide than having to describe a partial value function.

Another variant on the elicitation mode is whether priorities or preferences are expressed numerically or nonnumerically. Behavioural experiments suggest that decision makers with higher numeracy express values more easily when assisted by numerical techniques, whereas decision makers with higher fluency find value elicitation easier with nonnumerical techniques (Fasolo and Bana e Costa 2014). For instance, AHP has verbal, quantitative and graphical elicitation tools (Dolan 2008) so that it can be tailored to decision makers' abilities.

Second, the elicitation techniques adopted pose participants with tasks of varying levels of complexity. For instance, the pairwise comparisons required by AHP are easier for participants than the comparisons required by swing weighting (which need consideration of the range of values a criterion can take) or DCE, which require participants to weigh up options across multiple criteria. Though it should be noted that the relative simplicity of the AHP elicitation questions comes at the cost of needing to ask multiple such questions, and to do so separately for both scoring and weighting exercises. Furthermore, the cognitive challenge posed by the DCE choice sets will depend on the DCE design, and it is contingent on the researcher to ensure that such designs do not become overly complex.

Third, the 'support' provided to participants varies between the techniques. This is at least partly a function of whether a workshop or a survey approach is adopted. DCEs invariably adopt a survey-based approach, which are inevitably limited in the information they can provide participants and do not allow for interaction with or between participants. DCEs assume that stakeholders possess latent value functions that can be elicited through their responses to surveys. In contrast, the other techniques described above tend to be undertaken in a workshop context. This facilitates knowledge sharing between experts and participants, allows participants to clarify the tasks being posed and also facilitates discussion between participants. The latter is particularly valuable when participants are not expected to have well-formed preferences for the criteria.

4.3.3 Interpreting the Outputs from MCDA

Factors that will impact the interpretation of the outputs from an MCDA can be broadly organised into three groups. First, the meaning of results varies between weighting methods. Many of the methods discussed above adopt a simple weighting sum approach, which tend to produce results on a 0–1 scale, the meaning of which will vary with the design of the MCDA and will need careful explanation to stakeholders. For instance, where weighting methods generate estimates of trade-offs, rather than estimates of importance, changes in this scale have a more specific meaning and are thus easier to interpret. Subject to an exploration of the uncertainty in inputs, where trade-offs are elicited, the intervention with the higher score is preferred by stakeholders. DCE produces a different output. Given the DCE collects data on stakeholders' choices between hypothetical interventions, the models fit to this data predict the probability that stakeholders will chose one intervention rather than another.

Second, the transparency of the methods will impact the accessibility of the MCDA results to stakeholders. For example, stakeholder engagement with the results of MCDA is supported if weights are estimated instantaneously (i.e., in real time) when using direct rating or swing weighting methods. However, when using AHP, the results of the pairwise comparisons are converted into weights/scores using matrix calculations to estimate the eigenvector (and eigenvalue). Similarly, the weights and scores from DCE are estimated by performing statistical analysis using the choices from the stakeholders.

Third, the interpretation of the results should consider the impact of heterogeneity of and uncertainty in preferences. A choice needs to be made about whether the aim is to reach consensus among the stakeholders. Workshop-based methods tend to cover a smaller sample of stakeholders, but can be used to reach consensus among stakeholders, something that is not possible with survey-based methods.

The outputs from MCDA should also include sensitivity/robustness analysis to the uncertainty in the evidence. Some weighting/scoring methods allow direct incorporation of uncertainty evidence, while other methods need to elicit the weights/scores again in light of the uncertain evidence. For example, swing weighting can incorporate the evidence uncertainty directly in the partial value scores, while direct rating and AHP cannot.

A similar issue is the availability of a new 'alternative' after completion of the MCDA exercise. Again, swing weighting and DCEs can evaluate the overall value of the new alternative, given its performance on different criteria. However, when using direct rating methods, this new 'alternative' needs to be evaluated separately, and when using AHP, this alternative needs to be compared with all the rest of the initial 'alternatives'.

4.3.4 Practical Challenges

The practical challenges with eliciting the weights/scores in an MCDA can be broadly classified into (a) skill and resource constraints and (b) availability and time constraints.

Skill and resource constraints refer to the availability of personnel with specific skills, specialist software and analysis tools to support the MCDA process. It is important to consider whether the relevant expertise is available within the stakeholder's organisation, or whether specialist skills are required. Two types of resources can be distinguished. First, the facilitator skills required to run stakeholders workshops. Second, the analytical skills required to handle the data generated by the MCDA. For example, AHP and DCE need specialist analytical skills and software, while direct rating can be performed using standard spreadsheet calculations.

However, it is also worth noting that, while certain methods can be delivered using standard spreadsheet calculations, all methods can be supported by specialist software or advanced spreadsheet modelling skills, for instance, to support conducting sensitivity/uncertainty analysis.

Availability and time constraints refer to the challenges in coordinating stakeholders' input into the MCDA. This is largely a function of whether a workshop setting is used to elicit stakeholder inputs, or whether surveys are employed, and the number and duration of workshops required. The weighting/scoring methods will require different numbers of workshops, depending, for instance, on whether a consensus is necessary. The amount of stakeholder time required will also depend on the elicitation technique employed. For instance, AHP requires pairwise comparison to estimate the weights/scores which typically needs a significant time commitment. Swing weighting may also require substantial time to ensure consideration of ranges/swings. Direct rating and DCE may be performed more quickly.

4.4 Discussion

The increased interest in MCDA in healthcare has not yet been accompanied by the development of guidance to support those working in the field to select from the diversity of scoring and weighting to suit their needs. This poses several risks that may undermine the development and use of MCDA to support healthcare decision making. First, those designing MCDAs are insufficiently aware of the variety of techniques. Second, researchers may be aware of the alternative methods, but are unsure of which is most appropriate.

This paper identified a number of factors that can help those designing MCDA to distinguish between alternative scoring and weighting techniques and to determine those most appropriate to their needs. These are illustrated by applying them to describe the scoring and weighting methods adopted by four commonly employed MCDA techniques.

We would agree with the conclusions of other attempts to provide frameworks for understanding the differences between MCDA methods (Guitouni and Martel 1998; De Montis et al. 2005) that there is no 'best' MCDA method. This was summarised aptly by Guitouni and Martel (1998) who concluded that 'All methods have their assumptions and hypotheses, on which is based all its theoretical and axiomatic development – these are the frontiers beyond which the methods cannot be used'.

More specifically, the pertinence of the above features of scoring and weighting techniques will depend on the objective of the analysis, in particular whether the objective of the analysis is to rank options or to value them. The latter may be necessary for HTAs, where the objective may be to generate a method that can be applied repeatedly to different products or where the objective is to determine the price of an option. In this instance, it would be important to ensure that scores and weights have interval scale properties and are scaling constants. It is also likely that the time and resources required to undertake the necessary analysis would be available.

Other uses of MCDA in healthcare include, for instance, supporting SDM or authorisation decisions, in which instances a ranking will suffice. The implications for the required accuracy of the scoring and weighting techniques will depend on how marginal the ranking is. Where a decision on the ranking of options is not marginal, less accurate and less cognitive challenging techniques, such as direct rating or AHP, may be acceptable. Such approaches will be particularly valuable where the time available to undertake scoring and weighting exercises is limited, such as when working with patients to support prescribing. However, it is still important to be aware of the risks associated with these approaches, and appropriate steps should be taken to validate the results of the analysis. Further, the EMA have concluded that MCDA is particularly useful where decisions are marginal (European Medicines Agency (EMA) 2012). That is, it may be the case that MCDA tends to be applied where accuracy is a necessary feature.

Another important point that should be drawn from the above discussion is the importance of efforts to validate the results of MCDAs. The cognitive burden associated with collecting data in a manner that complies with the needs of MCDA – being scaling constants and having internal scale properties – suggested that it is not sufficient to just select the appropriate techniques. Effort is required to educate participants about how the data will be used and to validate that the results of the analysis correspond with stakeholders' understanding of how their inputs were intended to be used.

Given the relative merits of different scoring and weighting methods, it has been argued that no single method is reliable enough to adequately inform decision making in the context of high stake decisions. Rather, for truly important decisions, multiple methods should be used to test that they yield the same results – a process referred to as 'plural analysis' (Phillips 1984).

To the best of our knowledge, this is the first paper to address the appropriateness of scoring and weighting techniques to support different types of healthcare decisions; therefore, inevitably it is subject a number of limitations. First, while the study illustrates the difference in MCDA methods using four techniques selected to be representative of those used in healthcare to date, there are many other techniques available. Those designing MCDAs in healthcare should thus not restrict themselves to just those discussed in this paper. Further, the scoring and weighting components of MCDA methods can be combined in ways other than those illustrated in this paper. Second, the paper provides a conceptual discussion of the differences between techniques. This needs to be followed up with further empirical testing of the different performance of techniques. Third, this testing should include elicitation of decision makers' preferences for different methods, which is not covered in this paper, but will be crucial in determining the success of MCDA. Finally, the paper says nothing about the implementation of methods. Once appropriate methods have been selected, researchers should design and implement these methods in order to minimise the risk of bias (Montibeller and von Winterfeldt 2014).

References

Baltussen R, Niessen L (2006) Priority setting of health interventions: the need for multi-criteria decision analysis. Cost Eff Resour Alloc C/E 4:14. doi:10.1186/1478-7547-4-14

Belton V, Stewart TJ (2002) Multiple criteria decision analysis: an integrated approach. Kluwer Academic Publishers, The Netherlands

Ben-Akiva ME, Lerman SR (1985) Discrete choice analysis: theory and application to travel demand, MIT Press series in transportation studies. MIT Press, Cambridge

Bridges JFP, Hauber AB, Marshall D, Lloyd A, Prosser LA, Regier DA, Johnson FR, Mauskopf J (2011) Conjoint analysis applications in health–a checklist: a report of the ISPOR good research practices for conjoint analysis task force. Value Health 14:403–413

Communities and Local Government (CLG) (2009) Multi-criteria analysis: a manual see http://eprints.lse.ac.uk/12761/

de Bekker-Grob EW, Ryan M, Gerard K (2012) Discrete choice experiments in health economics: a review of the literature. Health Econ 21(2):145–172. doi:10.1002/hec.1697

De Montis A, De Toro P, Droste-Franke B, Omann I, Stagl S (2000) Criteria for quality assessment of MCDA methods. In: 3rd Biennial Conference of the European Society for Ecological Economics, Vienna

De Montis A, De Toro P, Droste-Franke B, Omann I, Stagl S (2005) Assessing the quality of different MCDA methods. In: Getzner M, Spash C, Stagl S (eds) Alternatives for environmental evaluation. Routledge, Abingdon/Oxon

Deal CL, Tony M, Hoybye C, Allen DB, Tauber M, Christiansen JS, Growth Hormone in Prader-Willi Syndrome Clinical Care Guidelines Workshop P (2013) GrowthHormone Research Society workshop summary: consensus guidelines for recombinant human growth hormone therapy in Prader-Willi syndrome. J Clin Endocrinol Metab 98(6):E1072–1087. doi:10.1210/jc.2012-3888

Devlin NJ, Sussex J (2011) In corporating multiple criteria in HTA: methods and processes.

Diaby V, Campbell K, Goeree R (2013) Multi-criteria decision analysis (MCDA) in health care: a bibliometric analysis. Oper Res Health Care 2:20–24

Dolan JG (1989) Medical decision making using the analytic hierarchy process choice of initial antimicrobial therapy for acute pyelonephritis. Med Decis Making 9(1):51–56

Dolan JG (1995) Are patients capable of using the analytic hierarchy process and willing to use it to help make clinical decisions? Med Decis Making 15(1):76–80

Dolan JG (2008) Shared decision-making--transferring research into practice: the analytic hierarchy process (AHP). Patient Educ Couns 73(3):418–425. doi:10.1016/j.pec.2008.07.032

Dolan JG (2010) Multi-criteria clinical decision support: a primer on the use of multiple criteria decision making methods to promote evidence-based, patient-centered healthcare. Patient 3(4):229–248. doi:10.2165/11539470-000000000-00000

Dolan JG, Isselhardt BJ, Cappuccio JD (1989) The analytic hierarchy process in medical decision making a tutorial. Med Decis Making 9(1):40–50

Dyer JS, Wendell RE (1985) A critique of the analytic hierarchy process. Department of Management, College of Business Administration and Graduate School of Business, Austin

European Medicines Agency (EMA) (2011) Benefit-risk methodology project. Work package 3 report: field tests

European Medicines Agency (EMA) (2012) Benefit-risk methodology project. Work package 4 report: benefit-risk tools and processes

Fasolo B, Bana e Costa C (2014) Tailoring value elicitation to decision makers' numeracy and fluency: expressing value judgements in numbers or words. Omega 44:83–90

Getzner M, Splash CL, Stagl S (2005) Alternatives for environmental valuation. Routledge, New York

Goetghebeur MM, Wagner M, Khoury H, Levitt RJ, Erickson LJ, Rindress D (2008) Evidence and value: impact on DEcisionMaking–the EVIDEM framework and potential applications. BMC Health Serv Res 8:270. doi:10.1186/1472-6963-8-270

Goetghebeur MM, Wagner M, Khoury H, Rindress D, Gregoire JP, Deal C (2010) Combining multicriteria decision analysis, ethics and health technology assessment: applying the EVIDEM decision-making framework to growth hormone for turner syndrome patients. Cost Eff Resour Alloc : C/E 8:4. doi:10.1186/1478-7547-8-4

Goetghebeur MM, Wagner M, Khoury H, Levitt RJ, Erickson LJ, Rindress D (2012) Bridging health technology assessment (HTA) and efficient health care decision making with multicriteria decision analysis (MCDA): applying the EVIDEM framework to medicines appraisal. Med Decis Mak : Int J Soc Med Decis Mak 32(2):376–388. doi:10.1177/0272989X11416870

Guitouni A, Martel J-M (1998) Tentative guidelines to help choosing an appropriate MCDA method. Eur J Oper Res 109:501–521

Haedrich G, Kuß A, Kreilkamp E (1986) Der analytic hierarchy process. Wirtschaftswissenschaftliches Studium 15(3):120–126

Hummel M, IJzerman M, van Manen J, Danner M, Gerber-Grote A, Volz F, Wiegard B (2013) Analytic hierarchy process (AHP) – pilot project to elicit patient preferences in the indication "depression". IQWiG Report

IJzerman MJ, van Til JA, Snoek GJ (2008) Comparison of two multi-criteria decision techniques for eliciting treatment preferences in people with neurological disorders. Patient: Patient-Cent Outcomes Res 1(4):265–272

Ivlev I, Kneppo P, Bartak M (2014) Multicriteria decision analysis: a multifaceted approach to medical equipment management. Technol Econ Dev Econ 20(3):576–589

Johnson RF, Lancsar E, Marshall D, Kilambi V, Mühlbacher A, Regier DA, Bresnahan BW, Kanninen B, Bridges JFP (2013) Constructing experimental designs for discrete-choice experiments: report of the ISPOR conjoint analysis experimental design good research practices task force. Value Health 16(1):3–13

Keeney RL (2002) Common mistakes in making value trade-offs. Oper Res 50(6):935–945

Keeney RL, Raiffa H (1976) Decisions with multiple objectives: preferences and value tradeoffs. Wiley, New York

Kelley T (1927) Interpretation of educational measurements. Macmillan, New York

Lancaster KJ (1966) A new approach to consumer theory. J Polit Econ 74(2):132–157

Lancsar E, Louviere J (2008) Conducting discrete choice experiments to inform healthcare decision making: a user's guide. Pharmacoeconomics 26(8):661–678

Lee WC, Hung FH, Tsang KF, Tung HC, Lau WH, Rakocevic V, Lai LL (2015) A speedy cardiovascular diseases classifier using multiple criteria decision analysis. Sensors 15(1):1312–1320

Liberatore MJ, Nydick RL (2008) The analytic hierarchy process in medical and health care decision making: a literature review. Eur J Oper Res 189(1):194–207

Manthey L (2007) Methoden der Präferenzmessung: Grundlagen, Konzepte und experimentelle Untersuchungen. Universität Jena, Norderstedt

Marsh K, Lanitis T, Neasham D, Orfanos P, Caro J (2014) Assessing the value of healthcare interventions using multi-criteria decision analysis: a review of the literature. Pharmacoeconomics 32(4):345–365. doi:10.1007/s40273-014-0135-0

McFadden D (1974) Conditional logit analysis of qualitative choice behavior. In: Zarembka P (ed) Frontiers of economics. Academic, London, pp 105–142

Miot J, Wagner M, Khoury H, Rindress D, Goetghebeur MM (2012) Field testing of a multicriteria decision analysis (MCDA) framework for coverage of a screening test for cervical cancer in South Africa. Cost Eff Resour Alloc : C/E 10(1):2. doi:10.1186/1478-7547-10-2

Montibeller G, von Winterfeldt D (2014) Cognitive and motivational biases in decision and risk analysis. LSE Working Paper

Mühlbacher AC, Bethge S (2015) Reduce mortality risk above all else: a discrete-choice experiment in acute coronary syndrome patients. Pharmacoeconomics 33(1):71–81. doi:10.1007/s40273-014-0223-1

Mühlbacher A, Bridges J, Bethge S, Nübling M, Gerber-Grote A, Markos Dintsios C, Scheibler F, Schwalm A, Wiegard B (2013) Choice-based conjoint analysis – pilot project to identify, weight, and prioritize multiple attributes in the indication "hepatitis C". IQWiG Report

Phillips L (1984) A theory of requisite decision models. Acta Psychol 56:29–48

Radaelli G, Lettieri E, Masella C, Merlino L, Strada A, Tringali M (2014) Implementation of EUnetHTA core model(R) in Lombardia: the VTS framework. Int J Technol Assess Health Care 30(1):105–112. doi:10.1017/S0266462313000639

Ryan M, Gerard K, Amaya-Amaya M (2008) Using discrete choice experiments to value health and health care. Springer, The Netherlands

Saaty TL (1977) A scaling method for priorities in hierarchical structures. J Math Psychol 15(3):234–281

Saaty TL (1980) The analytic hierarchy process: planning, priority setting, resource allocation. McGraw-Hill, New York

Saaty TL (1990) How to make a decision: the analytic hierarchy process. Eur J Oper Res 48(1):9–26

Saaty TL, Vargas LG (2006) Decision making with the analytic network process: economic, political, social and technological applications with benefits, opportunities, costs and risks. Springer, New York

Scholl A, Manthey L, Helm R, Steiner M (2005) Solving multiattribute design problems with analytic hierarchy process and conjoint analysis: an empirical comparison. Eur J Oper Res 164(3):760–777

Suedel BC, Kim J, Banks CJ (2009) Comparison of the direct scoring method and multi-criteria decision analysis for dredged material management decision making, 2009 U.S. Army Engineer Research and Development Center, Environmental Laboratory, 3909 Halls Ferry Road, Vicksburg, MS,39180-6199

Suner A, Çelikoğlu CC, Dicle O, Sökmen S (2012) Sequential decision tree using the analytic hierarchy process for decision support in rectal cancer. Artif Intell Med 56(1):59–68

Tanios N, Wagner M, Tony M, Baltussen R, van Til J, Rindress D, Kind P, Goetghebeur MM, International Task Force on Decision C (2013) Which criteria are considered in healthcare decisions? Insights from an international survey of policy and clinical decision makers. Int J Technol Asses Health Care 29(4):456–465. doi:10.1017/S0266462313000573

Thokala P, Duenas A (2012) Multiple criteria decision analysis for health technology assessment. Value Health: J Int Soc Pharmacoeconomics Outcomes Res 15(8):1172–1181. doi:10.1016/j.jval.2012.06.015

Tony M, Wagner M, Khoury H, Rindress D, Papastavros T, Oh P, Goetghebeur MM (2011) Bridging health technology assessment (HTA) with multicriteria decision analyses (MCDA): field testing of the EVIDEM framework for coverage decisions by a public payer in Canada. BMC Health Serv Res 11:329. doi:10.1186/1472-6963-11-329

Tu C, Fang Y, Huang Z, Tan R (2013) Application of the analytic hierarchy process to a risk assessment of emerging infectious diseases in shaoxing city in southern china. Jpn J Infect Dis 67(6):417–422

van Til JA, Renzenbrink GJ, Dolan JG, IJzerman MJ (2008) The use of the analytic hierarchy process to aid decision making in acquired equinovarus deformity. Arch Phys Med Rehabil 89(3):457–462

van Til J, Groothuis-Oudshoorn C, Lieferink M, Dolan J, Goetghebeur M (2014) Does technique matter; a pilot study exploring weighting techniques for a multi-criteria decision support framework. Cost Eff Resour Alloc: C/E 12:22. doi:10.1186/1478-7547-12-22

Velasquezl M, Hester PT (2013) An analysis of multi-criteria decision making methods. Int J Oper Res 10(2):56–66

Weernink MGM, Janus SIM, van Til JA, Raisch DW, van Manen JG, Ijzerman MJ (2014) A systematic review to identify the use of preference elicitation method in healthcare decision making. Pharm Med 28:175–185

Whitty JA, Lancsar E, Rixon K, Golenko X, Ratcliffe J (2014) A systematic review of stated preference studies reporting public preferences for healthcare priority setting. Patient-Patient-Cent Outcomes Res 7(4):365–386

Chapter 5
Dealing with Uncertainty in the Analysis and Reporting of MCDA

Catharina G.M. Groothuis-Oudshoorn, Henk Broekhuizen, and Janine van Til

Abstract The aim of this chapter is to provide guidance regarding the various types and sources of uncertainty that influence the outcome of a multi-criteria decision analysis (MCDA) model. For each MCDA step, i.e., structuring, scoring, weighting, and aggregating, we will describe sources of uncertainty and point to methods to deal with these uncertainties. Also the use of sensitivity analyses and the relevance of qualifying and quantifying uncertainty in MCDA will be discussed. The consideration of uncertainty is a difficult but important balancing act between capturing the complex uncertainties of the decision and keeping the MCDA comprehensible for decision makers.

5.1 Introduction

Multi-criteria decision analysis (MCDA) is no exact science. The output or outcome of any decision analysis depends on assumptions and decisions made while building the model and populating that model with criteria weights and performance scores. This is often referred to with the general term "uncertainty." Uncertainty can be regarded as the lack of complete knowledge or certainty about what the model should look like and what the correct inputs are (French 1995). There are many types and sources of uncertainty that influence the outcome of the MCDA model in different ways, each of which deserves specific attention while interpreting the results of an MCDA.

This chapter first describes the different types of uncertainty. Second, it will give an overview of how the different types of uncertainty play a role in the stages of an MCDA (Chapter 4). Uncertainties in the structuring, scoring, weighting and aggregating stages are reported separately, by discussing sources of uncertainty, (appropriate)

C.G.M. Groothuis-Oudshoorn (✉) • H. Broekhuizen • J. van Til
Department Health Technology and Services Research, MIRA institute, University of Twente, Drienerlolaan 5, 7522 NB Enschede, The Netherlands
e-mail: c.g.m.oudshoorn@utwente.nl

© Springer International Publishing AG 2017
K. Marsh et al. (eds.), *Multi-Criteria Decision Analysis to Support Healthcare Decisions*, DOI 10.1007/978-3-319-47540-0_5

reporting of uncertainty, and methods to study the influence of uncertainty on the outputs of the model. Finally, the use of sensitivity analyses and the relevance of qualifying and quantifying uncertainty in MCDA are discussed. Throughout the chapter we will point readers to further readings on the different topics.

Briggs and colleagues distinguished and defined four types of uncertainty in decision analytic modeling, namely, stochastic uncertainty, parameter uncertainty, heterogeneity, and structural uncertainty (Briggs et al. 2012). We use the example of a body weight scale to illustrate these different types of uncertainty. Stochastic uncertainty is the random, unexplained variability between different measurements of the weight of one person on a single weight scale of the same type and brand that occurs as a result of randomness, like the flipping of a coin or variation in the measurements of the weight of a single person if they are measured multiple times on the same device. Parameter uncertainty refers to the variability in the estimation of a parameter of interest as a result of different interpretation of the same measurement scale, for instance, the different readings of an analog weight scale by the same person on different days or by different persons (which cannot be attributed to actual differences in weight). The distinction between stochastic and parameter uncertainty is analogous to the difference between the standard deviation, a measure of variability of individuals in a population, and the standard error, i.e., a measure of precision of an estimated quantity. Like the standard error, parameter uncertainty can usually be reduced or eliminated by increasing the number of measurements. However, like the standard deviation, stochastic uncertainty cannot be eliminated but can only be better characterized, for instance, by describing the density of the random variation or the cumulative distribution. Heterogeneity is the between-person variability that can be explained by the persons' characteristics, e.g., for weight estimates this is the difference in weight between persons as a result of their differences in body composition. Structural uncertainty refers to the notion that the output of any model is conditional on its structural assumptions with regard to the best way to reach the goal itself, for example whether it is preferred to measure weight on an analog or a digital weighting scale.

As described in the previous chapters, four stages can be identified in an MCDA: structuring, i.e., establishing the decision context and building the model, weighting, scoring, and aggregating (recommendation and sensitivity analysis) (see Fig. 5.1). In each stage of an MCDA, the different types of uncertainty can be identified.

5.1.1 Problem Structuring

MCDA is mostly used in a group decision-making setting. Belton and Pictet distinguish three types of group decision-making models that can be employed during meetings in which judgments are elicited from decision makers: sharing, aggregating, and the comparing of judgments (Belton and Pictet 1997). In *sharing*

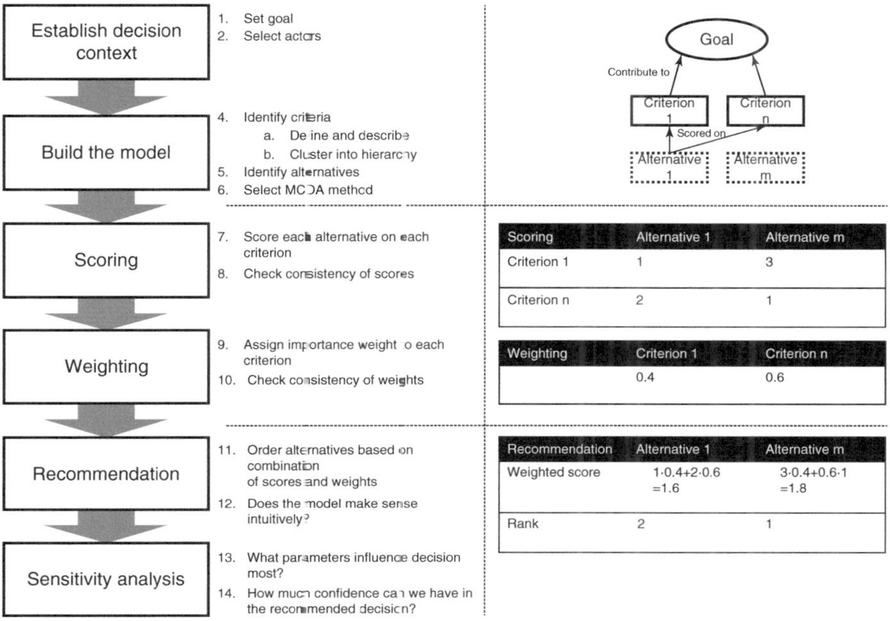

Fig. 5.1 Overview of the value-based MCDA decision-making process (*left*) and a simple numeric example (*right*)

of judgments, decision makers act as one decision maker for the purposes of the MCDA model. This implies that, even though initially there may be disagreement in the group about the judgments given, one value for each weight and performance score has to be agreed upon by the group at each stage, and only that judgment is used in the analysis. In contrast, in *aggregating judgments*, the individual judgments of each decision maker are retained throughout the decision-making process, and they are aggregated over decision makers in the final outcome, for example, by taking the mean of all individual judgments. In *comparing judgments*, the weights and performance scores of the decision makers are again retained throughout the decision analysis, and the individual judgments are actively compared during the final discussion to obtain insight into differences in opinion that may exist in between group members.

A similar but slightly different distinction in the way to handle differences in judgments is that between *statistical* aggregation and *behavioral* aggregation of judgments. Statistical aggregation is similar to Belton and Pictet's definition of aggregating: the group's individual judgments are combined into a mean judgment with a measure of variance to capture the differences between the decision makers. Behavioral aggregation is similar to Belton and Pictet's *sharing* of judgments: the group's single judgment is arrived at through a structured group process where the group can "share their knowledge and allow persuasive arguments to change their views" and therefore to revise their judgments (Phillips 1999).

The decision on which group decision model to use is a form of structural uncertainty, and moreover it influences the extent to which other types of uncertainty can be made explicit in later phases of the analysis. For instance, if at the first stage it is decided to use a sharing model where the weights and scores are set to single numbers despite possibly different judgments, the uncertainty around mean weight estimates (parameter uncertainty) and any differences between decisions makers (heterogeneity) cannot be studied. To clearly illustrate uncertainty in this chapter, we will use the statistical aggregating approach. We will illustrate the different stages of MCDA and the sources of uncertainty with a simplified case of a group decision in the medical context throughout this chapter (Text Box 5.1).

Text Box 5.1: Case Description
Six urologists within a private practice have a discussion on reducing unwanted practice variation in the choice of the first-line treatment for stage I prostate cancer patients in their practice. At present, they prescribe four alternative types of treatment: active surveillance, radical prostatectomy, external beam radiation therapy, and brachytherapy.

5.1.2 Uncertainty in Problem Structuring

The choice of criteria in an MCDA is a source of structural uncertainty. Criteria have to reflect the different points of view of the actors in the decision and enable comparisons of between the alternatives (Bouyssou 1990). To reduce structural uncertainty about whether all relevant criteria are included in the analysis, it is advised to combine the top-down and bottom-up approach to developing a set of criteria. Top-down approaches are where actors first agree on the relevance of particular consequences and then come up with examples of those often result in hierarchical value trees. Alternatively, bottom-up approaches often start with drawing up extensive lists of criteria from different sets, which can later be structured into hierarchies if desired. In the problem structuring stage, the value tree has to be determined and the final set of criteria has to be determined. Structural uncertainty about the shape of the value tree and the number and type of criteria to include can be made explicit by making detailed notes of all decisions made in this step and by including as many actors as needed to come up with a broadly supported value tree.

The goal of problem structuring is to come up with a clear, logical, and shared point of view of what decision criteria and decision structure best reflect the decision at hand and help the decision makers to achieve their objective. The final list of criteria should be as simple as possible, yet capture the complexity of the decision. There are no guidelines on what is the optimal number of criteria and/or decision structure. In some cases the type of MCDA or the cognitive limitations of the stakeholders put a limit on the number of criteria or favor a certain value tree structure. When in doubt about including a criterion, it is always wise to include it in the analysis, as some MCDA methods allow a criterion to be dropped in a later stage. The alternative of adding a criterion in a later stage is much more bothersome. Problem structuring is a skill that is acquired through experience. Flow charts, fish-bone diagrams, pro/cons lists, and quantitative techniques, such as the nominal group technique, can help groups come up with an adequate set of criteria and an adequate problem structure (Taner et al. 2007). However, it is known that the choice of criteria, MCDA method, and weight elicitation influences the outcome of the model. Besides extensive argumentation and good documentation of the way in which the decision problem was reflected in the choice of criteria, shape of the value tree, and choice of the MCDA method, the only way to explicitly study structural uncertainty is by testing the influence of the different options (i.e., different criteria sets, value trees, and MCDA techniques) on the outcome of the analysis. There are multiple examples of such tests in literature (van Til et al. 2014; IJzerman et al. 2012a, b).

Text Box 5.2: MCDA Model and Clinical Evidence

In the example, there are many criteria that potentially influence the choice of treatment in prostate cancer. The effectiveness of the treatment in prolonging life after diagnosis; the side effects of treatment, such as bowel problems, bladder problems, erection problems, and tiredness; and the process characteristics of treatment such as costs, duration, and frequency of follow-up needed all could influence treatment preference. For illustrative purposes, we limit the example to the four criteria mentioned in Table 5.1 and choose a simple multi-attribute rating technique (SMART) to demonstrate the different types of uncertainty in weighting, scoring, and sensitivity analysis.

SMART is a simple value-based MCDA method based on a linear additive value function. In our example, the model is $V_i = \sum_{k=1}^{4} w_k x_{ik}$, where V_i is the overall value of treatment i, w_k is the weight of the kth criterion as weighted using swing weighting, and x_{ik} is the performance of treatment i on k. The hypothetical clinical evidence for the example is given in Table 5.1.

Table 5.1 Bowel problems, incontinence, and erectile dysfunction as measured as probabilities of the event occuring in five years after treatment

	Active surveillance	Surgical removal	External beam radiation therapy	Brachytherapy
Sample size	1000	800	200	800
Survival (years)	10 [9.4–10.6]	15 [14.0–16.1]	12 [10.3–13.7]	12 [11.0–13.1]
Bowel problems	0 %	0 %	15 %	0 %
Incontinence	0 %	10 %	1 %	0.5 %
Erectile dysfunction	5 %	75 %	45 %	24 %

Based on Cooperberg et al. (2012), Hayes et al. (2013)

5.2 Uncertainty in Scoring

As described in Chapter 4, during the scoring stage either the available clinical evidence or expert judgment is used to judge the performance of the alternatives on the criteria, by transforming clinical performance (which may be measured on a variety of scales) to a common value scale. Both the clinical evidence and the expert judgments are possible sources of parameter and stochastic uncertainty, as well as heterogeneity (Durbach and Stewart 2012).

5.2.1 Performance Estimates

Preferably, performance of the alternatives on the different criteria is based on clinical data (including patient registries, cost databases, etc.). In our example, the average survival for the four treatments could be drawn from scientific literature. When clinical evidence is used as input in an MCDA model, often only the point estimates are used. However, the parameter and stochastic uncertainty surrounding these estimates of performance measurements can be used to explicitly model uncertainty in the MCDA. Parameter uncertainty in the performance estimates refers to the variability in the estimation of the outcome (for instance survival) as a result of the sampling (error). The standard errors or, equivalently, the confidence bounds of the point estimates obtained from clinical trial data can be used to represent the extent of the parameter uncertainty. Stochastic uncertainty, i.e., the unexplained variability in the clinical evidence, can be made visible by presenting the standard deviation or the range of the outcomes in the patient sample.

To demonstrate any heterogeneity in the clinical evidence in the model, one can calculate averages and standard deviations of outcome for different subgroups of patients. When clinical data is lacking, the performance estimates have to be based on expert judgments. Different expert elicitation techniques are available to do so (O'Hagan et al. 2006; Bojke et al. 2010; Bojke and Soares 2014). This introduces structural uncertainty to the model due to the differences in techniques. If clinical judgments are to replace clinical evidence, rather than just asking for point estimates of performance, experts should be asked to give distributions and/or confidence bounds for their estimates, if possible linked to patient characteristics. This enables analysts to take parameter uncertainty and heterogeneity into account.

5.2.2 From Performance to Value

In valuing performance, the performance of the alternatives on the natural scale (e.g., survival in years) is transformed to a score which represents the value of that performance on a scale ranging from zero (no value) to one (maximum value). One can determine the relative value of the performance estimates for the alternatives, or

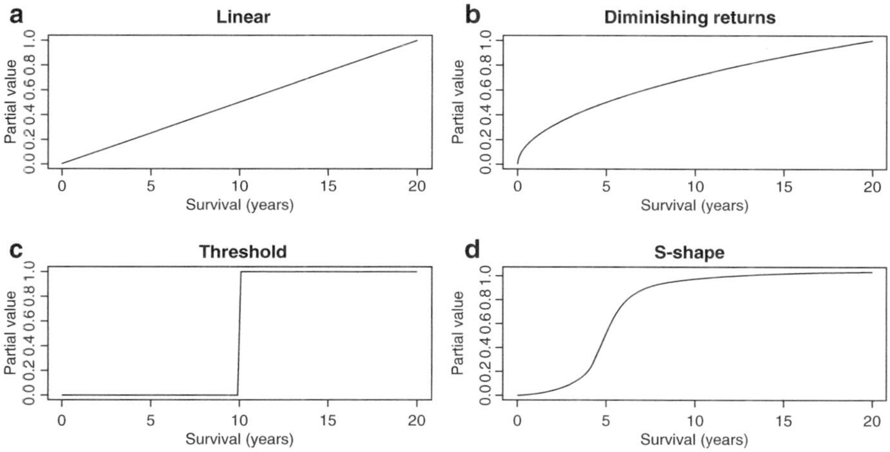

Fig. 5.2 (**a**) a partial value function where function scales linearly with increased survival. (**b**) a partial value function where there are diminishing returns with respect to survival, i.e. an increase from 0 to 5 years of survival is considered more valuable than an increase from 5 to 10 years of survival. (**c**) a partial function with a threshold. Here, all increases in survival less than 10 years are not considered valuable, but increases in survival of more than 10 years are considered valuable. (**d**) S-shaped partial value function. This can be seen as a smoothed version of the threshold function

one can map the performance to estimate value of all intermediate performances with the use of partial value functions. This can either be done "locally," meaning that the best and worst performance judgments of the alternatives on the criteria (as identified by experts) are used as the upper and lower bounds of the value function, or "globally," meaning upper and lower bounds are based on estimates of worst and best possible outcomes, irrespective of the performance of the included alternatives. For example, although a diagnostic test with sensitivity of 100 % is highly unlikely in clinical practice, 100 % sensitivity can be used as a theoretical best possible outcome.

One source of structural uncertainty in the valuation stage is the shape of the value function. Most commonly, a linear function is assumed (Fig. 5.2a). This is a simple function that linearly scales all performance values between the worst level W (partial value of zero) and the best level B (partial partial value of one):

$$v(x) = \begin{cases} 1, & x \geq B \\ \dfrac{x - W}{B - W}, & W < x < B \\ 0, & x \leq W \end{cases} \tag{5.1}$$

In such a linear value function, it is assumed that an increase in performance results in an equal increase in value independently from where on the performance scale this increase occurs. So for survival, it would mean that the value of increasing survival from 0 to 5 years is the same as the value of increasing the survival from 15 to 20 years. Confidence bounds for the value of performances can be obtained by applying the partial value function on the confidence bounds of the performances (see Table 5.2 for the example).

However, many other forms of the value function exist. For example, there can be diminishing returns to prolonging life, and for some people, living after a certain age might decrease the incremental value of this outcome (Fig. 5.2b). For other outcomes, a value function with a threshold that may vary between decision makers may be more appropriate where performance (outcome) switches from no value to maximum value (Fig. 5.2c), or there can be a combination of a linear function and diminishing returns: the S-shaped value function (Fig. 5.2d). It is common to agree upon the shape of the functional form on a group level.

If one wants to deviate from the linear function, additional inputs are needed from decision makers to determine the particular shape of the value function. For example, in the bisection method, the decision maker is asked to define the point on the attribute scale which is halfway in value terms between the two endpoints. From this a two-piece linear value function can be constructed (Belton and Stewart 2002). This process can be repeated multiple times until the decision makers are indifferent between further bisections. In MACBETH, a value function for a particular criterion is constructed from the pairwise comparisons of the performance of alternatives on that criterion using linear programming (Costa et al. 2012).

As value judgments may differ between decision makers, the final construction of a value function can consequently be based on averages of these judgments or based on another central measure (median, mode). By calculating a standard error and confidence intervals along with the average value, a measure for parameter uncertainty can be obtained. Stochastic uncertainty in the value judgments can be quantified by calculating a standard deviation of the value judgments.

Heterogeneity refers to possible differences in the value function or value of outcomes between different groups of decision makers that may be explained with their backgrounds. For instance, thresholds for survival might be different in urologists that mostly see older patients, compared to urologists that see relatively younger patients in their daily work. By constructing value functions for the different groups, one can see whether heterogeneity is present.

Summarizing, all types of uncertainty influence the values from the scoring step. Uncertainty (parameter, stochastic, or heterogeneity) in the evidence implies also uncertainty in the value function. The uncertainty in evidence and the uncertainty due to differences in value judgments can be quantified by calculating standard errors, standard deviations, or confidence bounds.

5.3 Uncertainty in Weighting

All inputs in the weighting stage are given by stakeholders (decision makers, patients, physicians, general public, etc.), which are therefore the main source of uncertainty in this stage. In the weights there can be structural uncertainty, parameter uncertainty, stochastic uncertainty, and heterogeneity.

Text Box 5.3: Calculating Partial Values
Assuming a linear value function in the urologists' case, the point estimates with confidence bounds of performance are transformed with Eq. 5.1 to the value estimates with confidence bounds (Table 5.2)

Table 5.2 Partial values in the urologists' case, with 95 % confidence intervals for the partial values for survival based on the confidence bounds reported in the clinical trial reports

	Active surveillance	Surgical removal	External beam radiation therapy	Brachytherapy
Average survival	0.50 [0.47–0.53]	0.75 [0.70–0.80]	0.6 [0.52–0.68]	0.6 [0.55–0.65]
Bowel problems	1	1	0.85	1
Incontinence	1	0.90	0.99	0.5
Erectile dysfunction	0.95	0.59	0.25	0.29

For example, the 95 % confidence interval for the average survival of patients under active surveillance is 9.4–10.6 years (Table 5.1), implying a confidence interval on the partial value from 0.47 to 0.53

Parameter uncertainty in weights is the variability in the estimation of a parameter of interest as a result of sampling. Although their underlying value may be the same, different decision makers will interpret a weighting scale differently and thus will come up with different weights. This can be reflected by calculating the mean weight along with the variance measure for each criterion over a group of decision makers. The parameter uncertainty is a function of the sample size and the underlying stochastic uncertainty. The larger the sample size n, the smaller the parameter uncertainty will be as it is a function of n with $1/\sqrt{n}$.

Individual weights are usually combined into an average weight over decision makers. The most commonly used method to combine individual weights is the arithmetic mean. However, in the analytic hierarchy process, the geometric mean is used to combine the weight estimates of different decision makers. The decision to use either the arithmetic mean or the geometric mean is important as it affects what method is appropriate for calculating the standard error around the mean weight.

Heterogeneity is the between-person variability that may be explained by the characteristics of the decision maker. For instance, erectile dysfunction as a result of treatment of prostate cancer may (or may not) be more important to a 40-year-old man compared to an 80-year-old man as the latter tends to have a less active sex life. It is important to have estimates of heterogeneity linked to background characteristics in MCDA, because the outcome of the analysis might be different for different (groups of) persons.

Stochastic uncertainty is the random, unexplained variability between different measurements of the weight estimates of one person. In most MCDA analyses, the magnitude of stochastic within-subject variability is not known as weight judgments are performed only once.

Heterogeneity is similar to stochastic uncertainty in that both cannot be reduced. The difference is that differences in weights as a result of heterogeneity of the subject need to be understood rather than minimized, while large random variability in weights is undesirable.

The choice of the weight elicitation technique induces structural uncertainty, as the use of different techniques can result in differences in weight estimates of the criteria, or may imply different (methodological) meanings of weights (Choo et al. 1999). Knowing that the exact weights vary based on the weight elicitation method stresses the need for sensitivity analysis on the final results. Previous research has shown that while exact weights might differ based on the weight elicitation method, the rank order of criteria is mostly maintained. In a few studies, it was shown that the differences in weights as a result of technique have a minor impact on the overall value of the alternatives. However, testing the range in which weights can vary before the rank order of alternatives changes (and to judge whether this extent of change is likely to happen as a result of the weight elicitation method) should be an important aim of sensitivity analysis (IJzerman et al. 2012a; van Til et al. 2014). To reduce structural uncertainty due to mismatches between the meaning of weights according to the MCDA model definitions and the decision makers' understanding of the weights' meanings, it is important to clearly explain the MCDA (elicitation) method to the decision makers.

Summarizing, all types of uncertainty influence the estimates of the weights. Parameter uncertainty can be made visible by presenting not only mean weights but also confidence intervals. Stochastic uncertainty and related structural uncertainty cannot be made explicit unless decision makers are asked to repeat their weight estimations with the same weight elicitation technique (stochastic uncertainty) or are asked to perform weight estimations with different weight elicitation techniques. Heterogeneity can be made visible by knowing and categorizing the decision makers and calculating mean weights (with confidence bounds) for the different subgroups.

5.4 Aggregation Methods

After the scoring and weighting steps are completed, performance values and criteria weights are (statistically) aggregated in an overall value. The most commonly used aggregation method is additive weighting, where the partial values on the different criteria are multiplied by their criteria weights and then summed up per alternative (see Chapter 4). The simplicity of additive weighting is attractive because it is easily understood by decision makers. From a theoretical perspective, other statistical aggregation methods might be preferred (see, e.g., Zhou and Ang 2009; Zanakis et al. 1998).

The choice of aggregation method is a form of structural uncertainty, since it can alter the model outcomes (Zhou and Ang 2009) and their interpretation. Moreover, because some approaches, such as the analytic hierarchy process, place very specific requirements on the performance and weight elicitation techniques, the choice of aggregation method is a decision that has to be made early in the MCDA (Choo et al. 1999; Liberatore and Nydick 2008).

Another type of structural uncertainty is the decision at which point to aggregate the results of different decision makers in the weighting and performance stage. In essence, there are two ways to do so. One can average individual performance values and individual criteria weights (with measures of variance) and use an aggregation approach (for instance, an additive model) to calculate one overall value (with measures of variance). Alternatively, one can calculate an overall value for each individual and average the multiple estimations of overall value (with measures of variance). As aggregation is based on the product of two values, both approaches result in different average overall values and different measures of variance. Moreover, in the former case, providing a measure of parameter uncertainty by calculating a standard error of the overall value is difficult as the overall value is a sum of products of averages. One way to calculate the variance (and thus the standard deviation) of a product is the delta method (Rice 2006).

Finally, irrespective of the exact statistical aggregation method used, the output of an MCDA model is a point estimate of the overall value of the different alternatives. The impact of uncertainties on the aggregated overall value can be made explicit by calculating standard errors, confidence intervals, or ranges of the overall value of a treatment based on the standard errors (for parameter uncertainty) or standard deviations (for stochastic uncertainty) in the performances and weights. By reporting not only the point estimate of the overall value of a treatment but also its standard error or confidence interval, the parameter or stochastic uncertainty in the overall value is made visible.

5.5 Sensitivity Analysis

The outcome of a value-based MCDA method is an overall value for each alternative. However, without information on the uncertainty surrounding the weight estimates and performance values, the stability of the overall value is not known. Therefore, the confidence with which the results of the MCDA can be interpreted is then also not known. If one or multiple types of uncertainty are taken into account, this will result in a distribution of values around the point estimates. The shape and spread of the value distribution provide information about the stability of the conclusions that can be drawn from the analysis.

Sensitivity analysis is the study of the impact of uncertainty throughout the decision-making process on its outcomes. Structural uncertainty occurs as a result of the choices made in problem structuring with regard to the shape of the value tree, the type and number of criteria included in the analysis, and the MCDA method chosen to perform the analysis (including the weight elicitation and value performance method). The impact of structural uncertainty on the outcome can only be made explicit by performing MCDA for the same problem with different value trees, criteria, and MCDA methods. This type of sensitivity analysis is a time-consuming process which is usually not performed.

A more common type of sensitivity analysis is studying the impact of parameter uncertainty in weights and performances or heterogeneity on the outcome(s) of an MCDA. When assessing the impact of uncertainty, one can do so throughout the whole MCDA process, identifying sources and measuring the amount of uncertainty at each stage separately and then studying its impact on the outcome(s) of the MCDA process. Alternatively, one can assess the impact of uncertainty on the overall value after the criteria weights and performance values are aggregated. Both are commonly termed "sensitivity analysis" in literature, and the latter is also sometimes termed "robustness analysis" or "post hoc sensitivity analysis." Although these two concepts are conceptually different, similar methods can be used during their application to demonstrate the uncertainty around the point estimates. In the next paragraphs, we will describe two commonly used methods for sensitivity analysis, namely, deterministic and probabilistic sensitivity analysis, and shortly touch upon some alternative methods.

In an earlier literature review in the healthcare context, 19 studies were identified where uncertainty was explicitly taken into account in the MCDA analysis (Broekhuizen et al. 2015a). In nine studies, the deterministic sensitivity approach was used, four studies used a probabilistic approach, and in other four studies (concerning environmental health issues), fuzzy set theory was applied. It seemed that in most MCDA-supported decisions, a deterministic sensitivity analysis was used because of its ease of use and because the increased insight in the stability of results was deemed sufficient. However, when the uncertainty in multiple model parameters needs to be considered simultaneously, approaches that use probability distributions should be applied.

Deterministic sensitivity analysis is the most straightforward method for (post hoc) sensitivity analysis. In deterministic sensitivity analysis, one parameter, that is a criterion weight or performance score, is varied at a time, and the impact of varying this parameter on the rank order of alternatives is observed. If the induced variation does not change the rank order of alternatives, i.e., the preference of one alternative over the other is preserved, the decision seems robust. Alternatively, one can assess the extent to which a parameter can be increased or decreased before the rank order of alternatives changes. The range in which the particular parameter is likely to change can be based on expert' judgments or the variation in available clinical data.

Recall that the urologists in the example took the confidence bounds for the average survival across treatments options from the literature. We already demonstrated in an earlier section that these can be transformed to confidence bounds on partial values. However, it might also be insightful to consider the impact of the range of partial values on the overall value of treatments. This can be done by inserting partial values for the lower and upper confidence bounds in the overall value function. This results in a confidence interval of the overall value in which the

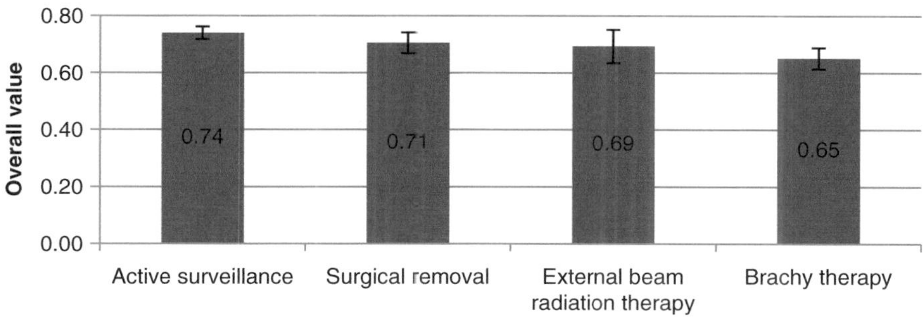

Fig. 5.3 Influence of parameter uncertainty in the survival estimates for the various treatments on their overall value in the urologists' example. Note the overlapping confidence bounds that indicate uncertainty regarding what treatment is more valuable

uncertainty depends only on the uncertainty present in the estimates for average survival (Fig. 5.3).

This deterministic sensitivity analysis reveals that there is overlap between the confidence bounds of overall values and that this depends (at least partly) on parameter uncertainty in the survival estimates. Furthermore, it seems that changing the survival estimates within confidence bounds can lead to rank reversals of alternatives. For example, it is possible that external beam radiation therapy has a higher overall value than surgical removal. The question remains, however, how likely it is that such a rank reversal between external beam radiation therapy and surgical removal occurs.

Deterministic sensitivity analysis can also be used to assess the impact of (uncertainty in the) criterion weights on the alternatives' overall value by manually varying the criterion weights one by one and observing how the overall values of the alternatives change. For example, if we increase the weight of survival and thereby decrease the weights of the other criteria (because weights add up to one), alternatives that have longer survival will increase in overall value compared to alternatives with a relatively shorter survival. One can vary each criterion weight from its lowest possible value to its highest possible value and observe the effect on overall value of the alternatives (Fig. 5.4). Alternatively, and more effectively, one can vary the weights within the confidence bounds resulting from parameter uncertainty and heterogeneity in preferences within the group and see whether this variation would change the outcome of the model.

Another particular deterministic sensitivity graph, popular in health-economic assessments, is the tornado graph. A tornado graph shows the impact on model outcomes of arbitrary fixed changes (e.g., −10 % and +10 %) in single model parameters. It is especially useful for determining which model parameter has the greatest influence on the outcome (Briggs et al. 2012).

The results of the analysis as presented in Fig. 5.4 will provide the urologist with more information on the robustness of their results. Active surveillance has the highest value when the mean criteria weights of the group of urologists are

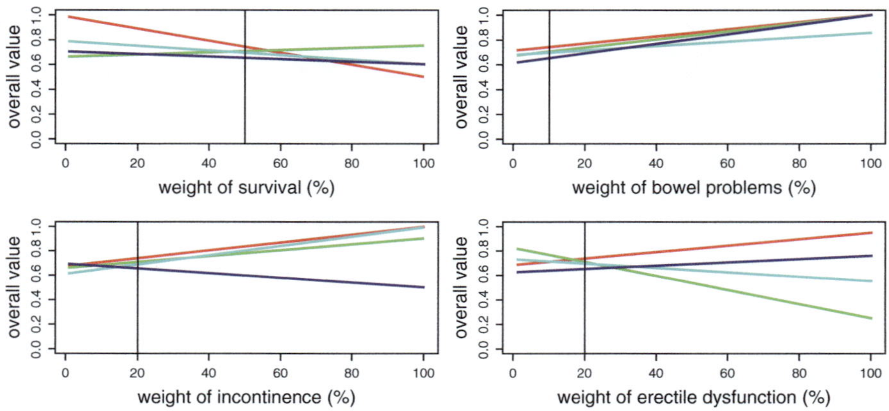

Fig. 5.4 Each of these three graphs shows how the overall value of treatments would vary, had the urologists chosen different (i.e., higher or lower) weights for each of the criteria. This overall value is on the vertical axes, the weights are on the horizontal axes, and the vertical black lines denote the point estimates of the weights. *Red* active surveillance, *Green* surgical removal, *Light blue* external beam radiation therapy, *Purple* brachytherapy

used. However, intersections between lines imply rank reversals between treatments based on changes in criteria weights. If, for example, the weight put on survival would increase above 58 %, surgical removal would have the highest value, making it the preferred treatment. However, the threshold, i.e., the weight for survival where a rank reversal between surgical removal and active surveillance occurs, is 8 % removed from the initial point estimate, and this falls within the variation of weights given by the individual urologists but not within the confidence interval of the average weight. The urologists must determine whether such an increase in weight is likely. For now, based on the deterministic sensitivity analysis, it seems that rank reversals are unlikely and that the preference for active surveillance is robust.

Although it is easy to implement, deterministic sensitivity analysis has two important drawbacks. First of all, only one model parameter (weight or performance score) is varied at a time. This is unrealistic because it assumes uncertainty in only one parameter, while actually multiple (or all) model parameters can be uncertain. Second, manually changing of model parameters, such as presented above or in a tornado graph, does not take into account the actual uncertainty in the model parameters. For example, if the observed range of a weight is between 40 % and 60 %, it does not make sense to investigate rank reversals that occur when the weight is 80 %. This is a relevant issue for the urologists, because their deterministic sensitivity analysis shows them that rank reversals occur at particular combinations of survival estimates, but they cannot quantify the likelihood with which this might happen.

Instead of a deterministic sensitivity analysis, a probabilistic approach could be used to gain insight into the impact of the combination in uncertainty in the clinical evidence, scores, and/or weights on the overall value of the alternatives. For example, in a study by Wen et al., two different methods (a delta-method approach and a Monte Carlo approach) for constructing a confidence interval of the overall benefit-risk score from an MCDA model were compared (Wen et al. 2014). The objective of the study was to provide suggestions for incorporating the uncertainty in performance data based on clinical evidence into the MCDA model when evaluating the overall benefit-risk profiles of different treatment options. In a study by Broekhuizen et al., the impact of uncertainty in the performance estimates based on clinical evidence was studied along with the uncertainty in criteria weights as given by patients (Broekhuizen et al. 2015b). In stochastic multi-criteria acceptability analysis (SMAA), uncertainties in preference data and clinical trial data are combined, and a non-informative (uniform) distribution based on the rank order of criteria is used for the weight distributions (Tervonen et al. 2011; van Valkenhoef et al. 2012). Finally, Caster et al. use qualitative data on the rank order of criteria and combine this with probability distributions for clinical data (Caster et al. 2012).

In a probabilistic approach, uncertainty in model parameters is represented with probability distributions. There are many different types of probability distributions. When data is available, the empirical distribution can be used or assumptions with regard to a parametric distribution must be made. A comprehensive review of methods for eliciting probability distributions from (groups of) experts can be found in (O'Hagan et al. 2006).

After selecting or eliciting a probability distribution that reflects the uncertainty in each model parameter, one can assess how the uncertainty in all these parameters translates to uncertainty in the overall value of the alternatives, for example, by means of a Monte Carlo simulation approach. This approach consists of sampling from the distributions of one or multiple model parameters simultaneously and then calculating the overall value of the alternatives for each of these (combinations of) sampled estimates. By repeating this process a large number of times (e.g., 1000 or more), it can give decision makers an idea about the likely distribution of overall value of each included alternative (Broekhuizen et al. 2015b).

In our prostate cancer example, a normal probability distribution is selected for survival because of the large sample sizes in the clinical trials. After parametrizing this distribution based on standard errors reported in the clinical paper and running the Monte Carlo simulations, the distributions for the overall values as presented in Fig. 5.5 are obtained.

The amount of overlap between these distributions is an indicator of the likelihood that the treatments are in the correct preference order, while the width of the curves is an indicator of how likely the point estimates of the values are. If there is much overlap between the value distributions of two treatments, and the value distributions are "wide" (such as with the light-blue line), there is more uncertainty about which treatment has the highest value. This uncertainty can be quantified by taking the percentage of Monte Carlo samples in which a particular treatment has the highest value. This is called the first ranking probability. One minus the first ranking probability is a surrogate of decision uncertainty as it estimates the probability that the alternative with the highest mean value does not have the highest rank (Table 5.3).

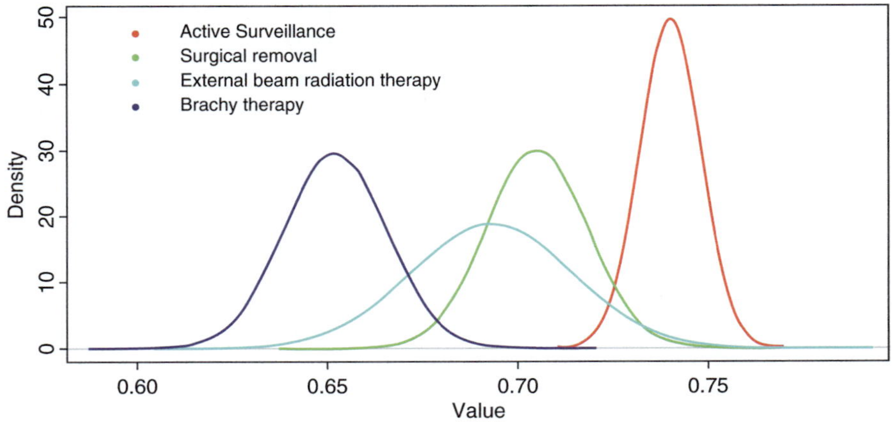

Fig. 5.5 Distribution of overall value of the alternatives in the urologists' case, when normal distributions based on clinical literature are assigned to the "survival" performance parameter. Estimated using a gaussian kernel density

Table 5.3 Ranking probabilities in the urologists' case, when the uncertainty in the survival estimates is represented with normal distributions (see Fig. 5.5) and after running 5000 Monte Carlo simulations

Probability of…	Active surveillance	Surgical removal	External beam radiation therapy	Brachytherapy
… being ranked 1st	97 %	1 %	2 %	–
… being ranked 2nd	3 %	68 %	29 %	–
… being ranked 3rd	–	31 %	64 %	5 %
… being ranked 4th	–	–	5 %	95 %

Please note that only uncertainty in survival is taken into account. When more parameters would be assigned probability distributions to reflect uncertainty, the probability of rank reversals may increase

Other approaches apart from deterministic and probabilistic approaches to incorporate uncertainty analysis in MCDA have been identified, namely, Bayesian frameworks, fuzzy set theory, and grey theory (Broekhuizen et al. 2015a).

Within the Bayesian framework, a distinction can be made between approaches based on Bayesian networks (Fenton and Neil 2001) and approaches based on Dempster-Shafer theory (Beynon et al. 2000). Fuzzy set theory aims to capture the ambiguity present in human language and judgment and is often combined with the AHP method of MCDA. Comparable to fuzzy set theory are approaches based on grey theory (Ju-Long 1982). With these approaches one can address all types of uncertainty except for structural uncertainty. The applicability of these methods for addressing uncertainty is sometimes strictly dependent on the specific form of MCDA used. For example, SMAA is a strictly probabilistic method (Lahdelma and Hokkanen 1998). Other MCDA methods like AHP, PROMETHEE, TOPSIS, and ELECTRE can be combined with (almost) all uncertainty approaches.

5.6 Summary and Conclusions

Uncertainty is introduced into an MCDA at the following stages: the problem structuring stage, the performance valuation stage, and the criteria weighting stage. Structural uncertainty is introduced as a result of methodological choices such as the MCDA method, structuring of the value tree, type of weight and performance elicitation techniques used, and aggregation method. Parameter uncertainty occurs because of sampling error. Stochastic uncertainty is the uncertainty as a result of random, unexplained variation and can be made visible by presenting, e.g., histograms/densities for the weights and performance values. Heterogeneity is the explained variation as a result of different background characteristics and values of the respondents. Often it is not possible or even desirable (in the case of heterogeneity) to reduce uncertainty, but the aim of this chapter was to explain how uncertainty can be made explicit throughout the decision process and to study its influence on the output of the MCDA.

We emphasized how the quantitative outcomes of the model depend on the way in which weight and performances are aggregated, while the interpretation of the output of the model depends also on the way in which the output is presented to the decision maker.

Through sensitivity analysis, the impact of uncertainty on the outcome of the decision analysis can be made explicit. We have demonstrated how different types of uncertainty in the inputs of the MCDA model influence its outputs and how uncertainty can be quantified with different measures of variability (standard deviation, standard error, range) or can be graphically displayed. Both deterministic sensitivity analysis and probabilistic sensitivity analysis were explained.

To fully analyze the impact of uncertainty in MCDA, additional efforts may be required from the decision makers in terms of additional model inputs (measures of variation, probability distributions, ranges of weights or scores) and from decision analyst in terms of analytic skills. A balance must be struck between increasing confidence of the decision makers in the output of the MCDA by demonstrating the impact of uncertainty and not losing confidence of decision makers in the MCDA itself by making the analyses too complicated.

References

Belton V, Pictet J (1997) A framework for group decision using a MCDA model: sharing, aggregating or comparing individual information? J Decis Sys 6(3):283–303. Available at: http://www.tandfonline.com/doi/abs/10 1080/12460125.1997.10511726. Accessed 18 Feb 2014

Belton V, Stewart TJ (2002) Multiple criteria decision analysis: an integrated approach, 2nd edn. Kluwer Academic Publishers, Dordrecht

Beynon M, Curry B, Morgan P (2000) The Dempster-Shafer theory of evidence: an alternative approach to multicriteria decision modelling. Omega 28(1):37–50

Bojke L, Soares M (2014) Decision analysis: eliciting experts' beliefs to characterize uncertainties. Elsevier Ltd. Available at: http://www.sciencedirect.com/science/article/pii/B9780123756787014061

Bojke L et al (2010) Eliciting distributions to populate decision analytic models. Value Health 13(5):557–564

Bouyssou D (1990) Building criteria: a prerequisite for MCDA. In: Readings in multiple criteria decision aid. Springer, Berlin, pp 58–80

Briggs AH et al (2012) Model parameter estimation and uncertainty: a report of the ISPOR-SMDM modeling good research practices task force-6. Value Health 15(6):835–842. Available at: http://www.ncbi.nlm.nih.gov/pubmed/22999133

Broekhuizen H et al (2015a) A review and classification of approaches for dealing with uncertainty in multi-criteria decision analysis for healthcare decisions. Pharmacoeconomics 33(5):445–455

Broekhuizen H et al (2015b) Estimating the value of medical treatments to patients using probabilistic multi criteria decision analysis. BMC Med Info Decis Making 15(1):1–10. Available at: http://dx.doi.org/10.1186/s12911-015-0225-8

Caster O et al (2012) Quantitative benefit-risk assessment using only qualitative information on utilities. Med Decis Making 32(6):E1–E15. Available at: http://www.ncbi.nlm.nih.gov/pubmed/22936214 [Accessed 3 Dec 2012]

Choo EU, Schoner B, Wedley WC (1999) Interpretation of criteria weights in multicriteria decision making. Comput Ind Eng 37(3):527–541. Available at: http://linkinghub.elsevier.com/retrieve/pii/S036083520000019X

Cooperberg MR et al (2012) Primary treatments for clinically localised prostate cancer: a comprehensive lifetime cost-utility analysis. BJU Int 111(3):437–450

Bana E Costa, C. A, De Corte J.-M, Vansnick J.-C (2012) Macbeth. Inter J Info Tech Decision Making 11(02):359–387. Available at: http://www.worldscientific.com/doi/abs/10.1142/S0219622012400068

Durbach IN, Stewart TJ (2012) Modeling uncertainty in multi-criteria decision analysis. Eur J Oper Res 223(1):1–14. Available at: http://linkinghub.elsevier.com/retrieve/pii/S0377221712003591. Accessed 27 Jan 2014

Fenton N, Neil M (2001) Making decisions: using Bayesian nets and MCDA. Knowl Based Syst 14(7):307–325. Available at: http://www.scopus.com/inward/record.url?eid=2-s2.0-0035505967&partnerID=tZOtx3y1. Accessed 18 Feb 2014

French S (1995) Uncertainty and imprecision: modelling and analysis. J Oper Res Soc 46(1): 70–79. Available at: http://www.jstor.org/stable/2583837

Hayes J et al (2013) Observation versus initial treatment for men with localized, low-risk prostate cancer. Ann Intern Med 158(12):853–860

IJzerman MJ, Van Til JA et al (2012) A comparison of analytic hierarchy process and conjoint analysis methods in assessing treatment alternatives for stroke rehabilitation. Patient 5(1): 45–56. Available at: http://www.ncbi.nlm.nih.gov/pubmed/22185216

IJzerman MJ, Til JA, Snoek GJ (2012) Comparison of two multi-criteria decision techniques for eliciting treatment preferences in people with neurological disorders. Patient Patient-Centered Out Res 1(4):265–272. Available at: http://dx.doi.org/10.2165/1312067-200801040-00008

Ju-Long D (1982) Control problems of grey systems. Syst Control Letters 1(5):288–294. Available at: http://linkinghub.elsevier.com/retrieve/pii/S016769118280025X

Lahdelma R, Hokkanen J (1998) SMAA-stochastic multiobjective acceptability analysis. Eur J Oper 2217(97):137–143. Available at: http://www.sciencedirect.com/science/article/pii/S037722179700163X. Accessed 26 Mar 2012

Liberatore MJ, Nydick RL (2008) The analytic hierarchy process in medical and health care decision making: a literature review. Eur J Oper Res 189(1):194–207

O'Hagan A et al (2006) Uncertain judgements: eliciting expert probabilities. John Wiley & Sons Ltd, Chichester. Available at: http://eu.wiley.com/WileyCDA/WileyTitle/productCd-0470029994.html

Phillips LD (1999) Group elicitation of probability distributions: are many heads better than one? In: Shanteau J, Mellors B, Schum D (eds) Decision science and technol- ogy: reflections on the contributions of ward edwards. Kluwer Academic Publishers, Norwell, p 313–330. Available at: http://eprints.lse.ac.uk/10520/

Rice J (2006) Mathematical statistics and data analysis. Thomson Brooks/Cole Belmont, CA, USA

Taner M, Sezen B, Antony J (2007) An overview of six sigma applications in healthcare industry. Int J Health Care Qual Assur 20(4):329–340

Tervonen T et al (2011) A stochastic multicriteria model for evidence-based decision making in drug benefit-risk analysis. Stat Med 30(12):1419–1428. Available at: http://www.ncbi.nlm.nih.gov/pubmed/21268053. Accessed 26 Mar 2012

van Til J et al (2014) Does technique matter; a pilot study exploring weighting techniques for a multi-criteria decision support framework. Cost Eff Res Allocation 12:22

van Valkenhoef G et al (2012) Multicriteria benefit-risk assessment using network meta-analysis. J Clin Epidemiol 65(4):.394–403. Available at: http://www.ncbi.nlm.nih.gov/pubmed/22197518

Wen S, Zhang L, Yang B (2014) Two approaches to incorporate clinical data uncertainty into multiple criteria decision analysis for benefit-risk assessment of medicinal products. Value Health 17(5):619–628. Available at: http://www.ncbi.nlm.nih.gov/pubmed/25128056. Accessed 21 Aug 2014

Zanakis SH et al (1998) Multi-attribute decision making: a simulation comparison of select methods. Eur J Oper Res 107(3):507–529

Zhou P, Ang BW (2009) Comparing MCDA aggregation methods in constructing composite indicators using the Shannon-Spearman measure. Social Indic Res 94(1):83–96

Part II
Applications and Case Studies

Chapter 6
Supporting the Project Portfolio Selection Decision of Research and Development Investments by Means of Multi-Criteria Resource Allocation Modelling

J.M. Hummel, Monica D. Oliveira, Carlos A. Bana e Costa, and Maarten J. IJzerman

Abstract The healthcare industry needs to carefully balance their research and development (R&D) project portfolios in terms of the diverse benefits, risks and costs of the technology they aim to develop. Although not common in healthcare, multi-criteria portfolio selection modelling can provide a structured and transparent approach to support decision-makers to share information on the performances of their R&D projects, to negotiate the necessary trade-offs to evaluate the projects and to arrive at a decision for an R&D project portfolio that decision-makers are committed to. In this chapter we illustrate how the Measuring Attractiveness by a Categorical Based Evaluation Technique (MACBETH) approach, assisted by the recent portfolio module of the M-MACBETH decision support system, was used to build a model to select a portfolio of robotic innovations for minimal invasive surgical interventions. We show how these projects were prioritized according to their value for money and how the value of the R&D portfolio was maximized under a budget constraint and under the presence of interdependencies between projects that could affect their benefits, risks and/or costs.

J.M. Hummel (✉) • M.J. IJzerman
Department of Health Technology & Services Research, MIRA, University of Twente, Drienerlolaan 5, 7522 NB Enschede, The Netherlands
e-mail: j.m.hummel@utwente.nl

M.D. Oliveira • C.A. Bana e Costa
Centre for Management Studies of Instituto Superior Técnico, Universidade de Lisboa, Alameda da Universidade, 1649-004 Lisbon, Portugal

© Springer International Publishing AG 2017

K. Marsh et al. (eds.), *Multi-Criteria Decision Analysis to Support Healthcare Decisions*, DOI 10.1007/978-3-319-47540-0_6

6.1 Introduction

Organizations developing healthcare technologies are under a growing pressure to fulfil stricter regulatory demands on the technologies' benefits and risks in the context of increasingly cost-constrained healthcare systems (Paul et al. 2010). In order to survive, organizations are facing multiple challenges in designing technologies with a high performance, without incurring unmaintainable research and development (R&D) risks and costs. Scarce resources need to be efficiently allocated to promising R&D projects.

Selecting a portfolio of R&D projects on healthcare technology that makes the best use of available resources is complex both at the technical and social level. In order to maximize the value of the portfolio, various trade-offs need to be made among the expected benefits and risks of the technologies, as well as the risks and costs for the developing organization. Since it is not likely that one and the same manager is most knowledgeable on all benefits, risks and costs, managers are to deliberate and assess these versatile trade-offs with their stakeholders (Philips and Bana e Costa 2007). Furthermore, budget constraints and interdependencies among R&D projects may complicate these assessments when selecting multiple projects (Stummer and Steinberger 2003).

Decision analytic methods can support health managers in making complex resource allocation decisions for R&D projects. They help decision-makers in selecting the most efficient portfolio of projects from a large set of projects, while taking into account relevant constraints, preferences and uncertainties (Salo et al. 2011). Multi-criteria decision analysis (MCDA) tools for resource allocation have been shown to be specifically helpful when the projects are to be evaluated by multiple evaluation criteria (e.g. benefits and risks) and when they compete for funding in a context of limited resources (Kleinmuntz 2007).

Various MCDA techniques have been used to assess the multiple benefits and risks of new technologies in the context of the healthcare system (Diaby et al. 2013; Marsh et al. 2014) and to prioritize the value of these technologies (Thokala and Duenas 2012). In particular the MCDA models based on the principles of value measurement – which we will name in this article as multi-criteria value models (MCVM) – have been recommended to assess healthcare technologies (Thokala and Duenas 2012). MCVM have been shown to support health policymakers in technology selection, to analyse market access options or to compare reimbursement systems (Baltussen and Niessen 2006).

When applying MCVM in the context of resource allocation to R&D projects, the benefits and risks of the technologies are assessed from the perspective of the R&D organization. Besides the benefits and lower risks, the R&D organization strives to deliver to healthcare to achieve market success, and other risks, such as technical or market failure, can be incorporated. Also in this context, diverse MCDA techniques have been applied to assist in building multi-criteria resource allocation models (e.g. Hurson and Ricci-Xella 2002; Vetschera and de Almeida 2012; Liberatore 1987).

Multi-criteria resource allocation models extend MCVM from assessing the value of single technologies to assessing the aggregate value of multiple technologies to develop within a restricted budget. The simplest and most common MCVM for resource allocation is to use a prioritization approach in which R&D projects are ranked by their value for money, i.e. by overall value divided by cost (Philips and Bana e Costa 2007). The costs typically include the R&D investments required to develop and market the technologies. However, this prioritization approach does not necessarily ensure the maximum total value for the budget available and cannot easily assist in cases in which there are interdependencies between projects. Our recommendation is to use the prioritization and the optimization approach together. Optimization implies, in the portfolio selection context, solving a mathematical programming problem to maximize the aggregated value of the projects without exceeding the budget constraint, while considering the constraints and synergies of combinations of R&D projects (Lourenço et al. 2012).

Several software packages assist the development of multi-criteria portfolio analysis, namely, Equity and HiPriority enable a prioritization analysis, Expert Choice Resource Aligner provides the optimization approach, while Logical Decisions Portfolio and PROBE enable both prioritization and optimization approaches (Lourenço et al. 2012). Even though there is an increasing trend in the use of multi-criteria resource allocation models in several contexts (for instance, in the pharmaceutical and oil and gas industries, as well as in the public sector (Salo et al. 2011)), they have, until now, only scarcely been applied by the healthcare industry.

This chapter illustrates how a multi-criteria resource allocation model can aid decision-makers in the healthcare industry to reflect on which R&D portfolio of healthcare technologies – or in our case study, robotic innovations that enable minimally invasive surgical interventions – should be selected under a budget constraint. We applied the *Measuring Attractiveness by a Categorical Based Evaluation Technique* (MACBETH) approach to conduct the portfolio analysis (Bana e Costa et al. 2005, 2012a). MACBETH is an interactive approach for building evaluation models that asks evaluators – either a decision-maker or a group of decision-makers – to judge the difference of attractiveness between options. MACBETH has sound theoretical foundations, being based on the principles of additive value measurement, and has been used in different managerial contexts in healthcare, including for the prioritization of community care programmes in (Oliveira et al. 2012) and for hospital auditing (Bana e Costa et al. 2012b). The recent portfolio module of the M-MACBETH decision support system (Bana Consulting 2005) enables multi-criteria resource allocation modelling. Following a decision-aiding perspective, we advocate that multi-criteria resource allocation models should express the viewpoints of managers of R&D organizations, and their development can help these decision-makers to discuss, negotiate and decide with the stakeholders on the R&D projects to invest in, bearing in mind the projects' benefits, risks and costs.

6.2 Case Study and Method

6.2.1 Case Study

Minimally invasive surgery has been applied to significantly lower the patient burden of disease and to reduce length of stay in hospitals (Mack 2001). In order to extend the application of minimally invasive procedures to new interventions and more complex interventions, robotic innovations are desired (Mack 2001; Gomes 2011). Nevertheless, the adoption of the currently available robotic systems has often failed due to unmet user needs in healthcare and to their high costs (BenMessaoud et al. 2011). For selecting a best portfolio of R&D projects for robotic systems, decision-makers need to consider multiple objectives, which include to maximize the benefits and to minimize the risks of the robotic innovations simultaneously for patients (BenMessaoud et al. 2011) and for healthcare professionals (Vander Schatte et al. 2009) and to minimize the costs for healthcare (Barbash and Glied 2010). Trade-offs among these (often) conflicting objectives need to be considered, as well as the costs to develop and market these innovations.

6.2.2 *Resource Allocation Modelling on Robotic Innovations with MACBETH*

Within MCDA, MACBETH is an interactive approach for building a model of quantitative values that requires only qualitative judgements of difference in value (Bana e Costa et al. 2012a). Central in this approach stands a questioning protocol in which the evaluator (a decision-maker or a decision-advising group) qualitatively pairwise compares projects, using a semantic scale – no, very weak, weak, moderate, strong, very strong and extreme difference in attractiveness – thus avoiding the difficulty of expressing value judgements numerically (Von Winterfeldt and Edwards 1986). Using linear programming (Bana e Costa et al. 2005), MACBETH assists not only in testing the consistency of the qualitative judgements expressed but also, when consistency is achieved, in proposing numerical value scales that are in accordance with the judgements. Within ranges that are compatible with the semantic judgements provided, decision-makers can fine-tune the proposed numerical values. This MACBETH procedure is used both to value the projects regarding each of the benefit and risk criteria and to weight these criteria. Then, the overall values of the projects can be calculated by a simple additive model, that is, by multiplying the value of the project in each criterion by the respective weight and summing up these products. An explanation of the mathematical algorithms behind MACBETH can be consulted in Bana e Costa et al. (2005, 2012a).

We developed a MACBETH resource allocation model by conducting two main activities: first to build an MCVM to evaluate the value of nine potential robotic R&D projects and then to analyse which combinations of projects maximize overall value for a given budget, by using both prioritization and optimization approaches for portfolio analysis. Both activities were enabled by means of the recent portfolio module of the M-MACBETH decision support system (beta version) (Rodrigues et al. 2015), following the next model building steps.

Step 1: Identifying Evaluation Criteria
The first step consists in identifying the key aspects, i.e. the benefits and risks that will be used as the evaluation criteria, to appraise the value of the robotic innovations.

It is well known in literature (Von Winterfeldt and Edwards 1986) that the application of an additive value model requires each criterion to represent an independent evaluation axis, i.e. the (partial) value of a project on one criterion should not depend on the performance of the projects on the other criteria. Preference independency may require the restructuring of the set of evaluation criteria, namely, by merging several interdependent aspects into one covering criterion. Each evaluation criterion is to be operationalized into an attribute (Keeney 2002) or descriptor of performance (Bana e Costa et al. 1999) which can either be a continuous or a discrete set of performance levels (either quantitative or qualitative). A detailed discussion on how to build attributes or descriptors of performance is available in Keeney (2002) or Bana e Costa and Beinat (2005).

In order to compare the potential value of the nine alternative robot-assisted surgical approaches, their foreseen benefits and risks were inserted as the evaluation criteria in the decision support system M-MACBETH (version 2.4.0) (Bana Consulting 2005). These criteria were adapted from the technological success factors that explain the probability of technical and commercial success, as distinguished by Cooper and Kleinschmidt (1995). For all criteria, quantitative or qualitative descriptors of performance were defined to measure the performance of the nine robotic innovations. In each descriptor, two reference performance levels were defined: a reference of “low (or neutral)” performance and a reference of “good” performance, with the substantive meaning of, respectively, a minimally and completely satisfying performance. These references of intrinsic value help to analyse whether each robotic project has an undesirable (worse than low) or a satisfactory (from low to good) or an outstanding (better than good) performance. This analysis could also be extended to consider all the criteria together, to appraise the intrinsic overall value of a project.

Step 2: Building the Evaluation Model
In this step, value scales and weights for the evaluation criteria are defined based on the elicitation of MACBETH value judgements.

A value scale enables the conversion of performance into a value score that measures the attractiveness or desirability of that performance. Weights harmonize the value scales across all criteria and enable the aggregation of value scales in an overall value scale that numerically represents the attractiveness or desirability of the alternatives.

Using the MACBETH protocol, value scales for each evaluation criterion were constructed to convert the foreseen performances of the robotic innovations into value scores. For each criterion, the evaluator was asked to judge the difference in attractiveness between pairs of performance levels, using the semantic categories of MACBETH. The MACBETH decision support system proposed numerical value scales that were compatible with the qualitative judgements on the differences in attractiveness of the robotic R&D projects. The reference descriptors of a "low" and a "good" performance of robotic innovations in each evaluation criterion worked as anchors in these value scales, being assigned a value of, respectively, 0 and 100. The evaluator was then asked to eventually adjust and validate the numerical value scale built for each evaluation criterion.

In order to weight the criteria, the qualitative swing weighting procedure of MACBETH was followed (Bana e Costa et al. 2012a; Oliveira et al. 2015). The evaluator was asked to consider the ranges between the low and good references of performance of the robotic innovations on the evaluation criteria. "Suppose a robot is expected to have a low performance on all criteria; on which criterion would a swing from low to good performance be most attractive?" The next most attractive swing was identified, until all performance swings were ranked. Following the additive value model, the ranking of the swings corresponds with the ranking of the weights of the criteria. It is worthwhile nothing that, therefore, a change on one reference level on one criterion may provoke a change in the ranking of the weights. As stated by Philips and Bana e Costa (2007), "a major error in multi-criteria modelling is the attempt to assign weights that reflect the 'importance' of the criteria without reference to any considerations of ranges on the value scales and how much each one of those ranges matters to the decision maker" (Keeney 2002). Next, the evaluator was asked to pairwise compare the global attractiveness of swings using the MACBETH categories. Again, the M-MACBETH decision support system provided numerical weights compatible with the qualitative judgements given by the evaluator. These weights needed to be analysed, eventually adjusted and validated.

Either in building value or weighting scales, M-MACBETH automatically detects inconsistent judgements and suggests ways to resolve inconsistencies (see details in Bana e Costa et al. 2012a).

Step 3: Valuing the Robotic R&D Projects

This step includes the appraisal of the performance of the projects on the criteria and the calculation of their (partial) value scores and overall value scores.

The robots range from more generic robots to facilitate multiple minimally invasive procedures (e.g. robot G having the da Vinci robot as a dominant competitor) to specialized robotics for enabling a specific procedure (e.g. robot F for knee surgery). On each evaluation criterion, the performance of each robot-assisted approach was established by assigning to it one performance level of the respective descriptor; then each performance was converted into a value score using the value scale defined for the respective criterion (see step 2); finally, the weighted average of the value scores is calculated to estimate the overall value of each project across all criteria.

Step 4: Structuring the Portfolio Analysis
This step includes the definition of the portfolio baseline and the modelling of synergies across projects as well as other constraints relevant for the analysis of candidate portfolios.

Proper portfolio decision analysis demands for the specification of a baseline value, that is, a so-called "do nothing" project. Only projects that are more attractive than the "do nothing" project are worthwhile to be considered as candidates for funding. This is important because the use of distinct baselines can affect the optimal portfolio (Morton 2015). There are different procedures to set the baseline value (Liesiö and Punkka 2014). In our case study, if a robotic innovation project was assigned a lower score than the baseline project, which has a "low" performance on all criteria, then that innovation project would not deserve to be funded and, consequently, would be discarded from the portfolio analysis (Bana e Costa et al. 2006). Besides the estimation of the benefits, risks and development cost of each innovation project, the R&D budget was defined and it was observed that the sum of the development costs of all the candidate projects exceeded the budget constraint. Furthermore, an analysis was conducted on the extent to which there were synergies between projects in terms of their benefits, risks and development costs.

Step 5: Analysing Portfolios Using Prioritization and Optimization Approaches
Step 5a: Prioritizing the R&D projects based on their value for money

The nine robotic technologies were prioritized with the M-MACBETH decision support system. These priorities were derived from their potential value for money, that is, by dividing the overall value of each robot innovation (see step 3) by the investment cost required to its development. The projects were ranked in order of decreasing priorities.

Step 5b: Optimizing the R&D project portfolio

With the optimization module of M-MACBETH, a mathematical programming problem was solved that identifies the optimal portfolio, that is, subset of projects that maximizes total value given the budget constraint and existing synergies between projects. Specifically, synergies in development costs of similar robotic technologies were modelled.

6.3 Results

Step 1: Identifying Evaluation Criteria
The criteria to evaluate the innovation projects included:

1. The health gains for patients, in terms of the additional quality-adjusted life years to be gained through the surgical intervention in comparison with current practice

2. Economic benefits to healthcare, in terms of the potential costs savings in comparison with current practice
3. Fit with the existing infrastructure and skills present within the existing healthcare system
4. Fit with the technological expertise and organizational resources of the developing organization
5. Market size in terms of the size of the target patient population of the robotic surgical interventions
6. Competition in the market, in terms of the amount of competing developers

Quantitative and qualitative descriptors of performance were defined to measure the performance of the R&D projects on the criteria (see Table 6.1). Criteria 1, 2 and 5 relate to the benefits of the innovations for the healthcare market, while criteria 3 and 4 relate to the developmental risks, and criterion 6 relates to the market risk. All criteria were framed positively, in the sense that a quality descriptor describing a low risk or a high benefit represented a high performance. The more specific operationalization of the qualitative descriptors, in this case all risk-related descriptors, is to be discussed and agreed upon by the evaluators.

Table 6.1 Criteria and types of performance descriptor

Evaluation criterion	Type of criterion	Type of descriptor	Descriptor of performance
QALY gain patient	Benefit	Quantitative	Quality of life years gained
Economic advantage healthcare	Benefit	Quantitative	Amount in euros
Fit with healthcare setting	Risk	Qualitative	5 qualitative performance levels
Fit with expertise and resources company	Risk	Qualitative	5 qualitative performance levels
Market size	Benefit	Quantitative	Number of patients
Market competitiveness	Risk	Qualitative	5 qualitative performance levels

Step 2: Building the Evaluation Model

Based on MACBETH's pairwise comparisons of the attractiveness of the performance levels, a value scale was created for each evaluation criterion, with 0 and 100 always assigned to the low and good reference levels, respectively. Figure 6.1 shows as an example the value curve of the first criterion: the gain in quality-adjusted life years per patient. Note in the horizontal axis that a half-a-year gain in quality-adjusted life years per patient is considered to be a low-performance outcome for a minimally invasive robot. An increase in 2.5 quality-adjusted life years is considered to represent a good performance. The S-shape of the value curve shows that an even higher QALY gain is not expected to much stronger increase the market need for the robot in healthcare and thus does not create much more value to the developers.

The MACBETH protocol for building weights led to the set of weights depicted in the second line of Table 6.2.

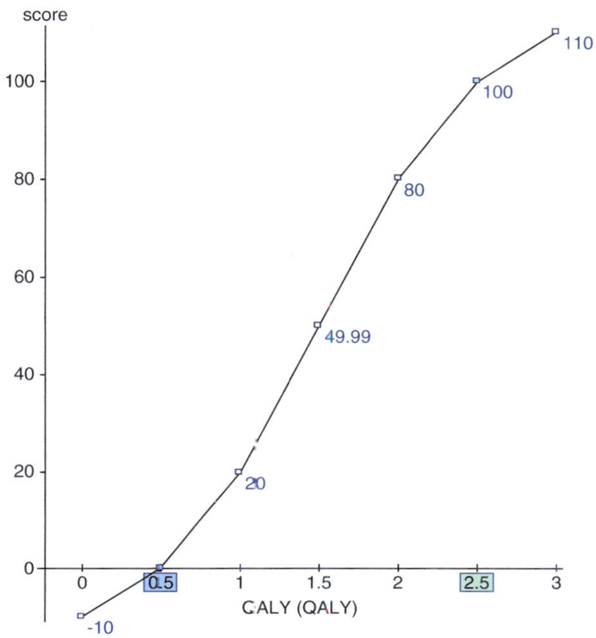

Fig. 6.1 Example of a value curve for the QALY gain criterion built in M-MACBETH

Table 6.2 Criteria weights and robot innovations' partial and overall value scores

	QALY gain	Economic benefit	Fit healthcare setting	Fit expertise and resources	Market size	Competitiveness	Overall value
Weight	*0.26*	*0.13*	*0.14*	*0.26*	*0.15*	*0.06*	
Robot A	102	−115	60	0	5	100	*27*
Robot B	27	116	120	−80	112	60	*39*
Robot C	−3	−102	0	0	11	60	*−9*
Robot D	−8	13	0	0	−6	60	*2*
Robot E	27	61	100	120	−7	−80	*54*
Robot F	14	19	100	100	−6	60	*49*
Robot G	102	−115	60	0	5	0	*21*
Robot H	6	−116	100	60	5	60	*20*
Robot I	39	47	−80	0	−6	120	*11*
Good allover reference	100	100	100	100	100	100	*100*
Low allover reference	0	0	0	0	0	0	*0*

Step 3: Valuing Alternative Robotic R&D Projects

The value scales were used to convert the performances of the robotic innovations into value scores. The performances on the criterion health gain, as estimated in step 1, were positive predictions of the gain in QALYs. These predictions were adapted from the first clinical evidence of similar robots, if available. For example, robot F is to facilitate a minimally invasive procedure for knee arthroplasty. By preventing pain and stiffness of the knee and slightly increasing the physical function of the knee, an improvement in quality of life of 0.06 was predicted during an average time span of 14 years. Resultantly, the predicted gain in health summed up to a QALY gain of 0.84. For more generic robots, the predicted QALY gain was averaged over the applicable procedures that most frequently occur in clinical practice. In this third step, the value scale helped to convert these QALY scores into partial values scores; in case of robot F, the QALY gain of 0.84 was converted in the rather low value score of 14.

Table 6.2 shows the partial and overall value scores of the nine R&D projects on the robotic surgical approaches. To appraise the overall intrinsic value of each project, Table 6.2 also includes two hypothetical robotic innovation projects, the reference good allover with "good" performance on all criteria and the reference low allover with "low" performance on all criteria, obviously with overall scores of 100 and 0, respectively. One can observe in Table 6.2 that several robots have a low or very poor performance on multiple criteria (leading to negative scores).

Step 4: Structuring the Portfolio Model

Investment synergies were incorporated in the portfolio model between two R&D projects: robots A and G. Both robots are more generic robots aiming to facilitate multiple minimally invasive procedures. Synergies are generated as the development of the two robots use a similar core technology. Accordingly, investment in this core technology would simultaneously benefit the two robots, only if both robots are included in the R&D portfolio.

Zero overall value and cost were inserted in M-MACBETH to establish the baseline for portfolio analysis, from which robot C was excluded due to its negative overall value score. This rejection of a project with negative overall value corresponded to the use of a "multi-criteria screening criterion", as defined by Bana e Costa et al. (2006).

Step 5a: Prioritizing the R&D Projects Based on Their Value for Money

The calculated overall values of the nine surgical approaches and the estimated development costs to deliver these products can be plotted in a cumulative cost versus cumulative value graph, by increasing order of the respective value for money ratios (Fig. 6.2). Each point in the graph represents a portfolio of projects, with increasing number of projects from left to right. The curve linking the points is the frontier of convex efficient portfolios, when neglecting interactions between projects. Under these conditions, for a maximum available budget of ten million euros, projects F, B, E, H and A would be selected, with a total cost of 9.2 million euros.

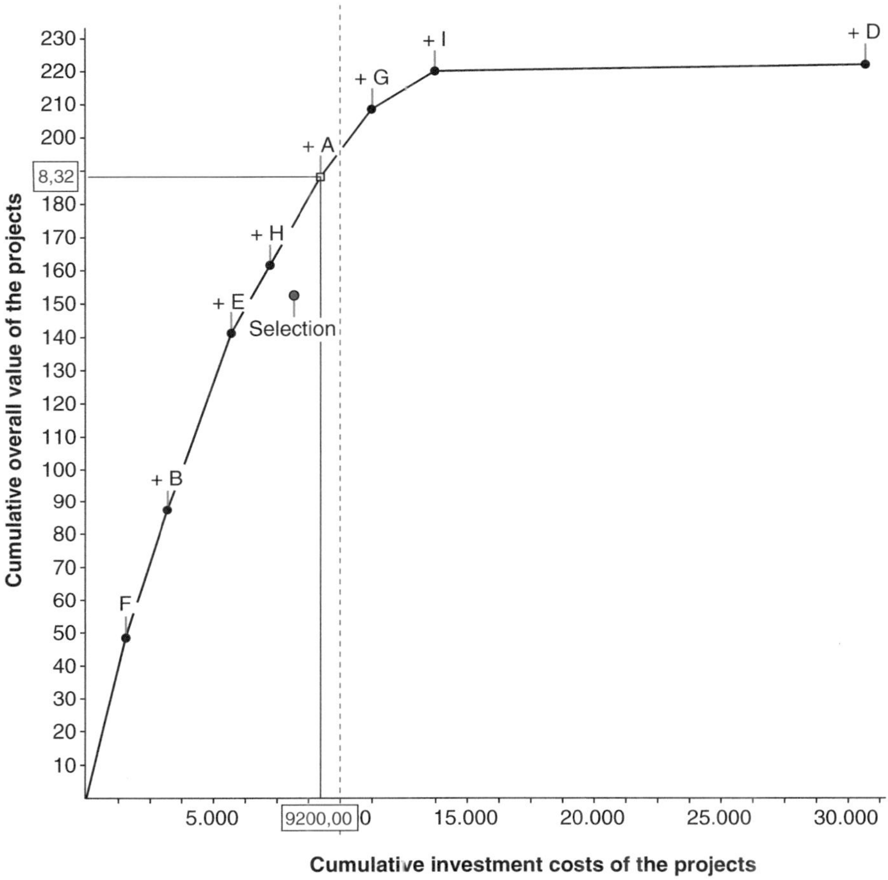

Fig. 6.2 Efficiency frontier and budget cut-off point (costs in 1000 euros units)

Step 5b: Optimizing the R&D Project Portfolio

When taking into account synergies in the development costs of robots A and G, robot G is now included and robot H is excluded from the optimal portfolio B, even though robot H has a higher overall value to cost ratio than robot G. This is shown by comparing the portfolio obtained with the prioritization approach in Fig. 6.2 with the portfolio obtained with the optimization approach in Table 6.1. Note that taken individually, one can include robots A or G in the portfolio, but when both are considered together, the costs change and robots A' and G' are the ones considered (Table 6.3).

The optimization of the project portfolio reduced the total costs from 9.2 to 9.1 million euros, while the aggregated value of the portfolio very slightly increased from 188 to 189 overall value units.

Table 6.3 Value for money of the R&D projects and portfolio

	Value	Cost	Value/cost ratio	In portfolio B
Robot A	27	2000	1.33	No
Robot B	*39*	*1700*	*2.28*	*Yes*
Robot E	*54*	*2500*	*2.17*	*Yes*
Robot F	*49*	*1500*	*3.24*	*Yes*
Robot G	21	2000	1.03	No
Robot H	20	1500	1.35	No
Robot I	11	2500	0.45	No
Robot A' (synergy)	*27*	*1700*	*1.33*	*Yes*
Robot G' (synergy)	*21*	*1700*	*1.03*	*Yes*
Aggregated value portfolio				*189*
Aggregated costs portfolio				*9100*

6.4 Lessons Learned and Discussion

The case study presented illustrates how a multi-criteria resource allocation model can support R&D investment decisions for multiple healthcare innovations. In multi-criteria portfolio analysis, candidate R&D projects can be selected for the R&D portfolio based on their foreseen values and costs. The number of candidate R&D projects can be reduced when minimum levels of performance levels for each benefit or maximum acceptable risks are demanded for the inclusion of a project in the portfolio. In our case, one R&D project was excluded due to its less than "low" overall value. Those performance thresholds are particularly relevant in case the amount of possible portfolios is high. In practice, the number of feasible portfolios can be enormous, exceeding by far the number of feasible portfolios in our illustration (Ghasemzadeh and Archer 2000). Of the appropriate candidate R&D projects to consider for the portfolio, the (convex) efficiency frontier graphically depicts these projects in order of descending priority, when priority is captured by the value for money ratio. For a preliminary analysis of portfolio by applying the prioritization approach, R&D project portfolios can be analysed following the order in the efficiency frontier, from left to right, until the available budget is exhausted.

Nonetheless, the prioritization approach does not necessarily ensure that the optimal portfolio is selected, that is, the subset of projects that maximizes cumulative value although respecting the budget constraint. Moreover, only the optimization approach enables to take into account the presence of synergies between projects. Note that the prioritization approach can lead leaving a significant part of the available budget unexploited when the budget cut-off point is further off from the total budget. In our illustration, altering the preliminary portfolio increased the total value that could be delivered for the total budget and diminished the portfolio costs, due to investment synergies between two R&D projects. These two projects aimed to develop robots that were based on a similar core technology, which generated cost savings. In general, interdependencies among projects can affect not only costs but also benefits and/or risks of the R&D projects (Eilat et al. 2006). Examples of cost interdependencies are the sharing of project resources that translate into overhead cost reductions for the single projects. Examples of benefit interdependencies are the use of competing technologies for which joint project benefits are reduced or the existence of complementary technologies in which one project can be developed only if another one is selected as well. An example of interdependent developmental risks is the existence of a critical mass of resource capital that can increase the likelihood of success of the R&D projects, which translates into lower project risks (Eilat et al. 2006). Due to these interdependencies among projects, proper tools to simultaneously analyse the value, costs and risks of combinations of R&D projects in alternative portfolios is necessary. Optimization modules can assist in proposing changes to the portfolio to maximize the overall value without exceeding the budget constraint (Lourenço et al. 2012). However, it should be noted that, contrary to the prioritization approach, the optimization approach does not guaranty the stability of the selected portfolio when an increase in the available budget is considered. That is why the combined use of the two approaches is recommended.

The combined approach illustrated provides a structured and transparent approach to support decision-makers to share information on the benefits, risks and costs of R&D projects competing for scarce financial resources, to negotiate the necessary trade-offs and to arrive at a decision for an R&D project portfolio the decision-makers are committed to. For our illustration, researchers constructed the multi-criteria resource allocation model being informed by literature and expert opinions. In empirical applications, it is a good practice to involve a constituency of (internal) stakeholders that need to be engaged to successfully realize the R&D projects. In fact, the adequate involvement of multiple stakeholders is paramount in constructing the value tree to capture the versatility of all relevant benefits, risks and costs (Montibeller et al. 2009). Moreover, stakeholders may have conflicting interests. Showing the decision-makers the consequences of changing the portfolio can support key stakeholders to discuss and negotiate the portfolios and to select a portfolio they are willing to engage to (Ghasemzadeh and Archer 2000). Philips and Bana e Costa (2007) have been successful in using a decision conferencing approach in multi-criteria portfolio analysis in real cases, showing that decision conferences can support communication between the stakeholders to develop a shared understanding of the issues involved in portfolio analysis and to make smarter decisions.

The R&D project portfolio analysis can be more advanced by analysing the uncertainty in the appraisal of value of the portfolio. In our illustration, we have implicitly dealt with this uncertainty, by including success factors that predict the probability of achieving commercial success as evaluation criteria and adapting these factors to the healthcare context. Accordingly, a higher score on these success factors predicts a higher probability of market success. There are other ways to deal with these uncertainties in development – for instance, to include as a risk criterion the probability that the benefits will not fully be achieved (Philips and Bana e Costa 2007) or the probability of success (e.g. Liberatore 1987). Or more generally, methods for uncertainty analysis can be applied (Broekhuizen et al. 2015). In optimizing the portfolio of R&D projects, sensitivity analyses can be conducted, or the robustness of the selected portfolio can be tested (Lourenço et al. 2012). A fuzzy approach has also been applied (Carlsson et al. 2007). For the case in our illustration, uncertainty analysis on the benefits would be a valuable addition, considering the contradictory findings on health gains evoked by the literature on the impacts of existing robotics for minimally invasive interventions.

Another elaboration of the multi-criteria resource allocation model described in this study would be the separate analysis and visualization of the individual benefits and risks of the portfolio to the developing organization. Furthermore, high- and low-risk projects could be balanced, minimum levels of benefit for different target groups of patients could be ensured, or other combinations can be optimized that make sense to the organization. With these elaborations, multi-criteria resource allocation modelling can be tailored to provide decision-makers the specific information they desire about R&D projects to facilitate the R&D project portfolio selection decision.

References

Baltussen R, Niessen L (2006) Priority setting of health interventions: the need for multi-criteria decision analysis. Cost Eff Res Allocation 4:14. doi:10.1186/1478-7547-4-14

Bana e Costa CA et al (1999) Decision support systems in action: integrated application in a multicriteria decision aid process. Eur J Oper Res 113(2):315–335

Bana e Costa CA, De Corte JM, Vansnick JC (2005) On the mathematical foundation of MACBETH. In: Figueira J, Greco S, Ehrgott M (eds) Multiple criteria decision analysis: state of the art surveys. Springer, New York, pp 409–442

Bana e Costa CA et al (2006) Prioritisation of public investments in social infrastructures using multicriteria value analysis and decision conferencing: a case study. Intl Trans in Op Res 13:279–297

Bana e Costa CA, De Corte JM, Vansnick JC (2012a) MACBETH. Inter J Info Tech Decision Making 11(2):359–387

Bana e Costa CA, Carnero CM, Oliveira MD (2012b) A multi-criteria model for auditing a predictive maintenance programme. Eur J Oper Res 217:381–393

Bana Consulting, M-MACBETH Version 1.1: User Manual (2005). Available at http://www.m-macbeth.com/help/pdf/M-MACBETH%20User's%20Guide.pdf

Barbash GI, Glied SA (2010) New technology and health care costs—the case of robot-assisted surgery. N Engl J Med 363(8):701–704

BenMessaoud C, Kharrazi H, MacDorman KF (2011) Facilitators and barriers to adopting robotic-assisted surgery: contextualizing the unified theory of acceptance and use of technology. Plos One 6(1):e16395

Broekhuizen H, Groothuis-Oudshoorn CG, van Til JA, Hummel JM, IJzerman MJ (2015) A review and classification of approaches for dealing with uncertainty in multi-criteria decision analysis for healthcare decisions. Pharmacoeconomics 33(5):445–455. doi:10.1007/s40273-014-0251-x

Carlsson C, Robert Fuller R, Heikkilac M, Majlender P (2007) A fuzzy approach to R&D project portfolio selection. Inter J Approx Reasoning 44:93–105

Cooper RG, Kleinschmidt EJ (1995) Benchmarking the firm's critical success factors in new product development. J Product Inno Manage 12(5):374–391

Bana e Costa CA, Beinat E (2005) Model-structuring in public decision-aiding. Operational Research working papers. LSEOR 05.79

Diaby V, Campbell K, Goeree R (2013) Application of multicriteria decision analysis in health care: a systematic review and bibliometric analysis. Oper Res Health Care 2(1-2):20–24

Eilat H, Golany B, Shtub A (2006) Constructing and evaluating balanced portfolios of R&D projects with interactions: a DEA based methodology. Eur J Oper Res 172:1018–1039

Ghasemzadeh F, Archer NP (2000) Project portfolio selection through decision support. Decision Support Syst 29:73–88

Gomes P (2011) Surgical robotics: reviewing the past, analysing the present, imagining the future. Robot CIM-INT Manuf 27:261–266

Hurson C, Ricci-Xella N (2002) Structuring portfolio selection criteria for interactive decision support. Eur Res Studies 5(1-2):69–93

Keeney RL (2002) Value-focused thinking: a path to creative decisionmaking. Harvard University Press, Cambridge, MA

Kleinmuntz DN (2007) Resource allocation decisions. In: Edwards W, Miles RF Jr, von Winterfeldt D (eds) Advances in decision analysis: from foundations to applications. Cambridge University Press, New York, pp 400–418

Liberatore MJ (1987) An extension of the analytic hierarchy process for industrial R&D project selection and resource allocation. IEEE Transactions Eng Manage 34(1):12–18

Liesiö J, Punkka A (2014) Baseline value specification and sensitivity analysis in multiattribute project portfolio selection. Eur J Oper Res 237:946–956

Lourenço JA, Morton A, Bana e Costa CA (2012) PROBE—a multicriteria decision support system for portfolio robustness evaluation. Decision Support Syst 54(1):534–550

Mack MJ (2001) Minimally invasive and robotic surgery. JAMA 285(5):568–572

Marsh K, Lanitis T, Neasham D, Orfanos P, Caro J (2014) Assessing the value of healthcare interventions using multi-criteria decision analysis: a review of the literature. Pharmacoeconomics 32(4):345–365. doi:10.1007/s40273-014-0135-0

Montibeller G, Franco A, E Lord E, Iglesias A (2009) Structuring Resource Allocation Decisions: A framework for building multi-criteria portfolio models with area-grouped options. European Journal of Operational Research 199:846–856

Morton A (2015) Measurement issues in the evaluation of projects in a project portfolio. Eur J Oper Res 245(3):789–796

Oliveira MD, Rodrigues TC, Bana e Costa CA, Sa de AB (2012) Prioritizing health care interventions: a multicriteria resource allocation model to inform the choice of community care programmes. In: Tanfani E, Testi A (eds) Advanced decision making method applied to health care. Springer, Milan, pp 141–154

Oliveira MD, Bana e Costa CA, Lopes DF (2015) Designing and exploring risk matrices with MACBETH. Inter J Infor Tech Decision Making. Forthcoming http://dx.doi.org/10.1142/S0219622015500170 pp. 1-37

Paul SM, Mytelka DS, Dunwiddie CT et al (2010) How to improve R&D productivity: the pharmaceutical industry's grand challenge. Nat Rev Drug Discov 9:203–214

Philips LD, Bana e Costa CA (2007) Transparent prioritisation, budgeting and resource allocation with multi-criteria decision analysis and decision conferencing. Ann Oper Res 154:51–68

Rodrigues T, Bana e Costa CA, De Corte J-M, Vansnick J-C (2015) M-MACBETH for multicriteria resource allocation, 27th European Conferences Operational Research (EURO 2015), Glasgow

Salo A, Keisler J, Morton AE (2011) Portfolio decision analysis: improved methods for resource allocation. Springer, New York

Stummer C, Steinberger K (2003) Interactive R&D portfolio analysis with project interdependencies and time profiles of multiple objectives. IEEE Transactions Eng Manage 50(2):175–183

Thokala P, Duenas A (2012) Multiple criteria decision analysis for health technology assessment. Value Health 15:1172–1181

Van der Schatte ORH, van't Hullenaar CDP, Ruurda JP, Broeders IAMJ (2009) Ergonomics, user comfort, and performance in standard and robot-assisted laparoscopic surgery. Surg Endosc 23:1365–1371

Vetschera R, de Almeida AT (2012) A PROMETHEE-based approach to portfolio selection problems. Computers Oper Res 39:1010–1020

Von Winterfeldt D, Edwards W (1986) Decision analysis and behavioral research. Cambridge University Press, Cambridge

Chapter 7
Benefit–Risk Assessment

Filip Mussen

Abstract While medicines have been assessed in terms of their benefits and risks since health authorities started requiring clinical studies in the 1960s, only recently more formal approaches for conducting benefit–risk evaluations have emerged. Both the European Medicines Agency (EMA) and the Food and Drug Administration (FDA) are in the process of implementing qualitative benefit–risk frameworks, but at the same time, the industry and some other stakeholders have started to pilot quantitative benefit–risk methods in regulatory settings. Multi-criteria decision analysis seems to emerge as one of the preferred quantitative methods, in particular for medicines with a complex multifactorial benefit–risk profile. In this chapter a number of case studies of the use of MCDA for benefit–risk assessment during drug development and for regulatory purposes will be described. Based on these case studies, technical and operational progress, learnings, and challenges will be discussed, and recommendations will be made when and how MCDA can be used for the benefit–risk assessment of medicines. These conclusions will be contextualized within the broader debate of the use of formal benefit–risk methods as decision tools mainly for regulatory purposes.

7.1 Introduction

7.1.1 The Purpose and Timing of Benefit–Risk Assessments

The purpose of benefit–risk evaluations of medicines is to describe if the favorable effects, with their uncertainties, outweigh the unfavorable effects, with their uncertainties (EMA 2010). In this respect, the European Medicines Agency (EMA) guidance defines a "favorable effect" as any beneficial effect for the target population (often referred to as "benefit" or "clinical benefit") that is associated with the medicine. Favorable effects most often pertain to improvements in clinical efficacy

---

F. Mussen
Janssen R&D, Pharmaceutical Companies of Johnson & Johnson,
New Brunswick, NJ 08933, USA
e-mail: fmussen@its.jnj.com

© Springer International Publishing AG 2017

K. Marsh et al. (eds.), *Multi-Criteria Decision Analysis to Support Healthcare Decisions*, DOI 10.1007/978-3-319-47540-0_7

but could also include other factors such as increased compliance and herd immunity. "Unfavorable effects" include any detrimental effects (often referred to as "risks," "harms," "hazards," both known and unknown) that can be attributed to the medicine or that are otherwise of concern for their undesirable effect on patients' health, public health, or the environment.

Benefit–risk evaluations of medicines are conducted at three distinct stages (Mussen et al. 2002). Initially during clinical development, pharmaceutical companies decide whether the preliminary benefit–risk profile of a compound warrants moving to the next stage of development, and if so what the clinical program of that next stage should encompass. During the regulatory approval process, first the applicant and subsequently the regulatory authorities evaluate whether the new medicine should be allowed on the market and with what labeling (indication, dose, etc.). Finally, during the post-approval phase, the benefit–risk profile is reevaluated at regular intervals as new efficacy and safety data emerge. At each of these stages, an MCDA benefit–risk model could be of value.

7.1.2 History of Benefit–Risk Assessment and Methodologies

The US Food, Drug, and Cosmetic Act first embraced the idea of benefit versus risk in 1962, when the Kefauver–Harris Drug Amendments required that firms had to show a drug's effectiveness before marketing. However, the first suggestion for benefit–risk methodology only appeared in 1987 (Walker and Asscher 1987). In 1998 CIOMS IV stated that "it is a frustrating aspect of benefit-risk evaluation that there is no defined and tested algorithm or summary metric that combines benefit and risk data and that might permit straightforward quantitative comparisons of different treatment options, which in turn might aid in decision making" (CIOMS IV 1998). The first formal initiative from a health authority emerged in 2007 when the EMA issued a report of the CHMP working group on benefit–risk assessment models (BRAMs) and methods (EMA 2007). This report included a review of the advantages and disadvantages of MCDA methods in terms of their usefulness for CHMP scientific assessments and was the start for further research and debate about the applicability of MCDA methods for regulatory benefit–risk decision-making. In the IMI PROTECT project, 49 benefit–risk assessment methodologies were critically appraised and classified. MCDA was among the methodologies that were recommended for further examination and testing in appropriate case studies (Mt-Isa et al. 2014). In addition, the recent draft Food and Drug Administration (FDA) CDRH guidance on patient preference information listed MCDA as one of the methods to elicit patient preferences (FDA 2015). Finally, the revised ICH guideline M4E(R2) and specifically the benefit–risk conclusions section of that guideline stipulate that applicants may use methodologies that quantitatively express the underlying judgments and uncertainties in a benefit–risk assessment (ICH guideline 2016).

7.2 Overview of the Development of an MCDA-Based Benefit–Risk Model

7.2.1 Introduction

MCDA involves a stepwise approach, and a typical MCDA model for benefit–risk evaluation includes the following steps (Mussen et al. 2007):

1. Establish the decision context.
2. Identify the alternatives to be appraised.
3. Identify the criteria:
    3.1 Identify criteria for assessing the consequences for each alternative.
    3.2 Organize the criteria by clustering them under high-level and lower-level objectives in the hierarchy (optional).
4. Assess the expected performance of each alternative against the criteria ("scoring").
    4.1 Describe the consequences of each alternative.
    4.2 Score the alternatives on the criteria.
    4.3 Check the consistency of the scores on each criterion.
5. Assign weights for each criterion to reflect their relative importance to the decision.
6. Calculate weighted scores at each level in the hierarchy and calculate overall weighted scores.
7. Examine the result and conduct a sensitivity analysis.

It should be noted that steps four and five can be reversed, i.e., assigning weights can be done before scoring the alternatives on the criteria.

While most MCDA models involve all above steps and quantify clinical judgment allowing benefits and risks to be fully quantified, other models only use the first three or four steps and are sometimes called partial MCDA models. A typical example of such a model is the BRAT framework (Coplan et al. 2011), which addressed the need for improved benefit–risk assessment by developing a structured, systematic, and transparent general platform for benefit–risk assessment. It consists of six steps (Fig. 7.1) and it facilitates the selection, organization,

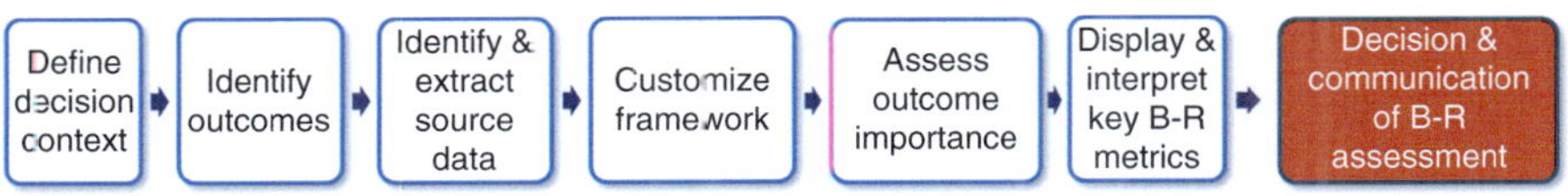

Fig. 7.1 Steps in using the Benefit–Risk Action Team (BRAT) benefit–risk assessment framework (Coplan et al. 2011)

summarization, and interpretation of data and preferences relevant to the benefit–risk decision and also serves as a tool to broadly communicate the rationale for the decision.

7.2.2 Establishing the Decision Context

Establishing the decision context is a prerequisite for a robust MCDA model (Mussen et al. 2007; Coplan et al. 2011) and pertains to four important aspects which should be well described, i.e.:

- The compound context, i.e., the specific therapeutic indication to be examined (e.g., a first- or second-line indication) as well as the intended patient population and the therapeutic dosage.
- The therapeutic context, i.e., a general review of the therapeutic value of the available medicines of the same and other pharmacologic classes for the same indication, as well as the identification of the unmet medical need. In contrast to the process of identifying criteria and scoring as described below, the goal of describing the therapeutic context is not to establish a direct comparison between the different treatments based on specific criteria, but rather to provide a general description to set the stage.
- The development context which should include an overview of the clinical studies that were conducted with the compound (design, comparators, etc.), of the safety database including the duration of exposure, and possibly of other data sources such as observational studies.
- The stakeholder context, i.e., whose values will be incorporated in the MCDA model. Options are including the values of the decision-makers such as experts from pharmaceutical companies or from health authorities, but alternatively values from customers such as prescribers or patients can be sought.

7.2.3 Identification of the Alternatives to Be Appraised

This step is usually rather straightforward in benefit–risk evaluations. The key question is whether the new compound should be allowed on the market and if so whether there should be any restrictions to its use. In order to make that evaluation, the new compound should be compared with the comparators used in the clinical program such as active comparators, placebo, standard of care, or no treatment. Comparisons can in theory also include other medicines for the same therapeutic indication but not used as comparators in the clinical program, although the validity and limitations of this kind of cross-study comparisons should be made explicit. From a technical perspective, the MCDA benefit–risk score or benefit–risk ratio generated for the new compound under discussion should be compared to the benefit–risk score or benefit–risk ratio of the active comparator(s), placebo, standard of care, or no treatment.

7.2.4 *Identification of the Criteria*

The identification of the relevant benefit and risk criteria is essential. Mussen et al. (2007) identified criteria based on a review of the EU, US, and ICH guidelines, complemented by a detailed review of the literature. Confirmation about the value of each criterion was sought by carrying out three pilot studies involving senior people from the industry and senior people from regulatory authorities who were asked to confirm the usefulness of each criterion for a benefit–risk assessment. The identified criteria are outlined in Table 7.1. It should also be noted that some of the criteria listed in the table can be labeled as uncertainty criteria (e.g., representativeness of the studied population for the population targeted in the label). How to address uncertainty is described in the next sections of this chapter.

Table 7.1 Benefit and risk criteria identified in Mussen et al. (2007)

Benefit criteria
1. Efficacy versus comparator and its clinical relevance (for each pivotal trial)
2. Design, conduct, and statistical adequacy of the trial (for each pivotal trial)
3. Clinical relevance of the primary endpoints (for each pivotal trial)
4. Representativeness of the studied population for the population targeted in the label (for each pivotal trial)
5. Statistical significance of the efficacy results (for each pivotal trial)
6. Evidence for the efficacy in relevant subgroups (for each pivotal trial)
7. Efficacy as per the results of the non-primary endpoints (for each pivotal trial)
8. Efficacy as per the results of the relevant non-pivotal trials and extensions
9. Anticipated patient compliance in clinical practice
10. Clustering (consistency) of results of the pivotal trials
Risk criteria
1. Overall incidence of adverse effects
2. Overall incidence of serious adverse effects
3. Discontinuation rate due to adverse effects
4. Incidence, seriousness, duration, and reversibility of specific adverse effects
5. Safety in subgroups
6. Interactions with other drugs and food
7. Potential for off-label use leading to safety hazards
8. Potential for non-demonstrated additional risk due to limitations of clinical trials and/or length of patient exposure
9. Potential for non-demonstrated additional risk due to safety issues observed in preclinical safety studies but not in humans
10. Potential for non-demonstrated additional risk due to safety issues observed with other medicines of the same pharmacological class

In all recent applications of MCDA to benefit–risk evaluation, the relevant benefit and risk criteria were identified on a case-by-case basis, and there has been little further work on identifying a general list of relevant criteria. While the above list was designed to address benefit–risk assessments for new products from the perspective of the regulatory decision-makers, this list can be used as a basis in other settings such as post-approval assessments and patient elicitation methods. For those kinds of decision problems, other relevant criteria such as those based on results from observational studies and patient reported outcomes might be added.

Having identified criteria, MCDA often requires refinement of the criteria list to ensure the criteria set complies with the analytical requirements of the additive models often employed in MCDA. Specifically, this involves ensuring that the criteria have the following properties: completeness, non-redundancy, non-overlap, and preference independence (Marsh et al. 2016).

Once the relevant criteria have been identified for a specific MCDA model, it is good practice to cluster them, in particular when there are many criteria. The easiest and most suitable way of organizing the benefit and risk criteria is constructing a value tree, which clusters the criteria in a clear hierarchical way (Fig. 7.2).

In 2013 the Food and Drug Administration published its benefit–risk grid highlighting the FDA's high-level decision factors (Table 7.2) (FDA 2013). This grid can be used to organize the criteria and the available data associated with those criteria. In addition to benefits and risks, three other decision factors are included in the grid, i.e., analysis of condition (a description of the natural course of the disease), current treatment options (a summary of their therapeutic value), and risk management (a description how the most important risks associated with the use of

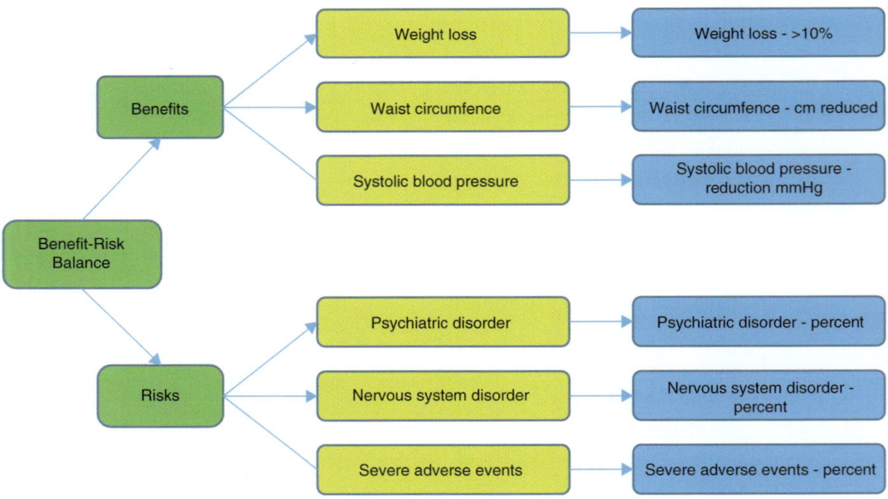

Fig. 7.2 Example of a benefit–risk value tree for rimonabant for weighting loss in obese or overweight patients (Hughes et al. 2013)

Table 7.2 FDA benefit–risk grid

Decision factor	Evidence and uncertainties	Conclusions and reasons
Analysis of condition		
Current treatment option		
Benefit		
Risk		
Risk management		
Benefit–risk summary assessment		

the medicine will be evaluated and mitigated). In particular "analysis of condition" and "risk management" can be included as high-level criteria in an MCDA model, in addition to "benefits" and "risks." Another interesting feature of this grid is that it allows describing uncertainty associated with each of the high-level criteria.

7.2.5 Scoring of the Criteria

Before engaging in scoring the alternatives on the criteria, data on the performance of alternatives is usually collected. It might be helpful to summarize the available performance measurements on each of the criteria, and the sources of information in a table, or a forest plot. One possible format is, for example, the so-called effects table (EMA 2012).

Scoring is the numerical assessment of the performance of alternatives against the criteria on a common interval scale (Mussen et al. 2007). To construct a scale, it is necessary to define two reference points and to allocate numerical values to these points. Several scoring methodologies are available, including methods to convert the natural scales used in clinical studies (e.g., the positive and negative syndrome scale (PANSS) used for measuring symptom severity of patients with schizophrenia) to a single standardized scale for all benefit and risk criteria. Straightforward scales can be developed and can easily be compared against each other when the benefit and/or risk is expressed in terms of a reduction of number of events (e.g., a reduction in mortality, a reduction in MIs, an increase in major bleedings). Conversion of the natural scales into a value function, in conjunction with swing weighting (see below), is usually the best approach for benefits measured in terms of the primary and secondary endpoints in the pivotal clinical studies and risks measured in terms of their frequency. Another scoring method which is easy to implement but somewhat less accurate is categorical value scales (Felli et al. 2009). Such a method can be used when there are no pertinent data available for a given benefit or risk, for example, when a new therapy is believed to provide increased adherence or ease of administration. Further details on scoring the criteria are provided in Chapter 4 of this collection.

7.2.6 Assigning Weights to the Criteria

In MCDA, weights are used to reflect the relative importance of criteria (Belton and Stewart 2002). Several weighting methods have been applied to benefit–risk assessment. The use of the swing weighting technique has been described in several benefit–risk models (Mussen et al. 2007; Felli et al. 2009). In swing weighting, the weight assigned to a criterion is essentially a scaling factor which relates scores on that criterion to scores on all other criteria. Thus, if criterion A has a weight which is twice that of criterion B, this should be interpreted that 10 value points on criterion A are valued the same as 20 value points on criterion B (Belton and Stewart 2002). Swing weighting requires judgments of the relative importance of the swing in performance on each criterion.

Sarac et al. used categorical weights and they proposed to assign to each benefit and risk criterion a weight/importance of 1 (low), 2 (medium), or 3 (high) (Sarac et al. 2012). Tervonen et al. used a ranking method (Tervonen et al. 2011). Experts were asked to identify the criterion that he or she considered to be most important, i.e., would foremost increase from the worst to the best value, then second most important, etc. Both methods require presumably less effort than swing weighting, but might generate less precise weights. That is, the precision achieved with swing weighting comes at the cost of greater cognitive burden on the part of stakeholders, with the risk of behavioral biases (Tervonen et al. 2015). In addition, in many real-life situations, decision-makers are not able to or do not want to give exact preference information (Tervonen et al. 2011).

Traditionally, weights are assigned by the decision-maker, which is either the pharmaceutical company developing a compound, or the regulatory authorities evaluating a compound. There is however an emerging trend of using patient perspectives to decide on the relative importance of criteria (FDA 2015; Ho et al. 2015). Further details on assigning weights to the criteria are provided in Chapter 4 of this collection.

7.3 Examples of MCDA-Based Benefit–Risk Models

Few prospective real-world examples of benefit–risk evaluations based on MCDA have been published. However, two groups have extensively tested MCDA for benefit–risk evaluation, i.e., the European Medicines Agency (EMA) and IMI PROTECT.

The EMA conducted a number of field tests using MCDA and applied it to a hypothetical medicine to illustrate the graphical displays (value tree, results of the weighted scores, sensitivity analysis) (EMA 2011). Fixed scales, with the endpoints defined by the best and worst performance which could realistically occur on the particular criterion, were developed to score the alternatives. Swing weighting was used to quantify the relative importance of the criteria. It was concluded that MCDA models could be a useful adjunct to the current EMA benefit–risk evaluation processes. They could not only serve to better explain licensing decisions to external stakeholders but also enable regulators to move away from "first do not harm" by incorporating patients' values into the decision-making process (Eichler et al. 2013).

In the IMI PROTECT project, MCDA was tested in the efalizumab, natalizumab, rimonabant, rosiglitazone, and telithromycin case studies (see: http://www.imi-protect.eu/). With regard to scoring the criteria, the data for each criterion were numerically transformed into utility scores. Swing weighting was generally used as weighting method. It was concluded that MCDA provides structured stepwise instructions with the capability of assessing and integrating multiple benefit and risk criteria, as well as comparing different alternatives. According to IMI PROTECT, MCDA is also the only approach that can formally deal with multiple objectives simultaneously. Another appealing feature of MCDA is that several software packages to perform the analysis are available.

In IMI PROTECT Work Package 6, a case study with efalizumab was used to test how MCDA-based approaches could be applied within the real-life conditions of post-licensing regulatory decision-making (Goetghebeur et al. 2016). Advanced statistical analyses and longitudinal modeling allowed providing effect estimates when relevant evidence was limited. A by-criterion benefit–risk evidence matrix was developed based on the EVIDEM methodology to contain the synthesized data for each criterion as well as scoring scales. As weighting method, hierarchical point allocation was used, which involves distributing weights (100 points at each level) across the criteria and sub-criteria of the value tree. This is a relatively straightforward direct weighting method which is appropriate if used together with categorical scoring scales. The constructed 11-category scoring scale was designed to conduct a comparative assessment ranging from "much better than comparator" (score +5) to "much worse than comparator" (score −5). Such constructed scales can address the issue of data heterogeneity, as they can accommodate different types of data which cannot be reduced to a single measure (e.g., based on different treatment durations). In addition, they allow both absolute data and relative data (e.g., odds ratios) to be used in the MCDA model. However, constructed scales require judgment on the data, in contrast to measured scales which represent a mathematical transformation of the data to a 0–100 scale. This model also illustrates how the benefit–risk balance evolves over time with different data sets at different time points. It was concluded that the combination of advanced statistical analysis and a pragmatic and straightforward MCDA model can be used for real-world decision-making and support transparent, consistent, and comprehensive benefit–risk assessments.

Other examples of MCDA-based benefit–risk models include the so-called BRAM (benefit–risk assessment model) which graphically presents contextual beliefs about benefits and risks in a framework conducive to focused discussion (Felli et al. 2009). Using the pharmacological class of statins as an example, Tervonen et al. made recommendations for addressing key methodological challenges with the use of MCDA (Tervonen et al. 2015). Guidance was provided how to define the decision problem, how to select a set of non-overlapping criteria (study endpoints), how to synthesize and summarize the available data (using network meta-analysis), how to translate relative measures obtained through evidence synthesis to absolute scales that permit comparisons between the criteria, how to define suitable scale ranges, how to elicit preference information, and how to incorporate uncertainty into the analysis using stochastic multi-criteria acceptability analysis (SMAA).

Vaccines are another area where decision analysis models could be useful, given the need to demonstrate a unequivocally positive benefit–risk profile in a healthy population of vaccine recipients. Phillips et al. developed a decision tree model shortly after the H1N1 influenza virus reached pandemic status in June 2009, with the purpose of using it in deliberations about approving vaccines soon based on limited data or waiting for more data (Phillips et al. 2013). Marcelon et al. developed an MCDA model to quantify the benefit–risk balance of the quadrivalent human papillomavirus vaccine for use in males, including for anal cancer prevention (Marcelon et al. 2016). Specific features of the model included a comprehensive value tree and effects table and the use of swing weighting and sensitivity analysis. The main challenges were agreeing on the value tree that reflects criteria specific to vaccines such as indirect effects, comparing immediate adverse effects to long-term benefits, extracting effect estimates on a comparable scale, and for some outcomes, identifying the correct comparator. It was concluded that MCDA can be used to transparently evaluate the benefit–risk balance of vaccines. Suggestions for further development of the model included standardizing some aspects of the value tree for vaccines (e.g., indirect effects), integrating uncertainty on the estimates into the model, and developing methods to solicit weights from other stakeholders such as vaccine recipients.

7.4 Outstanding Issues of MCDA-Based Benefit–Risk Models

An important concern about the use of MCDA in benefit–risk assessment pertains to dealing with uncertainty. There are three distinct but interrelated components of uncertainty in evidence (IOM 2014). The first component is clinical uncertainty, which refers to the fact that results from clinical studies cannot be necessarily extrapolated to the patient population for whom the therapy is intended, for example, because of strict inclusion or exclusion criteria in the clinical studies. Another source of clinical uncertainty is the limited number of patients treated and the limited duration of clinical studies. The second component of uncertainty is methodological uncertainty, which refers to the design (e.g., randomization method) and conduct (e.g., number of patients lost to follow-up) of clinical studies. The third component is statistical uncertainty. In a traditional MCDA model, alternatives are scored on the different benefit and risk criteria based on point estimates, and uncertainty associated with sample variation inherent to criteria measurements obtained in experimental or observational studies can be captured in the sensitivity analysis (and so can clinical and methodological uncertainty), but with some limitations. To overcome these limitations, Tervonen et al. developed a stochastic multi-criteria acceptability analysis (SMAA) and applied it to two second-generation antidepressants (Tervonen et al. 2011). Instead of using deterministic values, the criteria values in an SMAA model are assumed to be random variables with a joint density function. Chapter 5 provides more detail on uncertainty in MCDA.

Another major challenge is the complexity and diversity of data to be captured in benefit–risk evaluations, in particular in the post-licensing setting. A benefit–risk analysis often involves combining data from multiple sources, including randomized clinical studies and observational studies, with different designs, durations, comparators, and endpoints. A complicating factor in this respect is that the quantification of risks, which is characterized by multiple dimensions including incidence, severity, and reversibility, is far behind the quantification of efficacy (Quartey and Wang 2011). These challenges associated with the synthesis of data are however not limited to MCDA, but apply to all approaches to benefit-risk analysis.

Another area of ongoing debate is whose preference (scores and weights) should be used in benefit–risk assessment and which methods should be used to elicit them. The EMA's benefit–risk methodology project elicited preferences from agency staff using swing weighting methods (EMA 2011). Recent FDA guidance places the emphasis on eliciting patient preference for use in quantitative benefit–risk assessment and identifies a range of methods that could be used, including discrete choice experiment, best–worst scaling, analytical hierarchy process, and SMAA (FDA 2015). It also notes the lack of guidance on which methods are most appropriate and under which circumstances. Recent guidance from the International Society for Pharmacoeconomics and Outcomes Research discussed the difference between weighting methods and their relative merits (Marsh et al. 2016), and further detail on this topic is available in Chapter 4 of this collection, though we anticipate much more work on this topic in the near future. Of particular interest will be Topic 1 of the Innovative Medicines Initiative's fifth call, which is concerned with methods for eliciting patient preferences for benefit–risk assessment (http://www.imi.europa.eu/content/stage-1-16). This will involve a consortium of academics, industry, and regulators testing multiple methods over the coming 5 years.

7.5 Conclusion: The Place of MCDA-Based Benefit–Risk Models

MCDA has the potential to support the evaluation of the benefit–risk balance of drugs and devices. The use of so-called partial MCDA models has become a standard practice in regulatory submissions, especially in Europe. In such models, benefit and risk criteria are defined and arranged in, for example, a value tree, but values are not quantified so that no benefit–risk scores are calculated. Such models require little effort and may be sufficient for more straightforward benefit–risk decisions (Phillips et al. 2011). As a consequence, the EMA now utilizes a partial MCDA model in the form of an effects table.

In some instances it is valuable to also elicit scores and weights and undertake a full MCDA. The EMA concluded that a full MCDA model would be most useful for difficult or contentious cases. These could arise when the benefit–risk balance is marginal and could tip either way depending on judgments of the clinical relevance of the effects and in the case of many conflicting attributes (EMA, work package 4 report). The FDA has also recently taken steps toward greater use of full MCDAs, encouraging the collection of patient preference data to inform a quantitative benefit–risk analysis for devices (FDA 2015).

Because the features of each benefit–risk assessment are specific to the therapeutic and pharmacological class of the therapy which is being assessed, ideally a separate MCDA model should be developed for each therapeutic/pharmacological class. Work is ongoing to develop further guidance on which MCDA methods are most appropriate for benefit–risk assessment, addressing outstanding issues such as how best to measure performance on benefit and risk criteria, which weighting methods to employ, and how best to deal with uncertainty.

When deciding the MCDA approach, as with any method, there is a trade-off between the level of precision generated and the effort required. In general, value analysis methods such as MCDA provide high-quality decisions but at the expense of larger effort. If not implemented well, they also risk reducing the transparency of the decision-making process (Russo and Schoemaker 2002). The latter is very important in regulatory decision-making, and it must therefore be ensured that any MCDA model is used as a tool for, but does not substitute the decision-makers. In addition, the decision-makers will have to articulate their decision and the corresponding conclusions from the MCDA model in a language which is understandable for key stakeholders.

Bibliography

Bass R (1987) Risk-benefit decisions in product license applications. In: Walker SR, Asscher AW (eds) Medicines and risk/benefit decisions. MTP Press Limited, Lancaster, pp 127–134

Belton V, Stewart TJ (2002) Multiple criteria decision analysis: an integrated approach. Kluwer Academic Publishers, Boston

CIOMS Working Group IV (1998) Benefit-risk balance for marketed drugs: evaluating safety signals. CIOMS, Geneva

Coplan PM, Noel RA, Levitan BS, Ferguson J, Mussen F (2011) Development of a framework for enhancing the transparency, reproducibility and communication of the benefit-risk balance of medicines. Clin Pharmacol Therapeutics 89:312–315

Eichler HG, Bloechl-Daum B, Brasseur D, Breckenridge A, Leufkens H, Raine J, Salmonson T, Schneider CK, Rasi G (2013) The risks of risk aversion in drug regulation. Nat Rev Drug Discov 12:907–916

European Medicines Agency (2007) Report of the CHMP working group on benefit-risk assessment models and methods http://www.ema.europa.eu/docs/en_GB/document_library/Regulatory_and_procedural_guideline/2010/01/WC500069668.pdf

European Medicines Agency (2010) Benefit-risk methodology project – work package 2 report: applicability of current tools and processes for regulatory benefit-risk assessment http://www.ema.europa.eu/docs/en_GB/document_library/Report/2010/10/WC500097750.pdf

European Medicines Agency (2011) Benefit-risk assessment methodology project. Work package 3. Field tests. http://www.ema.europa.eu/docs/en_GB/document_library/Report/2011/09/WC500112088.pdf

European Medicines Agency (2012) Benefit-risk assessment methodology project. Work package 4. Benefit risk tools and processes. http://www.ema.europa.eu/docs/en_GB/document_library/Report/2012/03/WC500123819.pdf

Food and Drug Administration (2013). Structured approach to benefit-risk assessment in drug regulatory decision-making – draft PDUFA V implementation plan. http://www.fda.gov/downloads/ForIndustry/UserFees/PrescriptionDrugUserFee/UCM329758.pdf

Food and Drug Administration (2015) Patient preference information – submission, review in PMAs, HDE applications, and De Novo requests, and inclusion in device labeling. http://www.fda.gov/downloads/medicaldevices/deviceregulationandguidance/guidancedocuments/ucm446680.pdf

Felli JC, Noel RA, Cavazzoni PA (2009) A multiattribute model for evaluating the benefit-risk profiles of treatment alternatives. Med Decis Making 29:104

Goetghebeur MM, Wagner M, Nikodem M, Zyla A, Micaleff A, Amzal B (2016) Pragmatic multicriteria decision analysis (MCDA) combined with advanced pharmacoepidemiology for benefit-risk assessments of medicines adapted to the real-life constraints of regulators: development and case study. Ther Innov Regul Sci. 50:620-631

Ho MP, Gonzalez JM, Lerner HP, Neuland CY, Whang JM, McMurry-Heath M, Hauber AM, Irony T (2015) Incorporating patient-preference evidence into regulatory decision making. Surg Endosc 29:2984–2993

Hughes D et al (2013) IMI-PROTECT Benefit-Risk Group. Recommendations for the methodology and visualisation techniques to be used in the assessment of benefit and risk of medicines. http://www.imi-protect.eu/documents/HughesetalRecommendationsforthemethodologyandvisualisationtechniquestobeusedintheassessmento.pdf

International Council for Harmonisation (2016). Revision of M4E guideline on enhancing the format and structure of benefit-risk information in ICH – Efficacy M4E(R2)http://www.ich.org/fileadmin/Public_Web_Site/ICH_Products/CTD/M4E_R2_Efficacy/M4E_R2__Step_4.pdf

Institute of Medicine (2014) Characterizing and communicating uncertainty in the assessment of benefits and risks of pharmaceutical products: workshop summary http://nationalacademies.org/hmd/reports/2014/characterizing-and-communicating-uncertainty-in-the-assessment-of-benefits-and-risks-of-pharmaceutical-products.aspx

Marcelon L, Verstraeten T, Dominiak-Felden G, Simondon F (2016) Quantitative benefit-risk assessment by MCDA of the quadrivalent HPV vaccine for preventing anal cancer in males. Expert Rev Vaccines 15:139–148 http://www.ich.org/fileadmin/Public_Web_Site/ICH_Products/CTD/M4E_R2_Efficacy/M4E_R2__Step_4.pdf

Marsh K, IJzerman M, Thokala P, Baltussen R, Boysen M, Kaló Z, Lönngren T, Mussen F, Peacock S, Watkins J, Devlin N (2016) Multiple criteria decision analysis for health care decision making—emerging good practices: report 2 of the ISPOR MCDA Emerging Good Practices Task Force. Value Health 19:125–137

Mt-Isa S et al (2014) Review of methodologies for benefit and risk assessment of medication. http://www.imi-protect.eu/documents/ShahruletalReviewofmethodologiesforbenefitandriskassessmentofmedicationMay2013.pdf

Mussen F, Salek S, Walker S (2007) A quantitative approach to benefit-risk assessment of medicines – part 1: the development of a new model using multi-criteria decision analysis. Pharmacoepidemiol Drug Saf 16:S2–S16

Mussen F, Salek S, Walker S (2002) What is the best model for assessing the benefit/risk ratio of my product? In: VandenBurg M, Salek S, Wight LJ (eds) Dilemmas and solutions in global drug development: your questions answered. PJB Publications Ltd, London, pp IIC3 1–IIC3 15

Phillips LD, Fasolo B, Zafiropoulos N, Beyer A (2011) Is quantitative benefit-risk modeling of drugs desirable or possible? Drug Discov Today Technol 8:e3–e10

Phillips LD, Fasolo B, Zafiropoulous N et al (2013) Modelling the risk-benefit impact of H1N1 influenza vaccines. Eur J Public Health 23:674–678

Quartey G, Wang J (2011) Statistical aspects in comparative benefit-risk assessment: challenges and opportunities for pharmaceutical statisticians. Pharm Stat 11:82–85

Sarac SB, Rasmussen CH, Rasmussen MA, Hallgreen CE, Søeborg T, Colding-Jørgensen M, Christensen PK, Thirstrup S, Mosekilde E (2012) A comprehensive approach to benefit-risk assessment in drug development. Basic Clin Pharmacol Toxicol 111:65–72

Russo JE, Schoemaker PH (2002) Winning decisions – getting it right the first time. In: A currency book, 1st edn. Doubleday, New York

Tervonen T, van Valkenhoef G, Buskens E, Hillege HL, Postmus D (2011) A stochastic multi-criteria model for evidence-based decision making in drug benefit-risk analysis. Stat Med 30:1419–1428

Tervonen T, Naci H, van Valkenhoef G et al (2015) Applying multiple criteria decision analysis to comparative benefit-risk assessment: choosing among statins in primary prevention. Med Decis Making 35:859–871

Chapter 8
Advancing MCDA and HTA into Coverage Decision-Making

Hector Castro, Michele Tringali, Irina Cleemput, Stephan Devriese, Olivia Leoni, and Emanuele Lettieri

Abstract *Introduction*: Country- and region-specific health technology assessment (HTA) organisations for priority-setting and resource allocation have emerged around the world. Decision-making in healthcare is a continuum from evidence generation to deliberation and communication of the decision made, and HTA is only a part of this process whereby the available evidence is assessed to inform decision-makers about the most efficient use of resources. Besides the assessment, reimbursement decision-making also involves appraising the available evidence, while bearing in mind societal values and ethical considerations. Even in countries where formal HTA activities are ongoing, transparency levels of resource-allocation decisions vary reflecting competing interests of governments and other stakeholders.

Overview: While multiple publications have examined the role of HTA through the collection of data, there is still limited knowledge of how decision-makers use and value this evidence, as well as the challenge of incorporating other broader criteria in an explicit manner. Multi-criteria decision analysis (MCDA) has

H. Castro (✉)
Instituto de Evaluación Tecnológica en Salud (IETS), Bogotá, Colombia

T.H Chan Harvard School of Public Health, Boston, MA, USA
e-mail: hcastro@hsph.harvard.edu; dochecj@hotmail.com

M. Tringali • O. Leoni
Direzione Generale Salute Regione Lombardia, Milan, Italy
e-mail: michele_tringali@regione.lombardia.it; Olivia_Leoni@regione.lombardia.it

I. Cleemput • S. Devriese
Belgian Health Care Knowledge Centre, Brussels, Belgium
e-mail: Irina.Cleemput@kce.fgov.be; Stephan.Devriese@kce.fgov.be

E. Lettieri
Department of Management, Economics and Industrial Engineering at Politecnico, Milan, Italy
e-mail: emanuele.lettieri@polimi.it

© Springer International Publishing AG 2017

K. Marsh et al. (eds.), *Multi-Criteria Decision Analysis to Support Healthcare Decisions*, DOI 10.1007/978-3-319-47540-0_8

emerged as a tool to support decision-making in healthcare. MCDA supports decision-making by breaking down complex problems into multiple components and drawing on both qualitative and quantitative approaches to measure and then combine these components.

Objectives: The aim of this chapter is to demonstrate the potential of, as well as the challenges associated with, using MCDA for resource-allocation decisions by presenting case studies carried out by well-established institutions in Colombia, the region of Lombardy in Italy and Belgium.

Conclusion: Further research on merging MCDA and HTA to support better informed coverage decision-making, especially on methods, consistency and replicability of MCDA results may be of value for all countries.

8.1 Introduction

Health technology assessment (HTA) examines the consequences of the application of health technologies aimed at better informing decision-makers. As such, HTA has become a topic of great interest, albeit not without controversy. HTA advocates argue that it promotes efficiency of resource allocation, while critics state HTA is simply a means to restrict access to new and costly technologies (O'Donnell et al. 2009).

Over the past decades, different countries have established HTA organisations to better inform healthcare policies and clinical practice. HTA agencies have gained space in taxation-based and social health insurance systems. In fact, most high-income countries (HICs) utilise some form of HTA process to facilitate decision-making and priority setting within their health systems (Bulfone et al. 2009; Castro 2011). Recent examples of HTA agencies in the developing world have also emerged (Castro 2012).

HTA, although important, is only a part of the process of decision-making (Cleemput et al. 2012). Beyond scientific evidence, decision-making also requires value judgements (Eddy 1990; Tunis 2007; Cleemput et al. 2011). Neither HTA reports nor the results of cost-effectiveness analyses should be blindly used to make decisions.

While multiple studies and publications have examined the role of HTA as a data collection process (Heyse et al. 2001; Briggs 2001; Briggs et al. 2002; Hoch et al. 2002), there is still limited knowledge of how decision-makers used this data, as well as the challenge of incorporating other criteria in an explicit manner. Authors like Drummond and Sorenson (2009) have suggested a "divorce" of the evidence produced and decision-making process, since many HTAs and economic evaluations published in the literature have been performed with no specific decision-maker in mind.

Even in countries where formal HTA activities are ongoing, and in most low- and middle-income countries (LMICs), many resource-allocation decisions are still based on non-transparent choices that reflect competing interests of governments, donors and other stakeholders (Glassman et al. 2012). Frequently, decision-making is inconsistent and unstructured. Important criteria such as budget impact, equity and disease severity have not always been taken into consideration, and if they have, it is not often clear how they have impacted a final decision (Baltussen and Niessen 2006). This can lead to implicit and covert rationing through waiting lines, low quality and inequities (Glassman et al. 2012).

Multi-criteria decision analysis (MCDA) has emerged as a tool to support decision-making in healthcare (Miot et al. 2012) attempting to move beyond the evidence generation/collection phase of the process. MCDA methods are designed to help people make "better" choices when facing complex decisions involving several dimensions. "MCDA are especially helpful when there is a need to combine 'hard data' with subjective preferences or make trade-offs that involve multiple decision-makers" (Dolan 2010). In theory, MCDA allows a structured and objective consideration of the factors that are both measurable and value based in an open and transparent manner (Baltussen and Niessen 2006; Dolan 2010) thus could be considered an important step towards rational priority setting in developing countries (Baltussen et al. 2007; Miot 2012).

The aim of this chapter is to demonstrate the potential of, as well as the challenges associated with, using MCDA for resource-allocation decisions by presenting case studies carried out by well-established institutions in Colombia, the region of Lombardy in Italy and Belgium.

8.2 The Case Studies

8.2.1 Testing MCDA in Colombia

The Colombian Regulatory Commission for Health (CRES) operated until December 2012, as the coverage decision-making body. Arguably, CRES was disbanded because of a lack of "legitimacy", and the Ministry of Health and Social Protection (MoHSP) regained reimbursement decision-making powers. This institutional instability created the opportunity to test MCDA methods.

The MCDA framework Evidence and Value: Impact on Decision-Making (EVIDEM) developed by Goetghebeur et al. (2008) was the one used by CRES in Colombia before its disbandment when attempting to implement a more systematic priority-setting process. EVIDEM is an open-source generic framework intended to help judge the value of interventions from two perspectives: the value system of the evaluator (decision-maker) with regard to the importance of each criteria (weights) and the performance of an intervention on preselected decision-making criteria (scores).

EVIDEM includes core quantifiable and contextual qualitative criteria considered important in decision-making; this approach has been tested and used in several countries (Guindo et al. 2012; Goetghebeur et al. 2010, 2012; Tony et al. 2011; Miot et al. 2012). The framework also includes detailed protocols for the collection, analysis, synthesis and reporting of evidence for each decision criterion (by criterion

HTA report). Appraisals are transformed into a holistic MCDA value estimate which allows for ranking and cross comparison of healthcare interventions.

8.2.1.1 Methods

The methodological approach taken in Colombia is similar to the steps followed by previous applications of EVIDEM for coverage decision-making (e.g. Miot et al. (2012) in South Africa, Tony et al. (2011) in Canada) (Fig. 8.1).

During a preparatory stage, investigators conducted literature searches and produced HTA reports for each intervention of interest, followed by panel sessions of decision-makers to contextualise criteria to be used, establish a committee perspective (weighting of criteria), appraise each intervention (scoring and consideration of criteria) and discuss the results and process.

Selecting Criteria and Assigning Weights

During October 2012 CRES led an independent initiative aimed at selecting criteria for coverage decision-making during three workshops involving 11 senior decision-makers (academics, researchers and civil servants) with broad experience of working in the context of the local health system. Participants were asked to

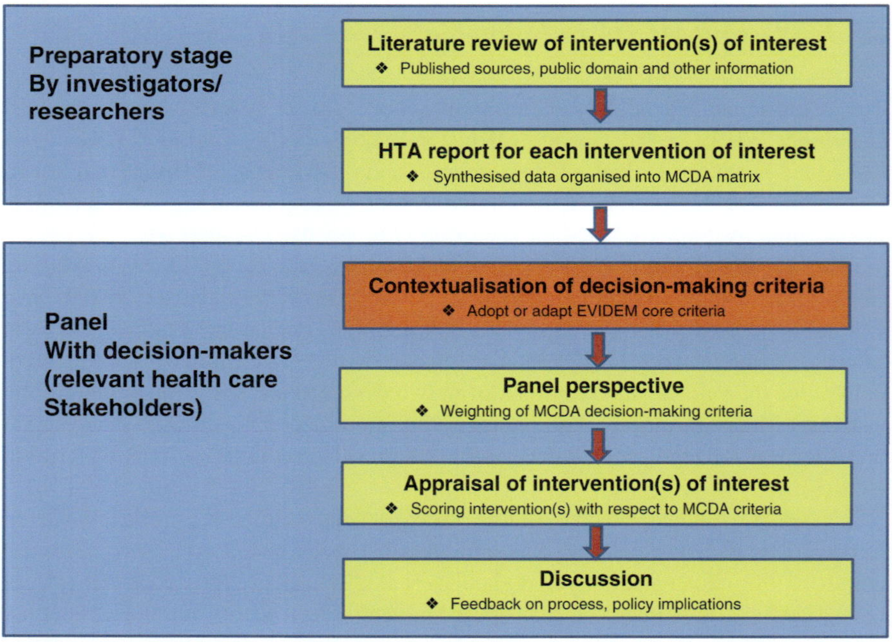

Fig. 8.1 Scheme of work for piloting EVIDEM (Source: Adapted from Goetghebeur et al. (2012))

identify additional contextual criteria considered relevant for resource-allocation in Colombia. After three voting rounds in two nominal group sessions, a final list with 15 criteria was produced, 13 from the EVIDEM core model and two added contextual criteria (bold) (Table 8.1).

Once the panel had agreed on the final criteria and their definitions, participants were asked to weight each criterion irrespective of any healthcare intervention. A participatory process was implemented by CRES, who organised meetings with various stakeholders (academics, patients associations, citizen councils and representatives from the medical societies) around the country and asked them to assign weights. A total of 201 citizens weighted each of the 15 criteria (CRES 2012).

Assembling the Evidence for Selected Technologies

Four technologies were selected for the pilot: primary prophylaxis (PP) for severe haemophilia A (SHA), zinc supply for diarrhoea prevention, anastrozole as first-line therapy for hormone receptor-positive postmenopausal women with metastatic breast cancer and ticagrelor + acetylsalicylic acid (ASA) for patients with acute coronary syndrome (ACS) without ST elevation and moderate to high cardiovascular risk. Technology selection was partly based on convenience with availability of published local HTA summaries for these interventions. In addition, all three non-haemophilia-related technologies were considered as potentially cost-effective, while prophylaxis was not. At the time of running the pilot, no reimbursement decisions had been made as to whether they would be publicly reimbursed.

The clinical practice guidelines by Perry et al. in 2012 (anastrozole), Florez et al. (zinc) (2013) and Senior et al. (ticagrelor) in 2013 were used to produce the HTA reports. In the case of PP, the HTA report was based on a recent cost-utility analysis (CUA) and a literature review (Castro et al. 2013). The adapted EVIDEM MCDA matrix was used to assemble the HTA information of the four technologies in Spanish. All reports contained the relevant information organised considering the criteria and weights developed by CRES in 2012.

Appraisal of Interventions and Discussion

Because CRES was dissolved before appraising the value of any intervention, a new focus group was organised as a mock reimbursement decision committee to appraise the value of the four interventions in August 2013. The focus group was designed to mimic a resource-allocation decision-making committee, 12 organisations were identified as containing potential sources of participants (government, insurers, providers, patients groups, academics, healthcare professionals, people's advocates and lay members). Senior policy-makers and "high profile individuals were selected to assure legitimacy and 'buy in' of the pilot".

Table 8.1 Final list of criteria and weights for the Colombian-modified version of EVIDEM

Criterion	Definition	Weight (%)
Disease severity	Severity of the health condition of patients treated with the proposed intervention (or severity of the health condition that is to be prevented) with respect to mortality, disability, impact on quality of life and clinical course (i.e. acuteness, clinical stages)	9.3
Size of population affected by disease	Number of people affected by the condition (treated or prevented by the proposed intervention) among a specified population at a specified time; can be expressed as annual number of new cases (annual incidence) and/or proportion of the population affected at a certain point of time (prevalence)	8.9
Improvement of efficacy/effectiveness	Capacity of the proposed intervention to produce a desired (beneficial) change in signs, symptoms or course of the targeted condition above and beyond beneficial changes produced by alternative interventions. Includes efficacy and effectiveness data, as available	8.7
Current clinical guidelines applicable in Colombia	Concurrence of the proposed intervention (or similar alternatives) with the current consensus of experts on what constitutes state-of-the-art practices in the management of the targeted health condition; guidelines are usually developed via an explicit process and are intended to improve clinical practice	7.7
Type of medical service (clinical benefit)	Nature of the clinical benefit provided by the proposed intervention at the patient level (e.g. symptom relief, prolonging life, cure)	7.3
Budget impact on health plan (POS)	Net impact of covering the intervention on the budget of the target health plan (excluding other spending)	6.9
Improvement of safety and tolerability	Capacity of the proposed intervention to produce a reduction in intervention-related harmful or undesired health effects compared to alternative interventions	6.6
Public health interest	Risk reduction provided by the proposed intervention at the population level (e.g. prevention, reduction in disease transmission, reduction in the prevalence of risk factors)	6.5
Improvement of patient-reported outcomes	Capacity of the proposed intervention to produce beneficial changes in patient-reported outcomes (e.g. QoL, improvements in convenience to patients)	6.3,
Current intervention limitations	Shortcomings of comparative interventions in their ability to prevent, cure or improve the condition targeted; also includes shortcomings with respect to safety, patient-reported outcomes and convenience	6.2
Attention to vulnerable groups of population	*Capacity of the proposed intervention to beneficial impact to vulnerable groups of populations as defined by law in Colombia (e.g. displaced, elderly, disabled, native American, mentally ill, etc.)*	5.7
Cost-effectiveness of intervention	Ratio of the incremental cost of the proposed intervention to its incremental benefit compared to alternatives. Benefit can be expressed as number of events avoided, life-years gained, quality-adjusted life-years gained, additional pain-free days, etc.	5.5

Table 8.1 (continued)

Criterion	Definition	Weight (%)
Completeness and consistency of reporting evidence	Extent to which reporting of evidence on the proposed intervention is complete (i.e. meeting scientific standards on reporting) and consistent with the sources cited	5.1
Relevance and validity of evidence	Extent to which evidence on the proposed intervention is relevant to the decision-making body (in terms of population, disease stage, comparator interventions, outcomes, etc.) and valid with respect to scientific standards and conclusions (agreement of results between studies). This includes consideration of uncertainty	5.0
Attention to differential needs for health/healthcare	*Capacity of the proposed intervention to beneficial impact to people in need of differential care (e.g. orphan disease, palliative care, end of life, etc.)*	4.3

Since traditionally resource-allocation decision-making occurs as a centralised process in the country, all eligible participants were located in Bogotá. The feasibility and usefulness of using and incorporating HTA and EVIDEM to inform resource-allocation decision-making were explored during a 2-h focus group held at the Health Technology Assessment Institute-IETS through a set of open-ended questions. All participants were asked to consent to participate and to be recorded for transcription and to declare potential conflicts of interest.

To appraise the healthcare interventions, respondents were presented with MCDA evidence matrices which prompted HTA summaries and ask to score each criteria individually on a four-point cardinal scale (0–3), where 3 represents the highest level of fulfilment of each decision criterion and 0 the lowest (EVIDEM v2.0). The calculation of the MCDA value estimates was done by combining normalised weights and scores for each individual using a linear model with 1 being the highest value for an ideal intervention and 0 the lowest. Averaged results compiled at the group level were presented to participants at the end of the session to promote discussion.

To promote discussion, participants were presented with a hypothetical scenario where only those two technologies with the highest scores were to be reimbursed by the healthcare system. Questions such as "was there enough information to make resource-allocation decisions in Colombia?" and "what changes or improvements could be added to the processes and methods presented in the pilot for future implementation"? were asked to participants to gather their inputs, concerns and expectations.

The focus group was recorded, transcribed *verbatim* and uploaded to ATLAS-ti7 to assist content analysis. In order to interpret emerging data rather than simply describing it, no preliminary hypothesis was considered. Labels such as sufficiency of information, methods concerns, methods comparison, validity of information, incorporation of HTA into decision-making and the specific value of each intervention were predefined as the relevant categories that served to inform the aims of this chapter.

8.2.1.2 Results

Seven people attended the invitation to participate. Participants represented a broad range of stakeholders within the Colombian health system, from members of the MoHSP, academics, insurers, patients and professional associations to lay members of society. All participants were skilled workers with at least one postgraduate degree. No representatives from hospitals or people's advocates participated in the meeting, although they were formally invited to attend. Scoring the four technologies of interest using the MCDA evidence matrix took an average of 11.15 min (range 7–18 min) per healthcare technology per participant.

MCDA value estimate calculation indicated that zinc ranked first (0.904) followed by anastrozole (0.822), PP for SHA (0.794) and ticagrelor (0.708) (Table 8.2). Perceived value of interventions varied across participants [zinc (0.782–0.986), anastrozole (0.698–0.934), PP (0.595–0.977) and ticagrelor (0.449–0.945)], reflecting the diverse perspectives and interpretation of presented evidence of participants.

Table 8.2 Results of the EVIDEM comparative value of interventions by criterion

Criterion	Weight (%)	Standardised scores per technology			
		Zinc	Anastrozole	PP FVIII	Ticagrelor
Disease severity	9.3	0.093	0.080	0.093	0.075
Size of population affected by disease	8.9	0.089	0.076	0.076	0.085
Improvement of efficacy/effectiveness	8.7	0.083	0.079	0.083	0.070
Current clinical guidelines applicable in Colombia	7.7	0.062	0.066	0.022	0.066
Type of medical service (clinical benefit)	7.3	0.059	0.063	0.059	0.063
Budget impact on health plan (POS)	6.9	0.066	0.046	0.049	0.049
Improvement of safety and tolerability	6.6	0.063	0.066	0.063	0.028
Public health interest	6.5	0.065	0.046	0.040	0.053
Improvement of patient-reported outcomes	6.3	0.063	0.036	0.051	0.024
Current intervention limitations	6.2	0.038	0.053	0.059	0.038
Attention to vulnerable groups of population	5.7	0.057	0.041	0.057	0.030
Cost-effectiveness of intervention	5.5	0.047	0.050	0.031	0.042
Completeness and consistency of reporting evidence	5.1	0.039	0.036	0.032	0.027
Relevance and validity of evidence	5.0	0.040	0.045	0.045	0.033
Attention to differential needs for health/healthcare	4.3	0.039	0.039	0.033	0.025
MCDA value per technology	100	0.904	0.822	0.794	0.708

In answer to the question *could EVIDEM be used in Colombia to assist resource-allocation decision-making*, participants found EVIDEM was a means of incorporating HTA into decision-making and also of prioritising different health interventions for resource-allocation. The final consensus was that a mixed methods approach including an appraisal based on an MCDA evidence matrix completed by a financial exercise with a detailed Budget Impact Analysis (BIA) examining the opportunity costs would be ideal for Colombia.

Participants also identified limitations regarding the adequacy of information presented in the EVIDEM summary. Some specific criteria represented more challenges than others for interpretation and valuation. Some doubts emerged when independently valuing each criterion. There was risk of double counting information (consideration of the same evidence in multiple criteria), since no strategy was considered to consistently synthesise HTA evidence to avoid it.

Another limitation of this pilot relates to language differences between the original EVIDEM tools used (matrix and by criterion), published in English and the non-validated Spanish versions presented to participants. The method used to elicit weights applied by CRES in 2012 clearly departed from the 1 to 5 scale originally used by EVIDEM, shall it had an impact on the final results could be as well an important limitation.

Since institutional HTA has been in place for less than 3 years in Colombia, there were still concerns and considerations among participants of the methods to conduct HTA, for instance, the validity of data used for modelling, the use of QALYs when conducting CUAs or the reliance on ICERs alone to inform decision-making but also on how to incorporate HTA results into decision-making. Nevertheless, the pilot is one of the first initiatives within the country to combine HTA and MCDA for more explicit priority setting.

8.2.2 Institutional HTA/MCDA Approach in Lombardy

Lombardy is a region in the north of Italy with 9.8 million residents served by a healthcare system involving 145,000 workers, 220 hospitals and 2700 pharmacies and an annual health budget of €17 billion. In 2008, the Lombardy Healthcare Directorate (LHCD) issued a policy for an HTA programme to maximise healthcare benefits to citizens by promoting more efficient and evidence-based healthcare resource-allocation and sustainable diffusion of technologies. The HTA programme was therefore based on principles of accountability, orientation to health outcomes, transparency in decision-making and sustainability.

Value for health is defined as health outcomes expected when the National Health Service (NHS) reimburses a health technology over other competing alternatives. The healthcare directorate started the programme with the naming of two representative committees (one for priority setting for emerging technologies and one for appropriateness of diffused technologies), alongside a policy for managing conflict of interest and a website platform to support it and collect contributions from hospitals, companies and experts. The programme mainly addresses prioritisation and appraisal tasks, while technical assessment is limited to the contextualisation of third-party HTA reports into an MCDA evidence matrix.

8.2.2.1 Historical Perspective and Rationale for Developing and Implementing an MCDA-Based Appraisal Process

The Lombardy government recognised an opportunity to strengthen the HTA programme taking into consideration methods developed by the European network of HTA (EUnetHTA) and the EVIDEM collaboration. EUnetHTA focuses on facilitating knowledge sharing, efficient use of resources and promoting good HTA practices in Europe. It publishes Core Models, guidelines and other resources to streamline assessment practices. The EVIDEM collaboration developed a pragmatic decision-making framework and some tools to help bridge MCDA and HTA in order to clarify appraisal practices.

The LHCD then developed an information framework incorporating adapted versions of both the EVIDEM set of criteria and the EUnetHTA Core Models (version 1.0); this was in order to build a complete, coherent and operational HTA-MCDA application aimed at structuring assessment reports for appraisal activities. A modified set of criteria from EVIDEM was inserted into the EUnetHTA framework under the top level (Domains) and also over the middle-level hierarchy (Topics). The EUnetHTA ontology structure was maintained, except from "Health problem relevance" and "Technology solution relevance" which were merged in the Lombardy's version as "Technical relevance", while "Effectiveness" was split into "Efficacy" and "Effectiveness" in order to comply with the original Lombardy regulation, issued 2 years before the publication of Core Models 1.0.

The Lombardy HTA-MCDA application ontology has been implemented as web-based tools for both the quantitative and qualitative stages of the prioritisation and appraisal process. This has helped to clarify processes and better communicate results to hospitals. It has been field tested internally and applied to most HTA projects from 2012 onwards (Migliore et al. 2014; Tringali et al. 2014).

8.2.2.2 The Appraisal Process

The process starts with a submission from hospitals, manufacturers, independent clinical experts or other bodies (e.g. the region itself or the Italian Agency for Healthcare research and quality-AGENAS). The framework is used by committed members formed by experts selected according to their expertise and declaration of vested interests. The framework contextualises participants on HTA reports and also provides the tools to support participants' personal judgement. Potential committees' decisions can be rejected, further assessed or directly approved for reimbursement within Lombardy NHS. Committees' decisions are usually translated into formal acts.

The appraisal stage proceeds as follows, developers present structured proposals to committee members and then HTA reports are produced internally or adapted from third parties by the region or local hospitals. For each appraisal each committee member is asked to judge on the relative importance of 8 general "domains" (for emerging technologies) or 15 more specific "criteria" (for diffused technologies, for which more information usually is available) through a personal weighting operation using an online form.

The weighting method is always a direct and anchored rating scale. For emerging technologies, each committee member is asked to assign eight to the domain considered as the most important and one to the least important one and then to distribute weights to the other domains to ensure differentiation among domains and avoid flattening of judgements towards a same level of perceived importance. Average weights by domain are obtained after summing up scores by participant and dividing them by number of participants. Alternative methods for weighting, like hierarchical point allocation or pair-wise comparison between individual domains/criteria, have been initially considered but put aside since committee's expertise with MCDA methods was still at an early stage, and the face validity of the simple eight-point scale weight elicitation method was deemed satisfactory (for more details on weighting methods, see Chapter 4).

The same process is applied by members of the appropriateness committee with 15 quantitative criteria. The individual weightings are then discussed online and during meetings, and each member can modify his/her own weightings. After these are approved, final weights are calculated and members are given access to the full documentation available.

Each member individually scores the performance of the proposed technology for each domains/criteria and with respect to available alternatives of care using an online form, with a predefined scoring system from 0 to 4, where 0 = absence of relevant information, 1 = comparative lesser value, 2 = comparative similar value and 3 or 4 = comparative (slightly or highly) better value. Members also provide a mandatory comment for each score. Uncertainty of scores was not initially modelled and was left to the discussion within committees, but a revision is planned with the introduction of a three-level classification of uncertainty for each assigned score.

Individual scores and comments are then elaborated into a judgement draft, in two parts

1. Priority (or appropriateness) index for the NHS. A linear additive model is used for the analysis of individual value contributions (normalised weights × scores) for each domain/criterion to provide an index from 0 to 1 representing the overall value of the technology as follows:
   (a) From 0 to 0.25 when the estimate's averages are among 0 and less than 1, in this case the intervention cannot be evaluated in a robust way.
   (b) Between 0.25 and 0.50 when the estimate's averages are among 1 and less than 2, here the relative value of the intervention is less or equal to the value of alternatives.

(c) Between 0.50 and 1 when the estimate's averages stand between 2 and 4 and the proposed intervention has a better overall comparative value than alternatives.

2. Qualitative analysis of comments written for each domain/criterion. Comments are categorised by two reviewers, with resolution of disagreement by consensus, and analysed within a descriptive report, where more frequent and robust arguments are proposed as possible motivations for the decision.

Both priority/appropriateness indexes for the NHS and categorised comments drafts are discussed and revised to verify the coherence between scores and comments, to eliminate ambiguities and to identify further areas of assessment. After revision, the index and the motivations are approved and sent to administration for consideration for policy-making.

For some of the appraised technologies, judgement was repeated by two or three independent subgroups of the committees in a blinded way to measure reproducibility of indexes; since this has always been very high, there have been no cases where there was a need to revise the final judgement. Intra-rater and inter-rater variability of committee members in expressing weights has also been explored and showed a high degree of consistency among voters (yet unpublished work). This internal analysis is now being replicated and extended by an independent academic group. Results of this analysis will help inform the updating of the regional HTA policy in the near future.

8.2.2.3 MCDA Outputs in Lombardy

From 2012 several diagnostic and interventional technologies have been prioritised, i.e. recommended or refused using the MCDA approach presented above in Lombardy. Figure 8.2 depicts the list of healthcare technologies prioritised for reimbursement during 2012–2014 in Lombardy (more information available at http://vts-hta.asl.pavia.it).

Most of the proposed technologies have been rejected; in other cases a positive appraisal was followed by reimbursement, sometimes with restrictions for an appropriate use, i.e. indication of specific centres, patient selection procedures and provisional tariffs linked to a conditional reimbursement (upon verification of prospected outcomes as registered in real-life patients).

Note that laser endo-microscopy and presepsin reached a similar value of the priority index, but different decisions were issued by the regional administration on the basis of the overall comments of the committee's members. XXX denotes a medical device for which an administrative appeal decision is pending against the rejection from reimbursement.

Figure 8.3 is an illustration from the final appraisal document for the trans-vascular aortic valve implantation (TAVI) for aortic stenosis procedure.

First, appropriateness indexes for the TAVI procedure in operable and inoperable patients were calculated through MCDA using 15 quantitative criteria by appraisal of

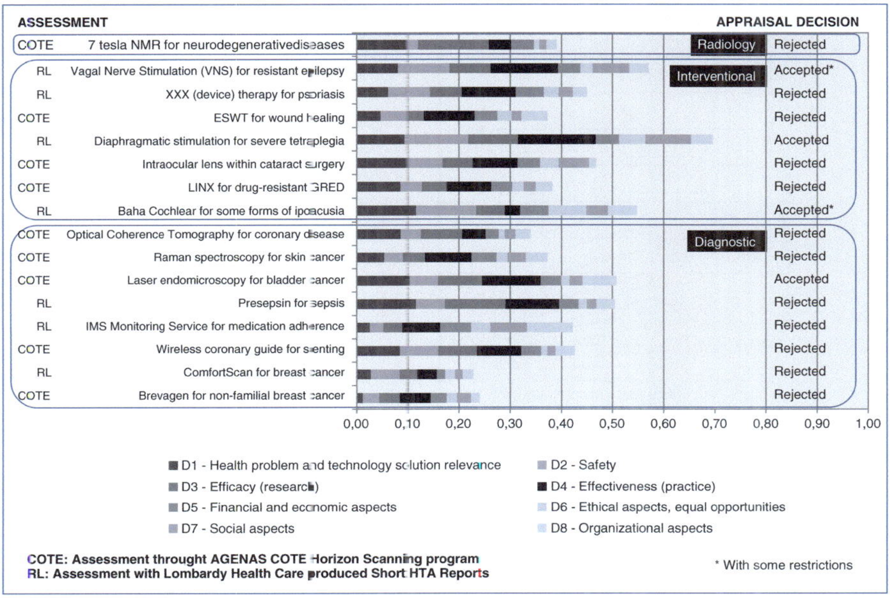

Fig. 8.2 Value of healthcare interventions for healthcare programming in Lombardy

committee members ($N=21$). The analysis of qualitative judgements expressed by the same members as negative, no or positive impact and related comments for six qualitative criteria helped to prepare a set of final recommendations for TAVI; which in this case were: audit of every case, revised criteria for authorisation of centres, team evaluation of frailty and comorbidities, clinical registry of pathology linked to the financing procedure and conditional repayment-payback if no positive outcome at 2 years (this policy act was issued in 2013).

8.2.2.4 Latest Developments in Lombardy and Future in Italy

During 2015 the Lombardy HTA-MCDA application ontology was revised to incorporate the content of the EUnetHTA Core Model version 3.0 (draft version as of September 2015) and most of the changes made in version 3.0 of the EVIDEM framework. The resulting updated list of domains and criteria in use is reported in Table 8.3.

The pioneering work of the Lombardy region is now explored by other regions in Italy as well as at the national level. Recently, a prescription for MCDA use was added to a national law for priority setting in the medical devices area highlighting the real-life value of this approach to support HTA, decision-making and communication with stakeholders.

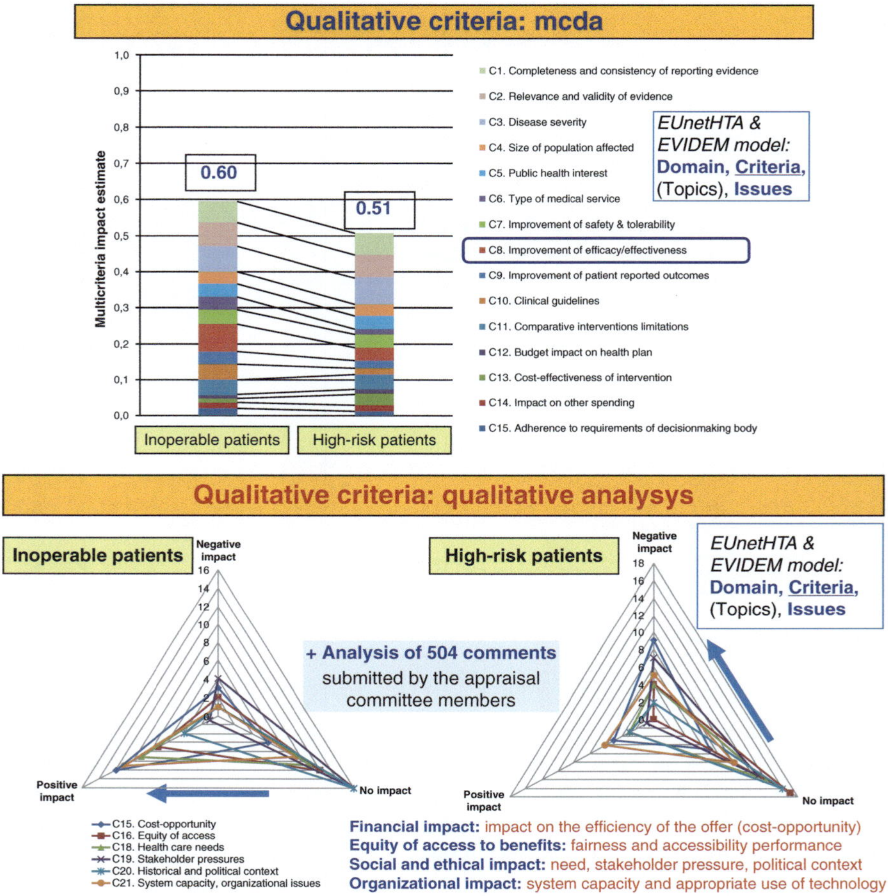

Fig. 8.3 Extract from the appraisal process for TAVI

8.2.3 *Developing an MCDA Approach for Coverage Decision-Making in Belgium*

Coverage decisions in healthcare in Belgium are taken by the Minister of Health, after advice from the National Institute for health and Disability Insurance (INAMI/RIZIV). This case study focuses solely on drug reimbursement decisions.

The Belgian drug reimbursement procedure underwent notable changes in 2001. The Drug Reimbursement Committee (DRC) was established to appraise the reimbursement requests from pharmaceutical companies and formulate advice to the minister of health.

The DRC consists of different stakeholders in the Belgian healthcare sector, including representatives from academia, physicians, pharmacists and sickness

Table 8.3 List of *domains* and *criteria*

Quantitative domains (D) and criteria (C)
D1 – health problem relevance
C01 – description of disease and of its severity
C02 – size of population interested
D2 – technology solution relevance
C03 – type of preventive benefit
C04 – type of therapeutic benefit
C05 – quality of evidence
D3 – safety
C06 – improvement of safety and tolerability
D4 – effectiveness
C07 – improvement of efficacy and effectiveness
C08 - improvement of patient-reported outcomes or patient-perceived health
C09 – comparative interventions limitations (unmet needs)
C10 – consensus in clinical guidelines and regulatory status
D5 – financial and economic aspects
C11 – budget impact on health plan (cost of intervention)
C12 – impact on other healthcare costs
C13 – impact on costs not related to healthcare
C14 – cost-effectiveness of intervention, opportunity costs and affordability
Qualitative domains (D) and criteria (C)
D6 – ethical aspects, equal opportunities
C15 – population priority and access (fairness)
D7 – organisational aspects
C16 – system and providers' capacity and appropriate use of intervention
D8 – social aspects
C17 – stakeholder pressures and barriers
D9 – legal aspects
C18 – legal requirements and adherence to mission of NHS

funds (voting members) and representatives from the ministries, pharmaceutical industry and INAMI/RIZIV (consultative members). Voting is done by a show of hands in the presence of consultative members. Individual representatives do not have to justify their vote.

The criteria that need to be taken into account during the appraisal process are defined by law. They include added therapeutic value, drug price and reimbursement basis, clinical effectiveness and likely impact of the product given the therapeutic and social needs, budget impact and cost-effectiveness. Criteria for assessing therapeutic value are also defined by law and include efficacy, safety, effectiveness, applicability and comfort. *Added* therapeutic value is recognised if the drug use in a given treatment demonstrates an impact on mortality, morbidity and/or quality of life. There is no explicit hierarchy in the criteria.

8.2.3.1 Transparency

The changes in the drug reimbursement procedures introduced in 2001 substantially enhanced the transparency and use of objective criteria compared to the period before the establishment of the DRC (Cleemput and Van Wilder 2009). However, issues of transparency remained. The appraisal phase remains a deliberation process in which formal as well as informal criteria are used. Moreover, the distinction between the assessment phase and the appraisal phase is not always very clear.

Primary assessment reports and decisions of the minister are published on the website of the INAMI/RIZIV, but it is not always clear which elements eventually led to the advice/decision as the main discussion points and arguments are not reported.

8.2.3.2 A Belgian MCDA Framework

In 2010, the Belgian Healthcare Knowledge Centre (KCE), an independent publicly financed policy research agency in Belgium, examined ways to improve the accountability for reasonableness of the drug reimbursement system (le Polain et al. 2010). First, it was recommended to make a stricter distinction between the assessment and the appraisal process. Assessment implies the collection of the evidence regarding the technology under consideration. Appraisal implies value judgements, e.g. related to the relative importance of each of the assessment elements. These value judgements should, in a democratic system, ideally reflect societal values and preferences. Second, KCE also presented a possible MCDA framework for making health technology appraisal processes more transparent (Table 8.4). The framework is meant to support decision-making regarding new interventions for different indications.

The framework consists of five questions, corresponding to five intermediate decisions. Each question needs to be answered using explicit decision criteria. The criteria must be (1) relevant and (2) weighted in accordance with the relative importance attached by the general public. The advantage of splitting up the decision process in intermediate questions is that it is cognitively easier for people to consider fewer criteria at once than to consider more criteria at the same time when making a choice (Ryan et al. 2001).

The questions are structured hierarchically, presuming that a new intervention can only be worthwhile reimbursing if there is a need for a better intervention, and the added value of the intervention is sufficient. However, it is not enough that there is a perceived need. Even if there is a need, the new intervention still needs to be better on other criteria considered as important. At a higher need, the better the intervention, meaning a higher propensity to pay for the new treatment with public resources (this on aspects that matter to patients).

The Belgian approach foresees the application of MCDA to each intermediate decision in the framework. In contrast to the examples described in the literature, the Belgian MCDA framework prescribes that criteria weights should come

Table 8.4 Key questions and possibly relevant criteria for a healthcare reimbursement appraisal process (MCDA framework)

Decision	Question	Possible criteria
1. Therapeutic and societal need	Does the product target a therapeutic and/or societal need	Therapeutic need: effective alternative treatments available or not available, severity of disease, inconvenience of current treatment
		Societal need: high/low prevalence; public expenditures related to the disease
2. Preparedness to pay out of public resources for a treatment	Are we, as a society, in principle, prepared to pay out of public resources for *a treatment* that will improve this indication?	Own responsibility, lifestyle-related condition
3. Preparedness to pay out of public resources for the treatment under consideration	Are we, as a society, prepared to pay out of public resources for *this particular treatment*, given that we in general would be prepared to pay for a treatment for this indication?	Safety and efficacy of the treatment compared to the alternative treatment(s); added therapeutic value; significance of health gains
4. Preparedness to pay more	Given that we are, as a society, prepared to pay for this particular treatment out of public resources, are we prepared to pay more for this treatment than for the best alternative treatment?	Added therapeutic value; potentially induced savings elsewhere in the healthcare sector; quality and uncertainty of the evidence; acceptability of patients cost-sharing; rarity of the disease
5. Willingness to pay (price and reimbursement basis	How much more are we willing to pay out of public resources for this particular treatment?	Added therapeutic value; budget impact/ability to pay; cost-effectiveness ratio; medical, therapeutic and societal need; quality and uncertainty of the evidence; limits to cost sharing

from the general public, because legitimacy in healthcare reimbursement decision-making presumes that societal preferences are taken into account. Because the public preferences for the reimbursement criteria were unknown, KCE performed a large population survey in 2014 to derive these weights. The remainder of this case report will discuss the methods and results of this survey and the application of its results into MCDA.

8.2.3.3 Deriving Preferences for Healthcare Reimbursement Criteria from the General Public

A random sample of 20,000 people, stratified by age and sex, was selected from the National Registry of all residents. People were invited to either fill out the web survey or request a paper version of the questionnaire.

The survey consisted of nine discrete choice questions, one moral reasoning exercise and a number of demographic questions. The part with the discrete choice questions was structured in three blocks:

1. Discrete choice questions for defining the relative importance of criteria for assessing therapeutic need, i.e. the need for a better treatment in a particular disease given the treatment already available, as determined by the quality of life under current treatment, the impact of the disease on life expectancy despite current treatment and the current treatment's inconvenience
2. Discrete choice questions for defining the relative importance of criteria for assessing societal need, as determined by the prevalence of the disease and the public expenditures per patient with that disease
3. Discrete choice questions for defining the relative importance of criteria for assessing added value of a new intervention relative to the best alternative intervention, as determined by the impact of that new intervention on all previous criteria

The criteria included in each block have been determined through literature review and expert workshops. With the objective of developing a generic MCDA in mind, the criteria were phrased to be relevant for all health conditions, i.e. not disease specific, hence allowing comparison across indications and potentially leading to optimal resource allocation. The criteria included in each block are presented in Table 8.5.

Responses of 4288 participants from the general public between 20 and 89 years of age (21.4 % out of 20,000 people invited, 89.2 % of respondents) were used for

Table 8.5 Criteria included in the survey

Therapeutic need	Added value of new treatment
Quality of life with current treatment ▪ 8 out of 10 ▪ 5 out of 10 ▪ 2 out of 10	**Impact on quality of life** ▪ improves the quality of life of patients ▪ does not change the quality of life of patients ▪ reduces the quality of life of patients
Life expectancy with current treatment ▪ no longer die from the disease ▪ die 5 years earlier than people without the disease ▪ die almost immediately from the disease, despite current care	**Prevalence of disease** ▪ cures fewer patients ▪ cures an equal number of patients ▪ cures more patients
Discomfort of current treatment ▪ experience much discomfort from current treatment ▪ experience little discomfort from current treatment	**Impact on discomfort of treatment** ▪ reduces the discomfort of treatment for the patient ▪ gives as much discomfort to the patient ▪ increases the discomfort of treatment for the patient
Societal need	**Impact on disease-related public expenditures per patient** ▪ reduces the disease-related public expenditures per patient ▪ does not change the disease-related public expenditures per patient ▪ increases the disease-related public expenditures per patient
Prevalence of disease ▪ is rare: less than 2000 people in Belgium have the disease ▪ is not so frequent: between 2000 and 10 000 people in Belgium have the disease ▪ is rather frequent: between 10 000 and 100 000 people in Belgium have the disease ▪ is very frequent: more than 100 000 people in Belgium have the disease	**Impact on life expectancy** ▪ does not change the life expectancy of patients ▪ increases the life expectancy of patients
Societal cost of disease per patient ▪ little public expenditures per patient ▪ much public expenditures per patient	

analysis. A multinomial logistic regression analysis was performed to analyse the data and in order to obtain level-independent but criterion-specific weights; a method based on log-likelihood differences between model specifications was used.

Depending on the block, respondents were asked to choose between two different patient groups (block on therapeutic need), two different diseases (block on societal need) or two different health interventions for the same disease (block on added value). With 24 different versions of the questionnaire, differing in the description of the scenarios between which to choose, and three choice sets for therapeutic need, 1 for societal need and 4 for added value, it was possible to obtain weights for each criterion included in a specific block.

The weights were calculated using the following algorithm:

1. Estimation of a multinomial logit regression – also referred to in literature as conditional logit – model for each block.
2. For each block, relative preference weights using the log-likelihood method were calculated:
   (a) Calculate the log-likelihood for the model.
   (b) Calculate the log-likelihood for the model minus one of the criteria, which represents the criterion of interest (=the reduced model).
   (c) Test if the reduced model is statistically equal to the full model with the likelihood ratio test. If the test rejects the equality hypothesis, consider the relative importance of the removed attribute to be different from zero.
   (d) Calculate the difference in log-likelihood between the full and each reduced model as a measure of relative importance of the attribute, and convert to a proportion.

This results in three sets of weights, one set for each block. The blocks are not combined in the Belgian model. The assessment of "overall need", encompassing therapeutic and societal need, remains a matter of judgement. If a disease scores high on both types of needs, it will represent as having higher needs than a disease which scores only high on one of the two. No attempts are made, however, to weight the societal needs (societal perspective) against the therapeutic needs (individual perspective) in this model.

8.2.3.4 Belgian Weights for Reimbursement Criteria

Therapeutic Need

The implicit weights given to the criteria included in the therapeutic needs domain are presented in Table 8.6. The general public gave the highest weight to the quality of life under current treatment. Therapeutic need is considered to be the lowest in people with a good quality of life given current treatment that do not die from their disease and experience little discomfort from their current treatment.

Table 8.6 Weights for criteria in the therapeutic need domain

Criterion	Weight
Life expectancy	0.14 (3)
Quality of life	0.43 (1)
Discomfort	0.43 (1)

Table 8.7 Weights for criteria determining the added value of new treatments

Criterion	Weight
Change in quality of life	0.37 (1)
Change in prevalence	0.36 (2)
Change in life expectancy	0.14 (3)
Impact on public expenditures	0.07 (4)
Impact on treatment discomfort	0.06 (5)

Societal Need

In the appraisal of societal need, people give more weight to the impact of a disease on public expenditures (0.65) than to the prevalence of the disease (0.35). They consider the need to be highest in very frequent diseases that cost a lot to society per patient.

Added Value

During the appraisal of the added value of new interventions, the citizens gave the highest weight to the intervention's impact on quality of life, followed by its impact on the prevalence of the disease and on life expectancy.

A general observation is that the value loss associated with something negative (higher expenditures, higher treatment discomfort, less patients cured) is higher than the value gain associated with something positive (lower expenditures, lower treatment discomfort, more patients cured). For example, the negative effect on the perceived added value of increasing public expenditures is higher (−0.43) than the positive impact of decreasing public expenditures (+0.23). Table 8.7 presents the weights for criteria determining the added value of new treatments.

Using the MCDA in Decision-Making

The framework described is not yet being applied in practice, but it is going to be used from 2016 onwards in the context of early temporary reimbursement decisions.

MCDA could be applied every time the reimbursement of a new treatment is requested. This involves (1) scoring diseases and treatments on the selected criteria, (2) weighting the scores and (3) summing the weighted scores. The clinical significance of the impact of a disease or treatment on a criterion is reflected in the scoring, while the extent to which that clinical significant or insignificant effect should matter for the decision is reflected in the weights.

The MCDA is applied as follows:

- *Step 1*: *Consideration of the condition targeted by the new treatment and the current treatment for the condition.*

  The committee members consider the condition targeted by the new treatment and score the criteria relating to therapeutic need and relating to societal need.

  For the scoring, the committee members should have an assessment report describing the existing scientific evidence regarding each criterion, as well as the evidence gaps. The members could consult external experts, e.g. in case of insufficient or inconclusive evidence.
- *Step 2*: *Consideration of the added value of the new intervention*

  The committee members score the criteria for added value for the new intervention for which reimbursement is being considered. The scores should be based on the best available scientific evidence.
- *Step 3*: *Weighting of scores for therapeutic need, societal need and added value*

  The scores are weighted with their respective public preference weights, as derived from the survey. This is done by multiplying the score with the weight. For each domain the weighted scores of the domain-specific criteria are summed.

  This, results in three scores: one for therapeutic need, one for societal need and one for added value of new treatment. Higher scores represent a higher level of priority in terms of therapeutic need, societal need or added value of treatment, depending on the domain considered. By repeating the MCDA for different decisions, a priority ranking of diseases and treatments will eventually be obtained.
- *Step 4*: *Deliberation about the resulting scores for therapeutic need, societal need and added value*

  The three total weighted scores allow the commission to consider in which quadrant of Fig. 8.4 the intervention is located. The higher the need and the higher the added value, the more likely it is that reimbursement can be considered. Whether it will be reimbursed is still a matter of willingness to pay, and this is something to be judged by the decision-makers. The process remains deliberative on this point. However, the number of interventions about which deliberation regarding willingness to pay is needed reduces (for interventions on the left of the *Y*-axis, no further discussion is needed, unless criteria have been missed in the MCDA).

  There might be criteria that are not included in the MCDA that also matter to the decision. Deliberation should include discussions about whether there are other criteria –not yet included in the MCDA – that are important and that would justify a change in the priority ranking in terms of need or added value. For example, it could be that policy-makers wish to give higher priority to prevention than to cure. If that is the case, preventive interventions might be moved up in the priority ranking. If additional criteria are considered important, they should be made explicit, and the committees should explain how these additional criteria modified the ranking of a disease or a treatment.

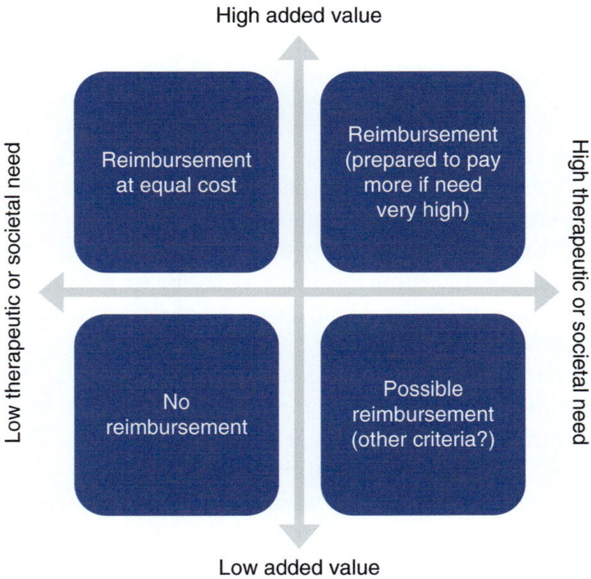

Fig. 8.4 Preparedness to pay (more) for a new intervention

Unlike many other MCDA approaches, the Belgian approach does not combine appraisal of need for a better treatment and added value of new treatments in one single weighted score. Although this might be considered a weakness, it could also be regarded as strength. The appraisal of need and added value requires a very different viewpoint: the first one encompasses disease-related criteria and the second technology-related criteria. It is hard to understand how such diverse criteria can be weighed against each other.

8.3 Discussion

Motivations for this chapter coincided with those of Tanios et al. (2013) on decision-makers' perceptions of the relevance and need of a wider range of criteria to assist decision-making and also Guindo et al. (2012) on the perceived importance of considering both normative and feasibility criteria for fair allocation of resources and optimised decision-making. Literature shows that country-specific HTA organisations and processes for priority setting have emerged globally. This emphasises the need of observing principles such as transparency, robust and appropriate methods for combining costs and benefits, explicit characterisation of uncertainty and active engagement with stakeholders (Drummond et al. 2008; Chalkidou et al. 2009; Pinchon- Riviere et al. 2010); however, there is still little information regarding what shall be considered as "good practice" whenever appraising the evidence to reach a final coverage decision.

All three case studies attempted to fulfil the methodological requirements of MCDA: (1) *completeness* (all criteria defining the value of interventions are considered), (2) *not redundancy* (no duplicates are allowed), (3) *mutual independency* (a criterion's score is independent from the score given to other criteria) and (4) *operationability* (criteria are unambiguously defined, assessment data are independently available and directionality of the scoring scale can be universally understood). However, it was very challenging to run an efficient and explicit process to ensure transparency and consistency of relevant factors and also fulfil the methodological requirements of MCDA; thus, limitations were expected to occur.

The methodological challenges posed by the use of MCDA for HTA reported in the literature were coincident with those of the case studies. For instance, in none of these cases, there was explicit account when dealing with uncertainty about MCDA estimates; perhaps, there is need to incorporate additional and more sophisticated statistical methods for dealing with this issue in the near future whenever presenting results to decision-makers. How to estimate opportunity costs remained as a challenge whenever using MCDA to assist coverage decision-making, should cost-effectiveness be kept as a single criterion to be contrasted against empirically estimated ICERs? Or should it be removed from relevant criteria to avoid double counting? In such cases inevitably some methodological trade-offs shall be made in the future. For a more comprehensive discussion of methodological challenges of MCDA, see Chapter 14.

It also emerged that when testing MCDA for cross comparison of interventions, it may not be possible to generate a generic MCDA framework for HTA that fits all needs of decision-makers, since it may be the case in which committee members may prefer a certain set of criteria regarding groups of similar interventions to assure more fair comparison among them. In the specific cases that looked at EVIDEM criteria, some would argue that it does not comply with core principles such as lack of overlapping or preferential independence while others may contend that the importance of this framework is to make explicit account of what is relevant to decision-makers and promote discussion. All these methodological considerations should be borne in mind for the robust incorporation of MCDA into coverage decision-making and for the agendas of future research. Limitations aside, all three case studies were an attempt to assure that after robust HTA has been conducted, transparent and systematic decision-making should be pursued.

Many lessons emerged, for instance, in Colombia and Lombardy on the need to provide more explanation to committee members before piloting; implementation needs some time for familiarising by decision-makers; this is similar to the findings reported by Goetghebeur et al. (2012). Provision of complete information together with homogeneity and coherence of reports could reduce uncertainty among decision-makers and improve consistency across committees and interventions. A final consensus was that a mixed approach including an MCDA evidence matrix completed with a detailed BIA would be ideal for Colombia – this is in line with the recommendations of the EVIDEM collaboration for the operationalisation of such MCDA framework (www.evidem.org/docs/2015/EVIDEM-v3-0-Decision-criteria-conceptual-background-definitions-and-instructions-June-2015b.pdf).

Lombardy government strengthened its HTA programme taking into consideration existing methods developed by EUnetHTA and the EVIDEM collaboration, implying no need to "reinvent the wheel". Lombardy also utilised web-based tools for quantitative and qualitative stages of the process; this may provide an opportunity to scale up deliberation to wider audiences within the same region or even within the country without representing major costs in the short run. However, commitment of additional resources, a revision of the procedures and a stricter link between HTA and other management programmes (i.e. revision of pathways of care, risk assessment) should be envisioned for the advancement of the forthcoming HTA policy act in this jurisdiction.

In the case of Belgium, it was mainly the objective of transparency and legitimacy of decision-making that triggered work on MCDA. It is only through the use and consideration of the relevant questions with the relevant criteria and their relative weights that the decision-making process can become more legitimate. Decisions about what the budget allows should be in line with what people consider important, both for individual patients as for the society as a whole. The Belgian approach is deliberative once the relevant values have been made explicit, but the deliberation process should be based on more consistent and transparent appraisals of criteria. Therefore, the process in Belgium should not stop at the point where it is at, and the scores calculated should be complemented with a deliberation process to depict potential additional considerations that shall be included. It was a common consideration that more research is still needed on how to deal with missing or low-quality evidence and also whenever there is need of deciding on early temporary coverage of products that have not yet obtained a marketing authorisation.

There was wide context variation; Colombia, for example, just recently incorporated HTA, and there is still need to upscale the use of MCDA during the appraisal stage of the decision-making process; thus, the pilot presented in this chapter is an illustration of the incipient efforts in this context. Belgium on the other hand incorporated robust evidence assessment for decision-making more than a decade ago, but it is the recent work of KCE which portraits the aims for a more explicit and legitimate process. The framework described in this case study is not yet in use, but it is expected to be implemented in 2016; hence although relevant, this could also be considered as a work in progress initiative.

It is the case of Lombardy, the one that probably represents the use of holistic MCDA in a more systematic and advanced stage at the moment, since it has been in place for over 3 years now. The pioneering work of the Lombardy region presented in this chapter is now being considered at the national level and for a broader focus than drugs and procedures. Of worth noting that each case study adopted a very different approach when attempting to merge MCDA and HTA for coverage decision-making, thus making fair comparison among them more complicated. Further comparative research on methods in the near future might be of value in assisting to identify which approach is the most appropriate.

8.4 Conclusions

All health systems face the challenge of managing finite resources to address unlimited demand for services; hence it is hoped that the content of this chapter could be of significant value to the field of public health and policy since non-explicit priority-setting processes, poor information, lack of policy on HTA, barriers to implementation, political agendas and limited resources are common findings in many countries (Youngkong et al. 2009).

It seems from these case studies and the growing interest on MCDA that structured and objective consideration of the factors that are both measurable and value based in an open and transparent manner may be feasible through the use of these frameworks. According to Mot et al. 2012, systematic and transparent approaches to priority setting are needed to produce decisions that are sound and acceptable to stakeholders. However, justifying advices towards the general public by making transparent what and how criteria is taken into account in the decision-making process is challenging but creates a societal ground for the decisions made; this is crucial for the continuing support of democratic systems with limited resources all around the globe.

The final results from the case studies may be applicable to wider contexts than Colombia, Lombardy and Belgium. MCDA can increase transparency and make value judgements explicit where before they remained implicit; this improves legitimacy and allows more consistency of results. Further research on merging MCDA and HTA to support better informed coverage decision-making, especially on methods, consistency and replicability of MCDA results, may be of value for all countries. Nonetheless, it is worth considering that values and decisions are expected to be dependent on committees' stability and composition, as well as contexts and competing technologies of interest.

References

Baltussen R, Niessen L (2006) Priority-setting of health interventions: the need for multi criteria decision analysis. Cost Eff Resour Alloc 4:14

Baltussen R, Ten Asbroek AH, Koolman X, Shrestha N, Bhattarai P, Niessen LW (2007) Priority-setting using multiple criteria: should a lung health programme be implemented in Nepal? Health Policy Plan 22:178–185

Briggs AH (2001) Handling uncertainty in economic evaluation and handling results. In: Drummond MF, McGuire A (eds) Economic evaluation in healthcare, merging theory with practice. Oxford University Press, Oxford, pp 162–180

Briggs AH, Goeree R, Blackhouse G, O'Brien BJ (2002) Probabilistic analysis of cot- effectiveness models; choosing between treatment strategies for gastroesophageal reflux disease. Med Decis Making 22:290–308

Bulfone L, Younie S, Carter R (2009) Health technology assessment: reflections from the antipodes. Value Health 12(Suppl 2):1–5

Castro HE (2011) Health technology assessment across borders and the role of NICE and NICE international on spreading the message on evidence based health policies. Organisational Policy Analysis Report (DrPH), London School of Hygiene & Tropical Medicine

Castro HE (2012) Agencias de Evaluación de Tecnologías Sanitarias: ¿Moda o Necesidad. Revista Via SALUD- Centro de Gestión Hospitalaria 16(1):12–17

Castro HE, Briceño MF, Casas C, Rueda JD (2013) The history and evolution of the clinical effectiveness of haemophilia type A treatment: a systematic review. Indian J Hematol Blood Transfus. Viewed May 8 2013, http://link.springer.com/article/10.1007%2Fs12288-012-0209-0

Chalkidou K, Tunis S, Lopert R, Rochaix L, Sawicki PT, Nasser M, Xerri B (2009) Comparative effectiveness research and evidence-based health policy: experience from four countries. Milbank Q 87(2):339–367

Cleemput I, Van Wilder P (2009) History of health technology assessment in Belgium. Int J Technol Assess Health Care 25(Suppl 1):82–87

Cleemput I, Neyt M, Thiry N, De Laet C, Leys M (2011) Using threshold values for cost per quality-adjusted life-year gained in healthcare decisions. Int J Technol Assess Health Care 27(1):71–76

Cleemput I, Franken M, Koopmanschap M, le Polain P (2012) European drug reimbursement systems' legitimacy: five-country comparison and policy tool. Int J Technol Assess Health Care 28(4):358–366

Dolan JG (2010) Multi-Criteria clinical decision support. A primer on the use of multiple criteria decision-making methods to promote evidence-based, patient-centered healthcare. Patient 3:229–248

Drummond MF, Sorenson C (2009) Nasty or nice? A perspective on the use of health technology assessment in the United Kingdom. Value Health 12(Suppl 2):S8–S13

Drummond MF, Schwartz JS, Jonsson B, Luce BR, Neumann PJ, Uwe Siebert U, Sullivan SD (2008) Key principles for the improved conduct of health technology assessments for resource-allocation decisions. Int J Technol Assess Health Care 24:244–258

Eddy D (1990) Clinical Decision-making: from theory to practice. Anatomy of a decision. JAMA 263:441–443

Florez ID, Lugo LH, Tamayo ME, Contreras JO, Sierra JM, Acosta JL, Lalinde MI, Granados CM, Lozano JM, Mejía AE, Atehortúa SC, Mejía ME, Ramírez CM, Quintero A- CINETS, Ministerio de Salud y Potección Social, Colciencias (2013) Guía de Práctica Clínica para la prevención, diagnóstico y tratamiento de la enfermedad diarreica aguda en niños menores de 5 años, Colombia. Viewed 16 Feb 2014. http://www.iets.org.co/reportes-iets/Documentacin%20Reportes/Gu%C3%ADa.Completa.EDA.2013.pdf

Glassman A, Chalkidou K, Giedion U, Teerawattananon Y, Tunis S, Bump J, Pichon- Riviere A (2012) Priority-setting institutions in health- recommendations from a Center from Global Development Working Group. Global Health 7(1):13–34

Goetghebeur M, Wagner M, Khoury H, Levitt R, Erickson L, Rindress D (2008) Evidence and value impact on decision-making- the EVIDEM framework and potential applications. BMC Health Serv Res 8:270

Goetghebeur M, Wagner M, Khoury H, Rindress D, Gregoire JP, Deal C (2010) Combining multicriteria decision analysis, ethics and health technology assessment: applying the EVIDEM decision-making framework to growth hormone for Turner syndrome patients. Cost Eff Resour Alloc 8:4

Goetghebeur M, Wagner M, Khoury H, Levitt RJ, Erickson LJ, Rindress D (2012) Bridging health technology assessment (HTA) and efficient healthcare decision-making with multicriteria decision analysis (MCDA): Applying the EVIDEM framework to medicines appraisal. Med Decis Making 32(2):376–388

Guindo LA, Wagner M, Baltussen R, Rindress D, van Til J, Kind P, Goetghebeur M (2012) From efficacy to equity: literature review of decision criteria for resource-allocation and healthcare decision-making. Cost Eff Resour Alloc 10(1):9–21

Heyse J, Cook J, Carides G (2001) Statistical considerations in analysing healthcare resource utilisation and costs data. In: Drummond MF, McGuire A (eds) Economic evaluation in healthcare, merging theory with practice. Oxford University Press, Oxford, pp 213–235

Hoch JS, Briggs AH, William A (2002) Something old, something new, something borrowed, something BLUE: a framework for the marriage of health econometrics and cost-effectiveness analysis. Health Econ 11:415–430

Le Polain M, Franken M, Koopmanschap M, Cleemput I (2010) Drug reimbursement systems: international comparison and policy recommendations. Health Services Research (HSR). Belgian Healthcare Knowledge Centre (KCE). KCE reports 147C, Brussels

Migliore A, Tringali M, Fortino I, Cerbo M (2014) The impact of EAA activities: from assessment to decision-making in Lombardia. EuroScan Newsletter 16:7

Miot J, Wagner M, Khoury H, Rindress D, Goetghebeur MM (2012) Field testing of a multi criteria decision analysis (MCDA) framework for coverage of a screening test for cervical cancer in South Africa. Cost Eff Resour Alloc 10(2), doi:10.1186/1478-7547-10-2

National Institute for Health and Clinical Excellence (2008) Guide to the methods of technology appraisal. London

O'Donnell JC, Sissi V, Pashos CL, Miller DW, Smith MD (2009) Health technology assessment: lessons learned from around the world- an overview. Value Health 12(Suppl 2):1098–2015

Perry F, Garcia O, Diaz S, Guzman L, Ángel J, Lehmann C, Sánchez J, Poveda C, Alba M, Sierra F, Peña E, González A, Medina E, Rosas ML, Martín H, Sánchez R, Moreno M, López MC, Murillo R, Rossi F, Acosta B, Cabarcas M, Zea D, Torres L, Serrano C, Rugeles J, Moran D, Arango N, Cuello J, Mejía A, Carvajal A, Ayala LE, García D, García MP, Ortegón M, Gamboa O, Muñoz A, Lozano T, Gamboa C, León E, Gil A, Instituto Nacional de Cancerología ESE, Instituto Nacional de Cancerología, Ministerio de Salud y Potección Social, Colciencias (2012) Guía de Práctica Clínica para la detección temprana, tratamiento integral, segumiento y rehabilitación del Cáncer de Mama, Bogotá, Viewed 24 Feb 2014. http://www.minsalud.gov.co/Documentos%20y%20Publicaciones/Gu%C3%ADa%20de20Pr%C3%A1ctica%20Cl%C3%ADnica%20%20de%20Cancer%20de%20Mama%20versi%C3%B3n%20completa.pdf

Pinchon- Riviere A, Augustovski F, Rubinstein A, Garcia Marti S, Sullivan SD, Drummond MF (2010) Health technology assessment for resource-allocation decisions: are key principles relevant for Latin America? Int J Technol Assess Health Care 26(4):421–427

Ryan M, Scott DA, Reeves C, Bate A, van Teijlingen ER, Russell EM, Napper M, Robb CM (2001) Eliciting public preferences for healthcare: a systematic review of techniques. Health Technol Assess 5(5):1–186

CRES- Unidad Administrativa Especial- Comisión de Regulación en Salud (2012) Metodología para la determinación de los criterios y categorías para la priorización de tecnologías en salud en el proceso de actualización del POS. Documento técnico proyecto POS – UPC 2012 – 2013. subdirección técnica, Bogotá. Viewed 18 Feb 2013. http://www.cres.gov.co/Portals/0/Convocatoria%20Participaci%C3%B3n%20Ciudadana%202012.pdf

Senior JM, Lugo LH, Acosta N, Acosta JL, Díaz J, Osío O, Plata JA, Saldarriaga CI, Trespalacios EJ, Toro JM, Pastor MP, Ciapponi A, Mejía AE, Atehortúa S, Ceballos M, Mejía ME, Ramírez C, Universidad de Antioquia, Ministeric de Salud y Potección Social, Colciencias (2013) Guía de Práctica Clínica para el Síndrome coronario Agudo. Viewed 25 Feb 2014. http://scc.org.co/wp-content/uploads/2013/07/GPC-SCA-Guia-para-Usuarios-MPS-Colciencias-UdeA.pdf

Tanios N, Wagner M, Tony M, Baltussen R, van Til J, Rindress D, Kind P, Goetghebeur MM (2013) International task force on decision criteria which criteria are considered in healthcare decisions? Insights from an international survey of policy and clinical decision-makers. Int J Technol Assess Health Care 29(4):456–465

Tony M, Wagner M, Khoury H, Rindress D, Papastavros T, Oh P, Goetghebeur MM (2011) Bridging health technology assessment (HTA) with multicriteria decision analyses (MCDA): field testing of the EVIDEM framework for coverage decisions by a public payer in Canada. BMC Health Serv Res 11:329

Tringali M, Strada A, Leoni O, Fortino I (2014) La Valutazione delle Tecnologie Sanitarie – HTA in Regione Lombardia. Economia & Politica del Farmaco (9). 2014 (Italian abstract only) http://www.economiasanitaria.it/index.asp?pagina=http://www.economiasanitaria.it/EPF/EPF00.asp

Tunis SR (2007) Reflections on science, judgment, and value in evidence-based decision-making: a conversation with David Eddy. Health Aff (Millwood) 26:500–515

Youngkong S, Kapiriri L, Baltussen R (2009) Setting priorities for health interventions in developing countries: a review of empirical studies. Trop Med Int Health 14:930–939

Chapter 9
Embedding MCDA in Priority-Setting Policy Processes: Experiences from Low- and Middle-Income Countries

Noor Tromp, Evelinn Mikkelsen, Roderik Viergever, and Rob Baltussen

Abstract This chapter addresses three policy issues related to the application of multi-criteria decision analysis (MCDA) for priority setting of health interventions in low- and middle-income countries (LMICs), namely, stakeholder involvement, institutionalization, and the impact of MCDA on policy decisions. Based on a literature review, we evaluate 11 case studies in the light of these issues. We found that there is no systematic approach for the involvement of stakeholders. Only four case studies implemented MCDA in an institutional context, and three studies evaluated the impact of MCDA on policy decisions. A detailed case study that explicitly integrated MCDA in the policy-making process for HIV/AIDS control in Indonesia is presented, and enablers and barriers of such an approach with regard to the three policy issues are outlined. The final part of the chapter provides recommendations of the future application of MCDA in policy processes. It provides methodological guidance on which stakeholders to involved and why. Recommendations are given on the institutionalization of MCDA and to improve the evaluation of the impact of MCDA on policy decisions.

N. Tromp (✉)
Department for Health Evidence, Radboud University Medical Canter, P.O. Box 9101, 6500 HB Nijmegen, Netherlands

Royal Tropical Institute (KIT), Mauritskade 63, 1092 AD, Amsterdam, Netherlands
e-mail: n.tromp@kit.nl

E. Mikkelsen • R. Baltussen
Department for Health Evidence, Radboud University Medical Canter, P.O. Box 9101, 6500 HB Nijmegen, Netherlands
e-mail: Rob.Baltussen@radboudumc.nl

R.F. Viergever
Department for Health Evidence, Radboud University Medical Center, P.O. Box 9101, 6500 HB, Nijmegen, Netherlands

Research4health, Utrecht, The Netherlands
e-mail: rviergever@research4health.org

© Springer International Publishing AG 2017

K. Marsh et al. (eds.), *Multi-Criteria Decision Analysis to Support Healthcare Decisions*, DOI 10.1007/978-3-319-47540-0_9

9.1 MCDA to Support Priority Setting in LMICs

Priority setting of health interventions is considered a complex undertaking in Western countries but is even more complex in LMICs due to the limited evidence base to inform decisions, the fragile institutional capacity, and the dominant influence of policy makers' opinions and international donor agencies (Kapiriri et al. 2007; Glassman et al. 2012; Chalkidou et al. 2013; Oliver et al. 2014). Without guidance, priority-setting processes tend to be ad hoc, historically based, and without inclusion of all relevant stakeholders (Baltussen and Niessen 2006; Kenny and Joffres 2008; Sabik and Lie 2008; Stafinski et al. 2011; Vuorenkoski et al. 2008; Youngkong et al. 2009). MCDA can be instrumental to improve the quality of decisions (by including all relevant criteria and being evidence based), to increase transparency and accountability of decisions, and to enhance the consistency of decisions both over time and across interventions (Baltussen 2015). MCDA has been defined as "a set of methods and approaches to aid decision-making, where decisions are based on more than one criterion, which make explicit the impact on the decision of all the criteria applied and the relative importance attached to them" (Marsh et al. 2014).

While priority setting of health interventions in LMICs by nature is explicitly embedded in policy-making processes, this is not fully recognized in the development of research methods. In MCDA, the emphasis is often on the technical aspects on the conduct of studies, e.g., on the best methods to elicit weights or on how to aggregate summary scores (Devlin and Sussex 2011). Relatively, little attention is paid to policy-related issues, namely, on the involvement of stakeholders in the analysis, to what extent MCDA exercise has been embedded in institutional policy-making processes, and how it has impacted policies. Involving all relevant stakeholders is a prerequisite to account for competing values at stake and to foster accountability and acceptance of decisions (Daniels 2008). The integration of MCDA in institutional processes is important to ensure that its results will actually be used (Daniels 2008). And last, measuring the impact of MCDA on decisions is essential to conclude whether it has actually contributed to policy changes (Sibbald et al. 2009; Kapiriri and Martin 2010).

This chapter is separated into three sections. First, it provides an overview of MCDA case studies in LMICs in the light of these three policy issues. Second, a case study from Indonesia will be presented that applies MCDA within a policy-making process for the priority setting of interventions in HIV/AIDS control. The barriers and enablers for such approach will also be discussed. Last, we will provide recommendations for future perspectives of MCDA.

9.2 Overview of MCDA Case Studies in LMICs

This section provides an overview of MCDA case studies in LMICs based on a literature review of Marsh et al. and an additional literature search in Pubmed. We will first describe the general characteristics of these case studies and subsequently review them against the three policy issues outlined above.

9.2.1 General Characteristics

Table 9.1 shows an overview of 11 peer-reviewed. Ten studies were articles included from a systematic review of Marsh et al. (2014). The review included all studies up till August 2013 and excluded studies that did not evaluate health-care interventions, such as MCDA, to assess the level of health needed in a locality. From the review, we only included studies conducted in LMICs as defined by the World Bank (2015). An additional nonsystematic search in PubMed (on 22 May 2015 with use of the search term "MCDA" and same inclusion criteria as Marsh et al. (2014)) resulted in one additional reference (Ghandour et al. 2015).

Most of the case studies (9 out of 11) were conducted at national level (Ghandour et al. 2015; Baltussen et al. 2006, 2007; Jehu-Appiah et al. 2008; Diaby and Lachaine 2011; Miot et al. 2012; Youngkong et al. 2012a, b; Holdsworth et al. 2013), while two report on an application in a hospital setting (Nobre et al. 1999; Erjaee et al. 2012). The national studies were conducted within the context of HIV/AIDS control (Youngkong et al. 2012a), noncommunicable diseases (cardiovascular disease (Ghandour et al. 2015), cervical cancer (Miot et al. 2012), and Obesity (Holdsworth et al. 2013)) and five compared interventions across disease areas (Baltussen et al. 2006, 2007; Jehu-Appiah et al. 2008; Diaby and Lachaine 2011; Youngkong et al. 2012b). The majority of these national level studies compared multiple interventions that led to a ranking, while one study evaluated whether a particular intervention (liquid-based cytology (LBC) as a cervical cancer screening tool) should enter a private health plan in South Africa (Miot et al. 2012). Two out of the 11 studies applied MCDA in multiple countries, one in Morocco and Tunisia (Holdsworth et al. 2013) and the other in Palestine, Syria, Tunisia, and Turkey (Ghandour et al. 2015). Out of the 11 studies three took place in Asia (in Thailand and Nepal) (Baltussen et al. 2007; Youngkong et al. 2012a, b), six in Africa (in Ghana, Cote d'Ivoire, South Africa, Morocco, and Tunisia) (Ghandour et al. 2015; Baltussen et al. 2006; Jehu-Appiah et al. 2008; Diaby and Lachaine 2011; Miot et al. 2012; Holdsworth et al. 2013), one in South America (Nobre et al. 1999), and two conducted research in the Middle East (Ghandour et al. 2015; Erjaee et al. 2012). Among the studies in a hospital setting, one reported on patient treatment options for *Helicobacter* infection among children in Iran (Erjaee et al. 2012), while the other on priority setting of health technologies for purchasement in a university hospital in Brazil (Nobre et al. 1999).

9.2.2 Findings on Policy-Related Issues

We have reviewed the 11 case studies in the light of three policy issues, and the detailed findings are presented in Table 9.1. Based on this review, we can make several observations.

Table 9.1 Overview of case studies of MCDA in LMICs and the findings for three policy-related issues: stakeholder involvement, institutional embedding, and impact on policy decisions

Year	Author	Country	Setting (level, disease area)	Policy issue 1: stakeholder involvement	Policy issue 2: is MCDA embedded in an institution?	Policy issue 3: has MCDA impacted on policy decisions?
1999	Nobre	Brazil	Hospital, ranking of eight health technologies for purchasement by hospital	*Stakeholders*: Medical doctors were selected as decision makers (DM), and two of them had experience in acquisition of equipment *MCDA steps*: 1. *Selection intervention options*: – (not reported) 2. *Selection criteria*: medical doctors ($n=4$) 3. *Criteria weights*: medical doctors ($n=4$) 4. *Scoring options*: medical doctors ($n=4$) 5. *Discussion performance matrix*: – (not reported)	No, methodological study to investigate whether fuzzy set approaches can be incorporated in MCDM	Not reported, likely not as it was a methodological study
2006	Baltussen	Ghana	National, ranking of 32 health interventions	*Stakeholders*: Policy makers (or people otherwise involved in decision-making in health), as being the representatives of the general population and having expertise and experience in the matter *MCDA steps*: 1. *Selection intervention options*: *authors* 2. *Selection criteria + related level*: based on review of criteria used in Uganda, plus discussion with a range of stakeholders (not specified) and policy makers 3. *Criteria weights*: health policy makers or people otherwise involved in decision-making in health ($n=30$) 4. *Scoring options*: author's paper 5. *Discussion performance matrix*: – (not done)	No, explorative study on how multiple criteria can be used in priority setting	No, explorative study

2007	Baltussen	Nepal	National, ranking of 34 health interventions to evaluate whether the lung health program should be a priority in Nepal	*Stakeholders*: Policy makers Health professionals People otherwise involved in regional health-care programs *MCDA steps*: 1. *Selection intervention options*: *authors* 2. *Selection criteria*: policy makers and people otherwise involved in regional health-care programs ($n=7$) 3. *Criteria weights*: policy makers and health professionals ($n=66$) 4. *Scoring options*: authors 5. *Discussion performance matrix*: – (not done)	No, authors state it was an explorative analysis and that the priority-setting process was not embedded in an organizational context	No, the results have not been discussed with a range of stakeholders, and this has limited the relevance of the results for actual policy making
2008	Jehu-Appiah	Ghana	National, ranking of 26 health interventions	*Stakeholders*: Policy makers (district and regional directors of the Ghana Health Survey) People otherwise involved in regional health-care programs *MCDA steps*: 1. *Selection intervention options*: *authors* 2. *Selection criteria*: policy makers and people otherwise involved in regional health-care programs ($n=7$) 3. *Criteria weights*: policy makers (district and regional directors of the Ghana Health Survey) ($n=63$) 4. *Scoring options*: policy makers 5. *Discussion performance matrix*: policy makers (directors) ($n=37$) made a simple rank order of the interventions as a validity check to the rank order based on MCDA	Yes, the priority-setting process was strongly embedded in the organizational context of the MoH to secure its integration in the third Five Year Program of Work (2007–2011)	Yes, anecdotal evidence shows that policy makers have used the present study findings as part of the development process of the third Five Year Plan of Work. This involved ranking of interventions, and other criteria (ethical budgetary concerns) were considered to determine priorities

(continued)

Table 9.1 (continued)

Year	Author	Country	Setting (level, disease area)	Policy issue 1: stakeholder involvement	Policy issue 2: is MCDA embedded in an institution?	Policy issue 3: has MCDA impacted on policy decisions?
2011	Diaby	Cote d'Ivoire	National, application of MCDA for drug reimbursement decisions	*Stakeholders*: A focus group of experts ($n=6$) including of three pharmacologists and a specialist in public health and health economics and two pharmacists A chairman and a secretary (pharmacist and physician, respectively, working for the MoH of Cote d' Ivoire) were responsible for, respectively, organizing and recording opinions of the focus group about drug reimbursement criteria) *MCDA steps*: 1. *Selection intervention options*: authors and then focus group ($n=6$) 2. *Selection criteria*: focus group, authors omitted criterion "social class" in later stage 3. *Criteria weights*: focus group 4. *Scoring options*: authors 5. *Discussion performance matrix*: – not reported	Yes, study conducted for the General Mutual Benefit Fund for Civil Servants and State Employees Cote d'Ivoire to improve drug reimbursement process. However, it was an exploratory study to see if MCDA could be used for priority setting	Not reported, likely not as it was an exploratory study if MCDA could be used for formulation of drug reimbursement list

2012	Miot	South Africa	National, (private health plan) evaluation of LBC as cervical cancer screening tool	*Stakeholders*: *Health-care funder* (private health plan) *Clinical policy and decision-making committee* of major health plan, consisting of experts including doctors (specialist and general practitioners), pharmacists, and nurses *MCDA steps*: 1. *Selection intervention options*: health plan 2. *Selection criteria*: health-care funder 3. *Criteria weights*: clinical policy and decision-making committee 4. *Scoring options*: clinical policy and decision-making committee 5. *Discussion performance matrix*: committee gave feedback on decision-making process and EVIDEM framework	Yes, within private health-care sector of South Africa, working with a clinical policy and decision-making committee of a major health plan	Yes, the EVIDEM process for LBC resulted in a consideration by the health plan to only fund for LBC up to the value of conventional Pap smears. A negotiation process was started with the pathology laboratories to review their tariffs for this diagnostic. The fee for LBC was reduced to an amount which was considered appropriate for full funding
2012	Youngkong	Thailand	National level, 40 HIV/AIDS interventions	*Stakeholders*: Policy makers People living with HIV/AIDs (PLWHA) Village health volunteers (VHVs) *MCDA steps*: 1. *Selection intervention options*: authors 2. *Selection criteria*: policy makers, PLWHA, VHVs 3. *Criteria weights*: policy makers, PLWHA, VHVs 4. *Scoring options*: authors 5. *Discussion performance matrix*: policy makers, PLWHA, VHVs	No, seems an explorative study on how deliberative processes can be included in MCDA	No, seems an explorative study on how deliberative processes can be included in MCDA

(continued)

Table 9.1 (continued)

Year	Author	Country	Setting (level, disease area)	Policy issue 1: stakeholder involvement	Policy issue 2: is MCDA embedded in an institution?	Policy issue 3: has MCDA impacted on policy decisions?
2012	Youngkong	Thailand	National level, ranking of 17 possible services for inclusion in national insurance scheme 2009-2010	*Stakeholders*: Project team including National Health Security Office (NHSO), the Health Intervention and Technology Assessment Program (HITAP), and the International Health Policy Program Research team including the Health Intervention and Technology Assessment Program and the International Health Policy Program Consultation panel 1: participants identified by their expertise and selected purposively to cover stakeholders who play an important role in the Thai health insurance system Consultation panel 2: policy makers and academics A working group: representatives of 7 groups (policy makers, health professionals, academics, patients and civil society, industry, lay people) The SCBP (the NHSO's subcommittee for development of benefit package and service delivery): policy makers, health professionals, civil society, and patient groups *MCDA steps*: 1. *Selection intervention options*: SCBP team approved subset of interventions 2. *Selection criteria*: research team (including authors), consultation panel 1 selected criteria, consultation panel 2 developed definitions and levels 3. *Criteria weights*: consultation panel 2 4. *Scoring options*: consultation panel 2 agreed on scoring scale, research team assigned scores 5. *Discussion performance matrix*: *SCBP team* decides on final inclusion of intervention options in benefit package *Note*: consultation panel 1 also decided which stakeholders should be involved in selection of intervention options and inclusion of criteria	Yes, research initiated by the National Health Security Office, the institute managing the Universal Coverage Scheme	Yes, the research team presented the results of the assessment of nine interventions to the SCBP for appraisal. They agreed to recommend three interventions for further consideration to be adopted under the UC scheme, because they were cost-effective and had low budgetary impact The final coverage decisions are not captured in the article

2012	Erjaee	Iran	Hospital, patient treatment options for *Helicobacter* infection	*Stakeholders*: Patient (child)/parents Medical doctor (physician) *MCDA steps*: 1. *Selection intervention options*: – (not reported) 2. *Selection criteria*: patient (child)/parent, physician 3. *Criteria weights*: likely patients and medical doctors (not well reported) 4. *Scoring options*: patient (child)/parent 5. *Discussion performance matrix*: in the end it is open to the parents or patient (child) to make the final decision regarding the selection of the best regime	No, illustrative case study to assess whether AHP can be used to include both qualitative and quantitative criteria, their effects on a regime, and patients' view in the selection of a proper regime	No, illustrative case. Authors also state that it is open to the patient (or the parents) to make the final decision regarding the selection of the best regime
2012	Holdsworth	Morocco, Tunisia	National, selection of interventions for national obesity policy	*Stakeholders*: Research team including representatives of the government, agri-food culture, health professionals, education sector, media, public interest NGOs, multilateral partners. Morocco $n = 37$, Tunisia $n = 45$ *MCDA steps:* 1. *Selection intervention options*: research team 2. *Selection criteria*: all above stakeholders 3. *Criteria weights*: – not reported 4. *Scoring options*: all stakeholder above 5. *Discussion performance matrix*: – not reported	No, not embedded in institution, aim of study was to explore the perspectives of key stakeholders and guide policy makers in their decision-making at national level	No, obesity was not recognized as a major public health priority; therefore convincing policy makers about the need to prioritize action to prevent obesity will be a crucial first step, particularly in Morocco

(continued)

Table 9.1 (continued)

Year	Author	Country	Setting (level, disease area)	Policy issue 1: stakeholder involvement	Policy issue 2: is MCDA embedded in an institution?	Policy issue 3: has MCDA impacted on policy decisions?
2015	Ghandour	Palestine, Syria, Tunisia, Turkey	National, rating cardiovascular disease interventions	*Stakeholders*: Different stakeholders for every country ($n=5$), e.g., directors health-care facilities, dean medical faculty, director CDC, academics, head of research lab *MCDA steps*: 1. *Selection intervention options*: 5 stakeholders per country, total set of 32 options which was shortlisted to by researcher to 10–20 per country based on situational analysis 2. *Selection criteria*: based on WHO framework, input from researchers, decision makers, key informants (not reported if these are the same as the five stakeholders). The authors excluded Burden of Disease and Cost-effectiveness criteria as data was difficult to find, and stakeholders were not familiar with the concepts 3. *Criteria weights*: authors (equal weights given) 4. *Scoring options*: five stakeholders 5. *Discussion performance matrix*: – (reported that this is important, not mentioned it has been done)	No, paper discusses the process and feasibility of using a simple MCDA approach to rank a list of CVD policies with key decision makers/ stakeholders All was part of the MedCHAMPS project, to advise on the policies most likely to be effective in reducing the burden of CVD and diabetes in these countries	Not reported, likely not as it was a research project conducted in four countries

With regard to stakeholder involvement, Table 9.1 shows that there is no systematic approach to the involvement of stakeholders as this differs across the studies and for the different steps of MCDA. Studies differed in the type of stakeholders that they included. On the one hand, in some studies, only medical doctors were involved as stakeholder, for example, in the case of purchasing of new technologies in a hospital (Nobre et al. 1999). On the other hand, for the selection of interventions for the Thai benefit package, multiple stakeholders in various consultation panels were included in different MCDA steps (Youngkong et al. 2012b). Most studies included policy makers (Baltussen et al. 2006, 2007; Jehu-Appiah et al. 2008; Youngkong et al. 2012a, b; Holdsworth et al. 2013) and the South African study on the inclusion of LBC cervical cancer screening tool in a private health plan also included the funder (Miot et al. 2012). Over time, we see a trend to increase the multidisciplinary of stakeholders involved. While in 2006 in Ghana, only policy makers were involved (Baltussen et al. 2006); in the studies from 2011, various parties were represented ranging from health professionals, civil society, industry, and lay people (Ghandour et al. 2015; Diaby and Lachaine 2011; Miot et al. 2012; Youngkong et al. 2012a, b; Holdsworth et al. 2013).

In many studies the authors were also involved in various steps of MCDA (Ghandour et al. 2015; Baltussen et al. 2006, 2007; Jehu-Appiah et al. 2008; Diaby and Lachaine 2011; Youngkong et al. 2012b). A clear rational for the involvement of particular stakeholders was often absent; however some studies state that this was based on their previous involvement in the implementation of the interventions under evaluation (Baltussen et al. 2006, 2007; Jehu-Appiah et al. 2008), their expertise in the field (e.g., in HIV/AIDS control (Youngkong et al. 2012a) or on the acquisition of hospital equipment (Nobre et al. 1999)), or their representation of the general public in the case of policy makers (Baltussen et al. 2006). Studies also differed in how they included different stakeholders. In some cases authors evaluated the performance of interventions (Youngkong et al. 2012a, b), while in others studies, this was done by academics that were not the authors (Youngkong et al. 2012b), policy makers (Jehu-Appiah et al. 2008), or a wider group of stakeholders (Ghandour et al. 2015; Miot et al. 2012; Holdsworth et al. 2013). In some studies multi-stakeholder panels and teams of focus groups were used in sometimes multiple steps of MCDA (Diaby and Lachaine 2011; Miot et al. 2012; Youngkong et al. 2012b; Holdsworth et al. 2013). For example, in South Africa the "clinical policy and decision-making committee" of the private health insurance plan was used and consisted of experts including doctors (specialist and general practitioners), pharmacists, and nurses (Miot et al. 2012). The committee was consulted for the weighting of criteria and scoring of the options and provided feedback on the decision-making process. In the case study on the Thai benefit package, even a project team, research team, two consultation panels, and a working group, all with multiple stakeholders, were involved in different steps of MCDA (Youngkong et al. 2012b).

We define institutionalization as an application of MCDA that is integrated in a real-world decision-making process within an institution; Table 9.1 shows that 4 (Jehu-Appiah et al. 2008; Diaby and Lachaine 2011; Miot et al. 2012; Youngkong et al. 2012b) out of the 11 case studies applied MCDA in an institutional setting. The study in Ghana was integrated in the development of the third Five Year (2007–2011) Program of Work of the Ministry of Health (Baltussen et al. 2007). The other three studies were embedded in health insurance and reimbursement decisions (Diaby and Lachaine 2011; Miot et al. 2012; Youngkong et al. 2012b). The study by Diaby et al. explored how MCDA could be used in Cote d'Ivoire to determine which drugs should be reimbursed under the General Mutual Benefit Fund for Cival Servant and State Employees (Diaby and Lachaine 2011). In Thailand, the case study was initiated by the National Health Security Office, the institute managing the Universal Coverage Scheme (Youngkong et al. 2012b). In South Africa the study was conducted for a major private health plan and closely worked together with the clinical policy and decision-making committee (Miot et al. 2012). These four studies seem to differ in their extent of embedding. In case of the Thai benefit package, the National Health Security Office initiated the research because they needed support in managing the Universal Coverage Scheme (Youngkong et al. 2012b). In Ghana, the MCDA research was strongly integrated in the development of the Five Year Program of Work (Jehu-Appiah et al. 2008). The case studies in Cote D'Ivoire (Diaby and Lachaine 2011) and South Africa (Miot et al. 2012) were to a lower extent embedded as the studies aimed to inform the institutions and were not part of an ongoing decision-making process within the institution.

The other seven studies reported to be either explorative studies to see whether multiple criteria could be taken into account in priority setting of health interventions (Baltussen et al. 2006, 2007) or remained research projects not embedded in institutions but aimed to advise decision makers (Ghandour et al. 2015; Holdsworth et al. 2013) or studied methodological issues of MCDA (Youngkong et al. 2012a; Nobre et al. 1999; Erjaee et al. 2012).

With regard to the third policy issue, impact on policies, Table 9.1 shows that among the 11 studies, three reported that MCDA had informed decisions (Jehu-Appiah et al. 2008; Miot et al. 2012; Youngkong et al. 2012b). In the case of Ghana, anecdotal evidence shows that policy makers used the study findings for the development of the third Five Year Plan of Work (Jehu-Appiah et al. 2008). This also involved ranking of interventions and considering multiple criteria (e.g., ethical and budgetary concerns) to determine priorities. In South Africa, the Evidence and Value: Impact on Decisions Making (EVIDEM) was field tested for decision-making on the funding of a screening test LBC for cervical cancer by a private health plan. The results of process led to the consideration by the health plan to fund for LBC up to the value of the conventional Pap smear test (Miot et al. 2012). A negotiation process was started with the pathology laboratories to review their tariffs for this diagnostic. The fee for LBC was reduced to an amount, which was considered appropriate for full funding. In Thailand, the research team presented the results of the assessment of nine interventions to the SCBP (National Health Security Office subcommittee for development of benefit package and service delivery) for appraisal (Youngkong et al. 2012b). The SCBP agreed to recommend three interventions for further consideration to be adopted under the Universal Coverage Scheme.

In three studies (Ghandour et al. 2015; Diaby and Lachaine 2011; Nobre et al. 1999), the impact on policy decisions was not reported by the authors; however it seems unlikely that they impacted policies due to the methodological focus of the research project. The other five studies reported that there was no impact on policy decisions, as they were exploratory and methodological MCDA studies (Baltussen et al. 2006, 2007; Youngkong et al. 2012a; Holdsworth et al. 2013; Erjaee et al. 2012). One of these witnessed that the disease area that MCDA was applied in (obesity) was not a priority for government in Morocco and concluded that this should be overcome before MCDA priority setting in this field.

Evaluation of an application of MCDA is instrumental to judge its impact on policy-making decisions. However, the majority of case studies have not rigorously done this, and often the authors conclude on the basis of their opinion that MCDA had improved the transparency and consistency of decisions. Only Miot et al. (Miot et al. 2012) in South Africa conducted a survey among the clinical and decision-making committee to evaluate the usefulness of the EVIDEM framework. The committee members favored the use of the EVIDEM process and were positive about its use. In addition, it was found to improve the understanding of the intervention, access to quality assessment of evidence, consideration of key elements of decision, transparency of decision, and understandability of decision by stakeholders.

In summary, we see that there is no systematic approach for inclusion of stakeholders in MCDA, not all case studies were embedded in an institution, and the majority of studies did not evaluate the impact on policy decisions. We analyzed a potential interaction in the case studies between the results on the three policy issues and the methods used in every MCDA step. On the basis of the overview of case studies, we could not identify any pattern, for example, in the methods used for criteria weighting and institutional embedding (policy issue 2).

9.3 The Application of MCDA in a Policy-Making Process: HIV/AIDS Strategic Planning at Provincial Level in Indonesia

This section reports on a case study of MCDA used within an explicit policy-making context, namely, the strategic planning process for HIV/AIDS control in West Java province, Indonesia. The implementation steps, the results, and the barriers and enablers for implementation will be described.

The MCDA approach applied here consists of five steps and these are presented in Fig. 9.1. The approach has a strong focus on the policy-making *process* as it integrates principles of the accountability for reasonableness framework (AFR) (Baltussen et al. 2013). The AFR framework has been applied in various Western countries and LMICs to guide priority-setting processes (Zulu et al. 2014; Byskov et al. 2014a) and is regarded as a highly relevant framework to incorporate ethics

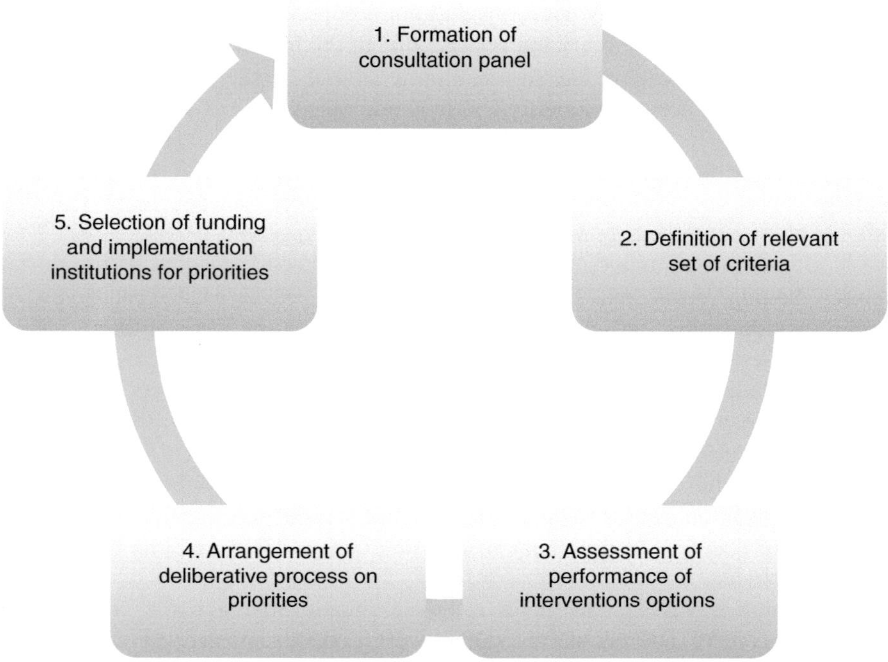

Fig. 9.1 The five steps of the integrated MCDA-AFR approach for priority setting of health interventions based on Baltussen et al. (2013)

in priority setting. The AFR framework outlines four conditions for fair priority-setting processes: relevance, transparency, appeal, and enforcement (Daniels 2008). This comprises involvement of all relevant stakeholders in the process and definition of the reasons for setting priorities (relevance), assurance of transparency of process and reasons for priority setting (transparency), ability for stakeholders to appeal to decisions (appeal), and inclusion of the first three conditions in institutional guidelines to assure that these can be enforced (enforcement).

9.3.1 *Implementation of MCDA During the Strategic Planning Process for HIV/AIDS Control in Indonesia*

Indonesia has one of Asia's fastest-growing HIV/AIDS epidemics with 610,000 people that were living with HIV/AIDS (PLWHA) in 2013 (AIDSdatahub 2014). The country is challenged by a funding gap of US$ 83 million for HIV/AIDS control, as only US$ 69 million was spent, while an estimated US$ 152 million was needed in 2012 (Indonesian National AIDS Commission 2009, 2012).

In Indonesia, West Java (46 million inhabitants) is among the provinces with the highest HIV prevalence, with an estimated 59,000 PLWHA in 2013 (West Java AIDS Commission 2013). The epidemic is concentrated in high-risk groups, with an estimated HIV prevalence rates of 23.2 % among people who inject drugs (PWID), 6.3 % among female sex workers (FSW), and 8.4 % among men having sex with men (MSM) in 2013 (Indonesian integrated biological and behavior survey 2013). The West Java provincial AIDS commission is responsible for coordination of HIV/AIDS activities and has a multi-sectorial design. Its members consist of representatives of different government sectors (like health, education, tourisms, and religious affairs), community-based organizations, and health-care facilities. The previous strategic planning process in 2008 (to develop the plan for 2009–2013) for West Java was evaluated based on qualitative interviews with involved stakeholders (Tromp et al. 2014b). The process appeared to be not systematic and not transparent. Stakeholders were not systematically involved and had limited options for appeal. Criteria were also not explicitly used for prioritizing interventions, and the use of data on the performance of interventions was limited. This resulted in a strategic document with a long list of interventions.

Here, we describe the implementation and evaluation of MCDA in a policy-making process to support the selection of interventions for the 5-year (2014–2018) HIV/AIDS strategic plan for West Java province in Indonesia. The strategic plan functions as a leading document for the allocation of domestic funding in the province. On the basis of this plan, the different government offices involved in HIV/AIDS control select the top priority interventions and search for funding either by making proposals for the local government budget or by searching for other sources as private or international donors. The total budget spent on HIV/AIDS control in West Java province is small (about US$ 1.7 million in 2010 [NASA 2009–2010]), and the strategic plan aims to increase this amount. This is especially important as the contribution of international funding for HIV/AIDS control is decreasing.

A project team ($n=6$) coordinated in 2013 the implementation of the MCDA and was formed by the West Java AIDS commission, Padjadjaran University in Bandung and Radboud university medical center in the Netherlands. The application of MCDA consisted of five steps (Baltussen et al. 2013). These are the formation of a multiple stakeholder consultation panel (step 1), the definition of the priority-setting criteria including weights to reflect their importance (step 2), a listing of HIV/AIDS intervention options by the consultation panel including the collection of data to assess their performance (summarized in a performance matrix that presents an overview of the performance scores of all intervention options on all criteria) (step 3), a deliberative process by the consultation panel on the performance matrix to reach consensus on the rank order of interventions (step 4), and implementation and funding institutions of high-priority interventions (step 5).

In step 1, the project team conducted a stakeholder analysis to determine which stakeholders are relevant in the context of HIV/AIDS control in West Java. On the basis of the stakeholder analysis, a consultation panel ($n=23$) was formed and consisted of government staff ($n=6$) from the health office, labor office, education office, and the coordinating body for family planning, staff from community organizations working on family planning and representing PLWHA and high at-risk groups ($n=4$), program managers from the West Java AIDS commission ($n=7$), and researchers with backgrounds in economics and epidemiology working on HIV/AIDS at Padjadjaran University ($n=6$).

In step 2, the consultation panel discussed criteria for priority setting of interventions in the strategic plan. Inputs for the discussion were the results of a local survey on the importance of criteria for priority setting (Tromp et al. 2014a), the WHO SUFA guidelines (World Health Organization 2012), and implicit criteria used during the development of the National and West Java strategic plans in 2008 and 2009, respectively (West Java AIDS Commission 2009; Indonesian National AIDS Commission 2009). Each consultation panel member received a paper to write down their top five criteria. The results were gathered by the project team and presented plenary to the consultation panel. In the end, the consultation panel agreed after a discussion to select the following four criteria for priority setting: "impact on the epidemic," "stigma reduction," "cost-effectiveness," and "universal coverage." The average criteria weights assigned by the consultation panel members on a scale from 0 to 100 were 34 for impact on the epidemic, 25 for stigma reduction, 18 for cost-effectiveness, and 23 for universal coverage.

In step 3, a larger group of seventy stakeholders proposed a set of 50 interventions (including new ideas) for the strategic plan. These stakeholders were not involved in the weighting of criteria. Scores for the performance of interventions on all criteria were assigned by the researchers within the project team, with 2 indicating high, 1 moderate, and 0 low performance. The scores were based on literature studies, projections of the Asian Epidemic Model for West Java, and expert opinion. To inform the consultation panel, the quality of evidence was indicated using a star system. Expert opinion for new ideas for interventions was indicated as lowest quality (one star), expert opinion for existing interventions as mediate quality (two stars), and the Asian Epidemic Model projections and scientific literature data as high quality (three stars). A total performance score was calculated per intervention by the sum of the weights times the scores per criterion. This was presented in a performance matrix that ranks the interventions based on the total score. The performance matrix shows that the *HIV testing and treatment package* has the highest performance score and is therefore the most attractive intervention to scale up in West Java, followed by *school-based education, information and education during Muslim Friday prayers, websites and social media interventions,* and *the citizen AIDS program. Harm reduction for PWID and mitigation interventions* had the lowest performance scores and were therefore considered less attractive to scale up as they performed least on the four criteria used for priority setting.

In step 4, during a deliberative process, the consultation panel reflected on the performance matrix. First, an interactive session was organized in which the stakeholders individually commented on the performance of each intervention presented on a poster. Only a few changes were made in the scores and this did not affect the overall rank order of interventions. Second, the consultation panel commented that due to ethical considerations, it was undesirable to not provide mitigation interventions (activities to reduce the economic and psychological burden of those living with HIV/AIDS) in West Java province and proposed to split up the performance matrix in three categories: prevention, treatment, and mitigation. In this way the strategic plan contained three separate performance matrices. The consultation panel decided that for the prevention and mitigation categories, the top five interventions should be prioritized. The treatment category consisted of only two interventions (antiretroviral treatment and opportunistic infection treatment), and the consultation panel agreed that both should be implemented.

In step 5, the implementation of prioritized interventions was discussed, and an evaluation of the use of MCDA within the strategic planning process was conducted. For the implementation, the consultation panel listed which stakeholders should fund and implement the prioritized interventions. The steps and results of the priority-setting process were included in West Java's 5-year (2014–2018) strategic document for HIV/AIDS control, which was approved by the governor early 2014.

For the evaluation of the process, an independent researcher conducted in-depth interviews with the consultation panel members ($n=21$). The results show that the members were overall positive about the process. All stated that they had learned from the process, especially regarding the new way of setting priorities, and most were satisfied by the way community organizations were better involved. They also stated that the new approach improved decision-making quality, especially regarding the use of criteria and evidence for decisions. Moreover they expressed it, increased the transparency of the process, and reduced the possibilities for corruption; however they doubted the impact in terms of increased funding for HIV/AIDS control. Aspects mentioned for improvement were a shorter time frame for the meetings and more education on the HIV/AIDS epidemic, HIV/AIDS interventions, and the MCDA and AFR principles. While the project team observed dominance of participants in the discussions, the interview respondents declared that they were fully able to give their opinion in the process.

In conclusion, Table 9.2 summarizes the analysis of these case studies against the three policy issues of this chapter. The consultation panel was systematically involved in all steps of MCDA. The application of MCDA was institutionalized within a policy-making context: it was integrated in the strategic development process organized by the AIDS commission of West Java. With regard to impact, the HIV/AIDS policy decisions were published in the 5-year strategic plan for HIV/AIDS control in West Java province that we based on the MCDA application. Whether it had an impact on the funding and implementation of decisions is uncertain due to the indirect funding systems for HIV/AIDS interventions and time delay to the allocation of funding, and this is not yet studied.

Table 9.2 Case study on the application of MCDA in policy context of strategic planning of HIV/AIDS control in Indonesia

Policy issue 1: Stakeholder involvement	Policy issue 2: Is MCDA embedded in an institution?	Policy issue 3: Has MCDA impacted on policy decisions?
Stakeholders: Consultation panel ($n=23$) consisting of government staff from the health office, labor office, education office, and the coordinating body for family planning ($n=6$), staff from community organizations working on family planning and representing PLWHA and high at-risk groups ($n=4$), program managers from the West Java AIDS commission ($n=7$), and researchers with backgrounds in economics and epidemiology working on HIV/AIDS at Padjadjaran University ($n=6$) *MCDA steps*: 1. *Selection intervention options*: large groups of stakeholders ($n=70$) (determined by consultation panel). Authors also added existing interventions and those were put forward by the international HIV/AIDS field (e.g., different ART policy options) 2. *Selection criteria*: consultation panel 3. *Criteria weights*: consultation panel 4. *Scoring options*: authors (based on literature review, mathematical modeling, and local expert opinion) and then approved by consultation panel 5. *Discussion performance matrix*: consultation panel	Yes, within the 5-year strategic planning process for HIV/AIDS control, organized by the West Java provincial AIDS commission	Yes, MCDA determined the 5-year strategic plan. Writing of the plan was integrated in MCDA steps. However, as this is only a guidance document and due to the indirect funding system for HIV/AIDS control, it is uncertain whether it determines HIV/AIDS resource allocation and eventually the implementation of interventions

9.3.2 Barriers and Enablers for the Application of MCDA in a Policy-Making Context

Box 9.1 reports the barriers and enablers of the application of MCDA in Indonesia in the light of the three policy issues. An important barrier to the equal involvement of stakeholders was the dominance in discussions of certain stakeholders from the constitution panel, while enablers were the multi-sectorial design of the AIDS commission and the familiarity with multi-stakeholder meetings. A barrier to the institutionalization of the approach was the acceptance and understanding of the staff of the West Java AIDS commission of the principles of MCDA. While the existing collaboration between the AIDS commission and the local university that wanted to implement MCDA was an enabler to institutionalize the approach. With regard to the third policy issue, the inclusion of the writing of the strategic development plan within the MCDA approach enabled to inclusion of the results in the strategic document. The indirect and fragmented funding system among multiple stakeholders for HIV/AIDS control was a barrier for impact of MCDA on changes in funding allocation.

Box 9.1 Barriers and Enablers for the Implementation of MCDA to Support the Selection of Interventions for the HIV/AIDS Strategy as Related to the Policy Issues Addressed in This Chapter

Policy issue	*Enablers*
Stakeholder involvement	Familiarity of the provincial AIDS commission with multi-stakeholder processes
	Existing collaboration between the local university researchers (coordinating the MCDA implementation) and stakeholders within the consultation panel (e.g., NGOs representing risk groups)
	Local researchers with expertise in HIV/AIDS, epidemiology and health economics that could be included in the consultation panel
Embedded in institution	Strong leadership by the provincial AIDS commission ("the institution") for the implementation of MCDA
	Existing collaboration between local university researchers (coordinating the MCDA implementation) and the provincial AIDS commission
Impact on policy decisions	The writing of the draft policy was part of the final step of MCDA
	The participation of the provincial planning board, responsible for the allocation of funding toward individual government institutions, in the fifth step of MCDA (Fig. 9.1) in which government institutions decide who proposes for funding from the planning board for the prioritized HIV/AIDS interventions
Others	None

Policy issue	*Barriers*
Stakeholder involvement	Dominance in discussions among stakeholders within the consultation panel
	Some relevant stakeholders (general public and religious leaders) were not included in the consultation panel
	Involvement of international donors was challenging as their decisions for the design and funding of interventions in the West Java province are made at foreign national government level (e.g., AusAID funding program)
	Identification and explanation of ethical reasons in deliberative process was difficult for consultation panel member and facilitator by the research team that led the discussion
	Limited understanding of principles of good governance, priority setting, cost-effectiveness, and HIV/AIDS control among majority of stakeholders in consultation panel
	Low attendance rates and replacement of stakeholders in meetings of the consultation panel
Embedded in institution	The role of the provincial government in HIV/AIDS control is poorly defined. Some say it should provide technical assistance for districts; others say it should provide general visions for which programs to implement across districts. Therefore, it is difficult to define
	The right institutional setting for implementation of MCDA The understanding of MCDA principles by the strategic planning coordinator at the institution was poor
Impact on policy decisions	There is no earmarked budget for HIV/AIDS control activities in Indonesia. The strategic document functions as guidance for provincial government institutions to propose for funding from the provincial government budget through the local planning board. It is therefore unsure whether prioritized interventions will receive funding
	The budget is also fragmented in Indonesia among government institutions from different levels, the private sector (CSR) and international donors (e.g., Global Fund)
	It is questionable whether the interventions prioritized in the performance matrix are relevant for the districts, as the local situation might be different and stakeholders may value other criteria as important
Others	Limited data available on the performance of interventions, especially for the new interventions suggested by stakeholders
	The mathematical model could not evaluate all intervention options, and an improved version was not finalized in time for the development of the final strategy

Similar findings have been reported by other scholars that implemented methods to improve priority setting (Youngkong et al. 2012b; Zulu et al. 2014; Hipgrave et al. 2014; Maluka 2011; Byskov et al. 2014b). With regard to stakeholder involvement, discontinuity of personnel and no perceived authority by those coordinating the process were reported as barriers. Trust among stakeholders is reported as an important enabler for equal involvement of stakeholders. For institutionalization, leadership and culture for openness are reported as key enablers.

Possible barriers and enablers should be identified before MCDA is implemented in a particular setting. And measures should be identified to overcome them.

9.4 Recommendations for Future Applications of MCDA

Based on the findings on the three policy issues and the reported barriers and enablers of the case study in Indonesia, we conclude this chapter with recommendations for the future applications of MCDA to support priority setting in LMICs.

9.4.1 Methodological Guidance on Which Stakeholders to Involve and Why

First we observe that improved methodological guidance is needed on the involvement of stakeholders in MCDA. For example, which stakeholders should be involved in which step of MCDA, how can the view of the public be included, how can ethical values be elicited, how can dominance be resolved in discussions, and how can heterogeneous preferences of stakeholders be aggregated. Various methods do already exist for the points addressed here. Nominal group techniques can be used to resolve dominance in discussions, and interactive evaluation may be used to elicit ethical considerations (Mitchell et al. 1997). In this section we provide further guidance on *which* stakeholder types to include and the underlying reasons *why* they should be included.

We distinguish the following reasons for *why* stakeholders could be included. First, stakeholders may be included in the priority-setting process because of their authority. These can be high-level politicians, academics, and policy makers. Second, stakeholders may be included to ensure fairness of the priority-setting process (Daniels 2008). According to the AFR framework, the priority-setting process should be transparent, and all stakeholders should have opportunity to appeal to decisions. Third, stakeholders may be included to achieve a comprehensive picture of all intervention options for priority setting and thereby also increase the acceptability of the outcomes of a priority-setting process. A broad group of stakeholders will improve the inclusiveness of the options. For example, we saw in the case of Indonesia that researchers gave input to the process to account for international debates on different strategies for antiretroviral treatment scale-up, while civil societies gave suggestions for interventions that would work in the specific context. The acceptability of decisions may also increase when the opinion of broad group of stakeholders is taken into account. Fourth, the inclusion of certain stakeholder types may improve the likelihood of implementation of priorities. For example, the inclusion of funders and policy makers may achieve this as they are deciding on funding and implementation of interventions. The media can be involved to inform citizens on the priority-setting process and outcomes, and this may hold institutions more accountable for actual implementation of the priorities. Fifth, stakeholder could be included to improve consensus and to align the views on priorities. For example, international donors may be included to align their programs with the preferences of local stakeholders. This is in line with the Paris Declaration that donors should align their efforts with countries' needs for development. Also views can be aligned between policy makers, researchers, and those working in the field of priority setting. In this way scientific knowledge and experiences from the field can inform policies.

To determine *which* types of stakeholders are relevant, a stakeholder analysis may be used (Dionne et al. 2015). This should leave room for those coordinating the implementation of MCDA to decide which stakeholders are most relevant in a particular context. We distinguish various types of stakeholders that can be included in priority-setting processes and propose that they vary on four axes (see Table 9.3). The first axis is the sector or discipline that the stakeholders belong to: patients, the general public, civil society, funders, the private sector, insurers, or the media. The

Table 9.3 Overview of type of stakeholders that may be included in a priority setting exercise

Axes	Description
1. Sector/discipline	Potential actors/stakeholders/participants (a) Patients (b) General public (c) Policy makers (d) Researchers (e) Practitioners, including various disciplines, e.g.: (i) Psychologists (ii) Medical doctors (iii) Nurses (iv) Social workers (v) Pharmacologists (vi) Rural health workers (vii) Hospital managers (f) Civil society (g) Private sector (h) Funders (i) Insurers (j) Media
2. Topical area of expertise	Actors with expertise in various areas: disease areas (such as HIV, cancer, maternal health), health system areas, and health-related areas (such as sociology and anthropology)
3. Specificity or broadness of expertise	Detailed van expertise: broad "helicopter view" experts vs. technical experts
4. Demographic expertise	Geographical expertise: actors with local vs. national vs. regional vs. global expertise Balanced gender representation

second axis consists of the area of expertise. Stakeholders might be included with expertise in various health areas, interventions, health system areas, or health-related areas (such as sociology or anthropology). The third axis is the specificity or broadness of a person's expertise. In some steps of the priority setting exercises, technical experts with narrow expertise on a specific subject may be included (e.g., in defining the intervention options), while in other steps, those with a "helicopter view" of the field may be more appropriate (e.g., in comparing the various intervention options across a set of criteria). The latter are often in higher-level positions, such as deans of universities, directors of organizations, and higher-level policy makers. The fourth axis represents the demographic characteristics of participants, for example, the gender or geographical origin of participants. Some stakeholders may be experts with regard to specific geographical areas, such as localities, countries, or regions.

9.4.2 Institutionalization of MCDA Including Capacity Building for HTA Research

To further improve the impact of MCDA on policy decisions, we also recommend to institutionalize and formalize its application. We define institutionalization as an application of MCDA that is integrated in a real-world decision-making process within an institution. The case study in Indonesia meets this definition as MCDA was implemented at the West Java AIDS commission, within their strategic planning process for HIV/AIDS control. Thereby, the results of the MCDA application directly determined the prioritization of interventions for the strategic plan. Institutionalization is also addressed by the enforcement condition of the AFR framework, which outlines that the conditions of good decision-making processes (in this case the principles of MCDA) should be formalized. This then enforces not only the use of MCDA principles in policy-making processes but also the outcomes of the MCDA into real-world policy decisions.

MCDA can be institutionalized at different locations in the health system, for example, at national level HTA institutes within their decision-making process on the reimbursement of new drugs (Miot et al. 2012; Dionne et al. 2015) or at decentralized level like the provincial AIDS commission in West Java in Indonesia within their strategic planning process. MCDA can also be implemented at the level of hospitals, within their decision-making process on the implementation of new technologies or within the decision-making process of doctors and patients on treatment options. The different levels of institutionalization depend on the organization of the health system. A country may have specific institutes with disease-specific policy-making processes, for example, for HIV/AIDS [(Jehu-Appiah et al. 2008), this Chapter], obesity (Holdsworth et al. 2013), or cardiovascular disease control (Ghandour et al. 2015). These decision-making processes may sometimes be limited to the development of policies only and are not always directly linked to funding allocation for interventions. This is illustrated by the case study on Indonesia in this chapter, where funding for HIV/AIDS control is fragmented among government institutions, private sector (corporate social responsibility budgets), and international donors.

In relation to this, we have learned from the Indonesian case study that capacity for health technology assessment (HTA) is necessary within these institutions or among those that coordinate the implementation of MCDA. Knowledge is needed on how to identify and select stakeholders for the consultation panel, how to use criteria for priority setting, how to collect and critically appraise evidence for different intervention options, and how to facilitate deliberative discussions. A key consideration is also to select methods as part of the application of MCDA that are appropriate to the cultural setting. While in some settings voting is an option to reach consensus, in some areas this is less appropriate (Tromp et al. 2014a). Again, a situational analysis on the context of the priority setting exercise is instrumental, and we recommend adding this as an initial and additional step in the integrated MCDA/AFR approach.

Various LMICs have established HTA agencies to different extents (Baltussen 2015). A study by Hernandez-Villafuerte et al. (2015) investigated the priority-setting readiness of 17 LMICs using a set of qualitative and quantitative indicator. Some countries have clearly established and centralized HTA institutions at different levels of maturity, in others HTA is applied in an unstructured or informal basis. It is unknown to which extent these HTA institutions already use the principles of MCDA in terms of using multiple criteria and involvement of multiple stakeholders in the priority-setting process. It would be recommended that the implementation of MCDA is institutionalized within these HTA agencies. Some LMICs are still setting priorities without any contribution of HTA.

9.4.3 Evaluation of the Impact of MCDA Approaches

In this chapter, we observed that most of MCDA research studies in LMICs did no impact on policy decisions. Related to this most of the studies did not evaluate the impact of MCDA. This seems also to apply to high-income countries. The aforementioned review by Marsh et al. could only identify two studies in high-income countries that assessed the impact of MCDA methods (Marsh et al. 2014). We therefore call for more impact assessment and guidance on how to do this. There are two frameworks published in the literature that provide guidance on how to evaluate priority-setting methods. The framework by Sibbald distinguished a set of process and outcome indicators (e.g., stakeholder satisfaction of the process' "decision-making quality" and "influence on resource allocation") and was validated for high-income settings (Sibbald et al. 2009). The framework by Kapiriri was developed particularly for LMICs and seems more comprehensive (Kapiriri and Martin 2010). It contains a broader set of indicators (including short- and long-term outcomes) and proposes indicators for the operationalization of the dimensions of good priority setting (Kapiriri and Martin 2010). However, it has not yet been tested in the field. The A4R framework is also often used to evaluate priority-setting processes and however is less explicit in indicators to determine success (Tromp et al. 2014b; Maluka et al. 2010). In addition, it is highly important to be able to understand the barriers and enablers of success for the application of MCDA. The application of the realist evaluation framework published by Pouwels and Tilly might be useful in this respect (Pawson and Tilly 2007). This framework assesses the context, mechanism, and outcome factors for the performance of MCDA in terms of improving priority-setting processes in health.

9.5 Conclusion

We have reviewed 11 case studies that applied MCDA in LMICs with a special focus on three policy-related issues. This revealed that there is no systematic approach to involve stakeholders in MCDA, that most of the applications of MCDA were not institutionalized, and that they had limited or unknown impact on policy decisions.

To further improve the application of MCDA in LMICs, we recommend developing methodological guidance on how to involve stakeholders in MCDA. Furthermore, the application of MCDA should be institutionalized, and capacity for HTA research should be strengthened in LMICs. Finally, MCDA case studies should include an evaluation component to assess the impact of MCDA on policy decisions. These aspects would further contribute to the success of MCDA studies and realize its potential to make real changes in policy making in health.

References

AIDSdatahub (2014) Indonesia country profile

Baltussen (2015) Question is not whether but how to use MCDA: value & outcomes spotlight, Jan/Feb 2015

Baltussen R, Niessen L (2006) Priority setting of health interventions: the need for multi-criteria decision analysis. Cost Eff Resource Allocat 4:14

Baltussen R, Stolk E, Chisholm D, Aikins M (2006) Towards a multi-criteria approach for priority setting: an application to Ghana. Health Econ 15:689–696

Baltussen R, ten Asbroek AHA, Koolman X, Shrestha N, Bhattarai P et al (2007) Priority setting using multiple criteria: should a lung health programme be implemented in Nepal? Health Policy Plan 22:178–185

Baltussen R, Mikkelsen E, Tromp N, Hurtig A, Byskov J et al (2013) Balancing efficiency, equity and feasibility of HIV treatment in South Africa -- development of programmatic guidance. Cost Eff Resource Allocat 11 26

Byskov J, Marchal B, Maluka S, Zulu JM, Bukachi SA et al (2014) The accountability for reasonableness approach to guide priority setting in health systems within limited resources--findings from action research at district level in Kenya, Tanzania, and Zambia. Health Res Policy Syst/BioMed Central 12:49

Chalkidou K, Marten R, Cutler D, Culyer T Smith R et al (2013) Health technology assessment in universal health coverage. Lancet 382:e48–e49

Daniels N (2008) Just health: meeting health needs fairly. Cambridge University Press, Cambridge

Devlin N, Sussex J (2011) Incorporating multiple criteria in HTA: methods and processes. Office of Health Economics, London

Diaby V, Lachaine J (2011) An application of a proposed framework for formulary listing in low-income countries: the case of Côte d'Ivoire. Appl Health Econ Health Policy 9:389–402

Dionne F, Mitton C, Dempster B, Lynd LD (2015) Developing a multi-criteria approach for drug reimbursement decision making: an initial step forward. J Popul Ther Clin Pharmacol 22:e68–e77

England R (2006) Coordinating HIV control efforts: what to do with the national AIDS commissions. Lancet 367:1786–1789

Erjaee A, Bagherpour B, Razeghi S, Dehghani SM, Imanieh IHM (2012) A multi-criteria decision making model for treatment of helicobacter pylori infection in children. HK J Paediatr (new series) 17:237–242

Ghandour R, Shoaibi A, Khatib R, Abu Rmeileh N, Unal B et al (2015) Priority setting for the prevention and control of cardiovascular diseases: multi-criteria decision analysis in four eastern Mediterranean countries. Int J Public Health 60(Suppl 1):S73–S81

Glassman A, Chalkidou K, Giedion U, Teerawattananon Y, Tunis S et al (2012) Priority-setting institutions in health. Global Heart 7:13–34

Guba EG, Lincoln YS. Fourth generation evaluation. Beverly Hills 1989

Hernandez-Villafuerte K (2015) International decision support initiative: mapping of priority setting in health for 17 low and middle countries acorss Asia, Latin America and Africa. Office of Health Economics

Hipgrave DB, Alderman KB, Anderson I, Soto EJ (2014) Health sector priority setting at meso-level in lower and middle income countries: lessons learned, available options and suggested steps. Soc Sci Med 102:190–200

Holdsworth M, El Ati J, Bour A, Kameli Y, Derouiche A et al (2013) Developing national obesity policy in middle-income countries: a case study from North Africa. Health Policy Plan 28:858–870

Indonesian integrated biological and behavior survey (2013) Ministry of Health. Jakarta

Indonesian National AIDS Commission (2009) Strategy of the national action plan for HIV/AIDS 2010–2014. Jakarta

Indonesian National AIDS Commission (2012) UNGASS. Republic of Indonesia Country report on the follow up to the 35 Declaration of Commitment on HIV/AIDS. Reporting Period 2010–2011. Jakarta

Jehu-Appiah C, Baltussen R, Acquah C, Aikins M, d'Almeida SA et al (2008) Balancing equity and efficiency in health priorities in Ghana: the use of multicriteria decision analysis. Value Health 11:1081–1087

Kapiriri L, Martin DK (2010) Successful priority setting in low and middle income countries: a framework for evaluation. Health Care Analysis 18:129–147

Kapiriri L, Norheim OF, Martin DK (2007) Priority setting at the micro-, meso- and macro-levels in Canada, Norway and Uganda. Health Policy 82:78–94

Kenny N, Joffres C (2008) An ethical analysis of international health priority-setting. Health Care Anal 16:145–160

Maluka SO (2011) Strengthening fairness, transparency and accountability in health care priority setting at district level in Tanzania. Glob Health Action 2011:4

Maluka S, Kamuzora P, San Sebastiån M, Byskov J, Olsen ØE et al (2010) Decentralized health care priority-setting in Tanzania: evaluating against the accountability for reasonableness framework. Soc Sci Med 71:751–759

Marsh K, Lanitis T, Neasham D, Orfanos P, Caro J (2014) Assessing the value of healthcare interventions using multi-criteria decision analysis: a review of the literature. PharmacoEconomics 32:345–365

Miot J, Wagner M, Khoury H, Rindress D, Goetghebeur MM (2012) Field testing of a multicriteria decision analysis (MCDA) framework for coverage of a screening test for cervical cancer in South Africa. Cost Eff Resource Allocat 10:2

Mitchell R, Agle B, Wood D (1997) Toward a theory of stakeholder identification and salience: defining the principle of who and what really counts. Acad Manag Rev 22(4):853–888

Mitton C, Donaldson C (2004) Health care priority setting: principles, practice and challenges. Cost Eff Resour Allocat 2:3

Nobre FF, Trotta LT, Gomes LF (1999) Multi-criteria decision making--an approach to setting priorities in health care. Stat Med 18:3345–3354

Oliver K, Innvar S, Lorenc T, Woodman J, Thomas J (2014) A systematic review of barriers to and facilitators of the use of evidence by policymakers. BMC Health Serv Res 14:2

Pawson R, Tilly N (2007) Realist evaluation. Sage Publications, Thousand Oaks

Sabik LM, Lie RK (2008) Priority setting in health care: lessons from the experiences of eight countries. Int J Equity Health 7:4

Sibbald SL, Singer PA, Upshur R, Martin DK (2009) Priority setting: what constitutes success? A conceptual framework for successful priority setting. BMC Health Serv Res 9:43

Stafinski T, Menon D, Philippon DJ, McCabe C (2011) Health technology funding decision-making processes around the world: the same, yet different. PharmacoEconomics 29:475–495

Tromp N, Prawiranegara R, Siregar A, Sunjaya D, Baltussen R (2014) Priority setting in HIV/AIDS control in Indonesia: the importance of multiple criteria perceived by multiple stakeholders. (submitted)

Tromp N, Prawiranegara R, Riparev Subhan H, Siregar A, Sunjaya D et al (2014b) Priority setting in HIV control in West Java Indonesia: an evaluation based on the accountability for reasonableness framework. Health Policy Plan 30:345–355

Tromp N, Prawiranegara R, Siregar A, Sunjaya D, Baltussen R. (2015) The importance of multiple criteria for priority setting of HIV/AIDS interventions. Int J Technol Assess Health Care 31:390–398

Vuorenkoski L, Toiviainen H, Hemminki E (2008) Decision-making in priority setting for medicines--a review of empirical studies. Health Policy 86:1–9

West Java AIDS Commission (2009) Strategy for HIV and AIDS program in West Java Province, Bandung, 2009–2013

West Java AIDS Commission (2013) West Java Asian epidemic model estimations. Bandung

World Health Organization (2012) WHO consultation on the strategic use of antiretrovirals (SUFA). 2nd expert panel towards programmatic guidance. Geneva

Worldbank list of countries (2015) http://data.worldbank.org/about/country-and-lending-groups

Youngkong S, Kapiriri L, Baltussen R (2009) Setting priorities for health interventions in developing countries: a review of empirical studies. Tropical Med Int Health 14:930–939

Youngkong S, Teerawattananon Y, Tantivess S, Baltussen R (2012a) Multi-criteria decision analysis for setting priorities on HIV/AIDS interventions in Thailand. Health Res Policy Syst/ BioMed Central 10:6

Youngkong S, Baltussen R, Tantivess S, Mohara A, Teerawattananon Y (2012b) Multicriteria decision analysis for including health interventions in the universal health coverage benefit package in Thailand. Value Health 15:961–970

Zulu JM, Michelo C, Msoni C, Hurtig A-K, Byskov J et al (2014) Increased fairness in priority setting processes within the health sector: the case of Kapiri-Mposhi District, Zambia. BMC Health Serv Res 14:75

Chapter 10
MCDA for Resource Allocation at a Local Level: An Application in the UK

Brian Reddy, Praveen Thokala, and Alejandra Duenas

Abstract *Introduction*: Resource allocation at a local level involves making difficult decisions about investment and, particularly in a time of economic stringency, about disinvestment. These complex decisions are influenced by a number of local, political and contextual factors. The use of MCDA can support the local decision-makers to allocate their resources in a rational manner, based on explicit consideration of their priorities.

Overview: This chapter provides an overview of methods for decision-making of relevance to health priority setting in local authorities. These methods have typically been developed in health-care independent of MCDA but share a number of similarities. Priority-setting approaches which draw on MCDA techniques include option appraisal, Portsmouth scorecard, prioritisation matrices, programme budgeting and marginal analysis (PBMA), sociotechnical allocation of resources (Star) and discrete choice experiments (DCEs). Whilst these applications are all based on MCDA, they vary significantly in terms of scientific rigour, robustness and time and other resources required.

Case Study: The case study (entitled SYMPLE) describes the MCDA approach used to inform a prioritisation process for smoking cessation interventions across four local government areas in South Yorkshire.

B. Reddy (✉)
School of Medicine, Trinity College Dublin, Dublin, Ireland
e-mail: reddybr@tcd.ie

National Centre for Pharmacoeconomics, Dublin, Ireland

P. Thokala
University of Sheffield, Sheffield, UK
e-mail: p.thokala@sheffield.ac.uk

A. Duenas
IÉSEG School of Management (LEM-CNRS), Paris, France

© Springer International Publishing AG 2017

K. Marsh et al. (eds.), *Multi-Criteria Decision Analysis to Support Healthcare Decisions*, DOI 10.1007/978-3-319-47540-0_10

Discussion: A number of MCDA methods exist for local resource allocation, ranging from quick and simple methods (e.g. direct methods) which can be performed in a couple of weeks and are based on subjective opinion to more complex methods like the HELP tool which was based on DCEs and robust evidence (systematic reviews, modelling and survey of general population) but took significantly longer to implement. The local decision-makers need to choose the appropriate method based on their resource/time constraints, scientific validity and significance and broader context of the decision problem.

10.1 Introduction

Resource allocation at a local level involves making difficult decisions about investment and, particularly in a time of economic stringency, about disinvestment. In the UK, local authorities have some leeway in how they deploy the public health budget although certain activities (e.g. implementing the national health check programme and providing sexual health services) are mandatory. They hold overall responsibility for promoting the impact of health interventions on their populations and simultaneously for addressing health inequalities across the range of their activities. Priority setting at a local level is informed by national guidelines and by local political and contextual factors and influences, including the extent of stakeholder and public engagement in identifying and agreeing priorities. However, there is no formal process for prioritising public health investment or for ranking interventions. Local authorities are likely to adopt a range of different approaches in practice to prioritise between possible actions, depending on their respective circumstances and preferences.

This chapter provides an overview of methods for decision-making of relevance to health priority setting in local authorities. Section 10.2 describes the priority-setting approaches which draw on multiple criteria decision analysis (MCDA) techniques including option appraisal, programme budgeting and marginal analysis (PBMA), socio-technical allocation of resources (Star) and other MCDA approaches incorporating discrete choice experiments (DCE). MCDA techniques are an extension of decision theory 'for appraising alternatives on individual, often conflicting criteria and combining them into one overall appraisal' (Keeney and Raiffa 1993). Section 10.3 includes a discussion on different techniques for weighting criteria and the different ways of gathering data on the alternatives' performance. Section 10.4 describes a case study of MCDA approach used for smoking cessation intervention prioritisation in four primary care trusts (PCTs) in South Yorkshire. The case study highlights that applications of MCDA may vary significantly in terms of scientific rigour, robustness and time and other resources required. The final section presents the conclusions, which state that the local decision-makers need to choose the appropriate method based on their resource/time constraints, scientific validity and significance and broader context of the decision problem.

10.2 Overview of MCDA Methods for Priority Setting at Local Level

This section provides an overview of methods used to support health priority setting by local authorities. The priority-setting approaches that draw on MCDA techniques include option appraisal, Star, PBMA and techniques using DCE approaches.

10.2.1 Option Appraisal, Portsmouth Scorecard and Other Prioritisation Matrices to Guide Deliberations

Option appraisal is widely used in government for comparing the costs and benefits of different options for investment. It is concerned with value for money in achieving stated objectives and involves a process of defining objectives, examining options and weighing up the costs, benefits, risks and uncertainties of those options (HM Treasury 2003; Government 2011). It therefore encourages a systematic approach to evaluate prospective ways to meet outcomes, achieved through exploring the relative costs and benefits of a particular option and making a comparison with other options against the same set of evaluation criteria.

Such approaches have been used to:

- Evaluate and consider the management, organisation and delivery of mental health services in Ashton, Leigh and Wigan, including those delivered by the local authorities in that area (Ashton, Leigh and Wigan PCT 2005)
- Support health service redesign for children with complex needs in Aberdeen, including consideration of services delivered by Aberdeen City Council (Aberdeen City 2010)
- Evaluate the costs and benefits of alternative systems of coronary heart disease monitoring in Scotland (Perry et al. 2000).

Prioritisation matrices, tailored to the specific decision-making setting, with varied criteria and weighted scoring systems, have been commonly developed by PCTs for their own use, although largely for prioritising new developments. These methods have the advantage of not requiring sophisticated quantitative analysis, and modified versions have been developed to inform decisions over clinical and non-clinical interventions in a number of localities across England (Robinson et al. 2011; Robinson 2011). It has been argued (Robinson et al. 2009) that these approaches are easy to understand and the criteria can be adapted to suit the priority-setting context. It is also argued that the tool can be used as a vehicle to engage different stakeholder groups in the priority-setting process (Robinson et al. 2009), to facilitate deliberation and potentially further stakeholder participation. A related approach, which incorporates more formal performance matrices, is the ‘Portsmouth scorecard’. In this approach, each option is scored against selected criteria, and total scores are calculated and discussed. Each criterion has a maximum score, and there are thresholds for scoring within each category, as seen in Table 10.1. Allowing decision makers (or other stakeholders) to assign these points using their subjective judgement is what distinguishes it from other performance matrix-style approaches, making it a 'quick and dirty' approach that will suffice in many scenarios. It usually involves calculating a single index score for each intervention and then ranking interventions accordingly (Williams et al. 2011; Austin et al. 2007). Interventions are placed in rank order (highest scoring interventions take priority). Typically, scorecards are designed to assess requests for investment through the collection of information on clinical and cost-effectiveness, numbers of patients who would benefit, clinical engagement in the proposal for investment and risks of not funding the intervention (Williams et al. 2011).

Table 10.1 Portsmouth scorecard

Factor	Very low	Mid-scale	Very high	Score	Out of
Magnitude of benefit (health gain)	Under 3 points Limited improvement in health or life expectancy	20 points Moderate improvement in health or life expectancy	40 points Large improvement in health or life expectancy		40
Addresses health inequality	Under 3 points Does not address a health inequality	20 points Partially addresses a health inequality	40 points Fully addresses a health inequality		40
Strength of evidence of clinical effectiveness	Under 3 points Limited or no evidence (case series, experimental)	20 points Modest evidence (cohort studies)	40 points Good evidence (meta-analysis, RCTs)		40
Cost-effectiveness	Under 3 points > £20,000 per QALY	20 points £10–20,000 per QALY	40 points <£10,000 per QALY		40
National and local priority	Under 3 points None	20 points Two targets Identified as need in the CSP/ JSNA	40 points Must do, Major need in CSP/ JSNA		40
Number who will benefit (not the number treated)	Under 3 points 10	20 points 1000	40 points 10,000		40
Affordability	Under 3 points >£100,000	10 points <£50,000	20 points Cost saving to the PCT		20
Total score for option				(Sum of above scores)	260

Austin et al. (2007)

10.2.2 Socio-Technical Allocation of Resources (Star)

This method comprises a pragmatic approach to priority setting, combining value for money (VFM) analysis with extensive stakeholder engagement through decision conferencing. The approach was initially developed through work carried out with the Isle of Wight (see Box 10.1 below) and Sheffield PCT (Airoldi et al. 2011, 2014), which has since been developed into socio-technical allocation of resources (Star) toolkit in collaboration with the Health Foundation (Airoldi et al. 2014; Airoldi 2013; Health Foundation 2012). This technique used MCDA approaches to facilitate local governments in deriving their own appropriate 'efficient frontier' to weigh up costs and benefits (however they defined these) and given the total budget available. The approach used a decision conference setting; to do so, an impartial facilitator works iteratively with stakeholders to generate an explicit model intended to help those present to think more clearly about the relevant issues (Phillips and Bana e Costa 2007).

Box 10.1: Star in Action

Airoldi et al. (2011) describe a research study conducted in collaboration with and for the Isle of Wight PCT in 2008.

This process included (i) a schedule of meetings, (ii) the design of a social process to engage key stakeholders and a technical process developed upon CEA principles to formulate a list of key priorities, (iii) guidance on utilising information from available demographic and epidemiological data to support the evaluation of interventions, (iv) the facilitation of meetings with stakeholders, (v) the analysis of results and (vi) the production of a final report setting out the key findings and recommendations.

Twenty-one proposed initiatives to improve quality of life and reduce health inequalities on the island were summarised in a single template which set out the intervention operationally; assessed expected cost; estimated the number of beneficiaries, identified the profile of an average beneficiary, including consideration of impact on health equalities; and set out the health benefit (Airoldi et al. 2011).

The information was used to generate a priority list in which interventions were ranked according to value for money. This ranking was a cost-effectiveness ranking similar to a cost/QALY league table.

Following the decision conference, a report was drafted which was used to feed into the PCT's prioritisation of £1million of additional resources. The analysis influenced the PCT's decision to approve an operational plan to fund the interventions with the highest value for money.

An Excel-based tool is used alongside a facilitated stakeholder workshop, and the results are presented using visual aids such as VFM triangles and efficiency frontiers. A key focus of the sociotechnical approach is for the problem and potential solution to be 'owned' by the stakeholders rather than having it 'imposed on them by outside agencies' (Williams et al. 2011).

10.2.3 Programme Budgeting and Marginal Analysis (PBMA)

PBMA is a structured deliberative process, involving multiple stakeholders, who make investment and disinvestment recommendations. The incremental costs and benefits of interventions under consideration are estimated (programme budgeting/PB) and the benefits arising from investments and disinvestments at the margin compared (marginal analysis/MA), in order to maximise impact and minimise costs (Donaldson and Mitton 2009). PB enables commissioners to assess data on spending as a whole and in relation to different practices, allowing for discussion over variations in patterns of expenditure. MA draws on economic concepts such as opportunity cost to explore the assessments of costs and benefits from various activities involved in a particular programme area. Stakeholders normally meet on a number of occasions and agree on final investment/disinvestment decisions based upon dialogue and compromise. The steps involved in PBMA are outlined in Table 10.2.

The primary concern in PBMA is with assessing costs and benefits at the margins, and the focus is on what can be gained from an increase in resources or lost from a reduction (Williams et al. 2011; Donaldson et al. 2010). PBMA can be used to address some of the barriers associated with the use of economic evaluation through the adoption of 'more flexible, accessible and locally appropriate' techniques to inform prioritisation (Robinson et al. 2011). PBMA has been promoted as a pragmatic approach to applying the economic principles of marginal analysis and opportunity cost to local resource allocation decisions. It can highlight some of the tensions related to priority setting locally and lead to improved cohesion and greater stakeholder ownership of the decision-making process (Bohmer et al. 2001; Ruta et al. 2005).

10.2.4 MCDA Using Discrete Choice Experiments (DCEs)

DCEs can be used during the weighting stage of an MCDA process. They are a stated preference method used for studying the preferences of patients and other stakeholders (Bridges 2003). DCE participants are offered a series of vignettes, each containing two options scored on multiple criteria and asked to choose which one they would prefer. Based upon these decisions, the implied weightings of the importance of each criterion can be deduced using multinomial regression. They

Table 10.2 Stages in a PBMA priority-setting exercise (Peacock et al. 2009)

1. *Determine the aim and scope of the priority-setting exercise*
Determine whether PBMA will be used to examine changes in services within a given programme (micro/within programme study design) or between programmes (macro/between programme study design)
2. *Compile a 'programme budget*
Resources and costs of programmes will need to be identified and quantified, which, when combined with activity information, becomes the programme budget
3. *Form a 'marginal analysis' advisory panel*
A panel of 8–30 people, made up of key stakeholders (managers, physicians, nurses, finance personnel, consumers, community representatives, etc.) is formed to advise priority-setting process. Marginal analysis involves attempting to broadly maximise the total impact from the available programme budget
4. *Determine locally relevant decision-making criteria*
Elicited from the expertise of the advisory panel (e.g. maximising benefits, improving access and equity, reducing waiting times, etc.), with reference to national, regional and local objectives, and specified objectives of the health system and the community
5. *Identify options for (a) service growth (b) resource release from gains in operational efficiencies (c) resource release from scaling back or ceasing some services*
The programme budget, along with information on decision-making objectives, evidence on benefits from service, changes in local health-care needs and policy guidance, is used to highlight options for investment and disinvestment
6. *Evaluate investments and disinvestments*
Evaluate in terms of costs and benefits and make recommendations for (a) funding growth areas with new resources (b) moving resources from 5(b) and 5(c) to 5(a)
7. *Validate results and reallocate resources*
Re-examine and validate evidence and judgements used in the process and reallocate resources according to cost-benefit ratios and other decision-making criteria

have increasingly been used over recent years in health-care settings (Reed Johnson et al. 2013).

In 2009, the Health England Leading Prioritisation (HELP) online tool was developed (Health England) from a project commissioned by Health England to help prioritise preventive interventions. An MCDA approach was employed for comparing interventions across a range of attributes, such as cost-effectiveness, and impact on health inequalities. The MCDA involved the following steps:

1. Identifying interventions to evaluate
2. Identifying criteria against which to evaluate the interventions
3. Measuring the interventions against the criteria
4. Combining the criteria scores to produce a ranking of each intervention

First, the list of interventions included in the analysis was selected by reviewing NICE recommendations, conducting stakeholder workshops and identifying whether the interventions meet national priorities. Secondly, criteria against which to evaluate interventions were identified using a review of previous prioritisation methods, stakeholder workshops and stakeholder surveys. Third, the performance of the interventions on the criteria was gathered from reviews of evidence of effectiveness and cost-effectiveness, construction of decision models to estimate the cost per QALY gained and analysis of affordability, reach and inequality score. Fourth, a DCE was undertaken to elicit the relative importance that decision-makers place on different criteria; a total of 1117 questions were answered by 99 respondents. Multinomial regression analysis was run using the conditional logit model, and the 17 interventions were then ranked by the probability of each intervention being funded using the results of the DCE.

10.2.5 The South Yorkshire Multi-criteria Decision Analysis Prioritisation for Local Effectiveness (SYMPLE) Approach

In Section 10.4, a case study is described, showing the approach used to prioritise between a range of interventions aiming to reduce tobacco prevalence across four local government areas (boroughs). A standard linear additive MCDA model was chosen as the most appropriate approach for this decision problem. This is the most commonly used approach in health care (Marsh et al. 2014). Only one half-day was available to bring the expert group together—so a simple approach was necessary—ruling out other potentially more time-intensive methods such as the paired comparison techniques. The total scores were calculated for each intervention, using a weighted sum method, which can then be used to prioritise between the interventions. The final decision was to be made by each borough's Director of Public Health (DPH), so the MCDA modelling can be considered as a tool to help quantify the benefit associated with each approach. The case study shows that modelling, in practice, in local government circumstances can be difficult for a range of reasons, such as lack of evidence, limited resources and the need to incorporate multiple stakeholders.

10.3 Discussion

All the different MCDA methods highlighted in Sect. 10.2 follow the same general principles of identifying criteria, weighting them, valuing the different options on the criteria and combining all this information to support prioritisation. In practical terms, however, techniques operate at different levels of complexity and the choice of appropriate technique for a given problem should also be partly determined by available time, data and skills. As seen in Sect. 10.2, approaches range from simple scorecards to computer-based modelling. There are a number of different techniques for weighting criteria, which can be used as part of any MCDA method. These include:

- Direct rating. A numerical figure is assigned from a given range to weight criteria (such as 0–10). This is easy to use; however, there is some criticism in that the stakeholders do not consider all the information with this method.
- Swing weighting. This requires the identification of the most important criterion by thinking about the difference between the best and worst performance on each criterion, given the alternatives under consideration. Criteria that under normal circumstances would be considered critical a priori may not end up important in the context of the model if similar levels are present in each of the alternatives, and vice versa. This is relatively straightforward to use and has explicit consideration of the scales of the different criteria (widely considered the 'gold standard' method).
- Paired comparison analysis. This establishes choices across or within programmes. It can be used for ranking options, and stakeholders choose between paired comparisons: options are ordered from 'most often preferred' to 'least often preferred'. This is relatively simple for non-experts but can lead to inconsistent preferences and, depending on the number of criteria, can take a long time.
- Conjoint analysis and discrete choice experiments (DCE). These use survey-based methods for eliciting trade-offs that stakeholders are willing to make. The HELP tool, as noted above, used DCE to prioritise across programmes. It was used to weight and combine five criteria scores (cost-effectiveness, proportion of the population eligible for the intervention, distribution of benefits across the population, affordability and certainty) to produce a ranking of each intervention. This approach can be used to collate the views of large numbers of people independently but does not necessarily facilitate deliberations or consensus building in smaller groups.

Another aspect of consideration for priority setting is the availability of evidence. As seen in Fig. 10.1, data on the alternatives' performance on each of the criteria can be gathered in a variety of ways, ranging from evidence synthesis to expert opinions. These include:

- Evidence synthesis, for example, building economic models and data analysis. This approach is explicit and transparent and may reveal counterintuitive relationships between criteria but needs time, resources and specialist skills which might not be available in-house.
- Internal data collection, such as current patterns of expenditure. Wherever available, these should be accessible, reliable and understandable by relevant stakeholders. However, there might not be enough information in the organisation regarding the performance of options against the criteria.
- Published evidence, including literature reviews. This is quick to use; however, there might not be enough information in the literature with regard to the performance of all options against the criteria.
- Subjective judgement, such as expert input. This is useful in public health settings where there is insufficient evidence. However, the criticism of using subjective opinion rather than objective information remains.

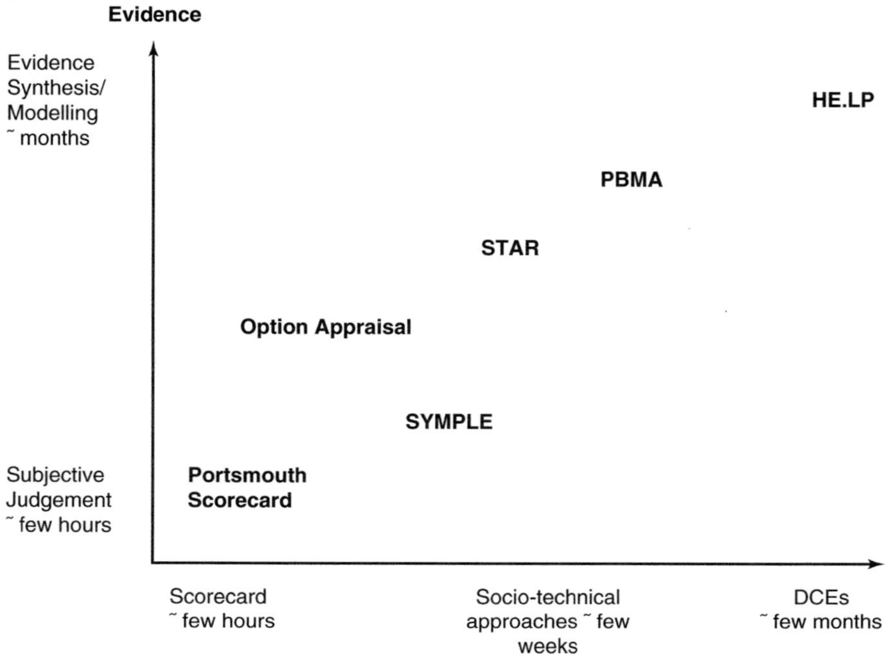

Fig. 10.1 Field showing range of possible MCDA-based approaches, described by evidence requirements and resource/time use

Other factors also play a role in which approach to choose. MCDA approaches have different advantages and disadvantages depending on who will be included as part of the decision-making process. DCE facilitates large numbers of people to be involved independently of each other and for general conclusions to be drawn on this basis. Star, on the other hand, uses a decision conferencing approach which necessitates that only a small number of decision-makers are involved, to allow them to converge on a single answer. Depending on the exact approach used, option appraisal and PBMA tend to follow a similar Delphi-style technique to elicit viewpoints and arrive at final decisions. Baltussen et al. (2010) also argue that PBMA is useful for choosing between a small set of alternatives in a specific context, but those studies that aim to inform prioritisation discussions on a larger scale are better suited to more formal MCDA techniques—though they also find that defining whether a study uses a PBMA approach or not is itself sometimes unclear. But the exact nature of the decision problem needs to be matched with an appropriate MCDA technique, given the necessary involvement of decision-makers given the specific context, making drawing definitive conclusions difficult.

Whilst all the methods seen in earlier sections are all based on MCDA principles, they vary significantly in terms of scientific rigour, robustness and time and other resources required. The choice of MCDA method for our study was based on the resource/time constraints, the scientific validity and the significance and broader context of the decision problem. In choosing the appropriate level for any given problem, researchers should consider such factors carefully. The case study reports on why we chose the techniques we did, the role of the stakeholders in doing so at each stage and a practical example of how one can go about designing such a technique given a particular decision context.

10.4 Case Study: Using MCDA to Inform Local Government Investment in Public Health

In this section, a case study is presented to describe the prioritisation process for a range of interventions to reduce smoking prevalence in South Yorkshire. We have called this the South Yorkshire Multi-criteria Decision Analysis Prioritisation for Local Effectiveness (SYMPLE).

Each of four boroughs in the South Yorkshire areas had a Tobacco Control Commissioners (TCC). These TCCs had been liaising for some years and hoped to identify an appropriate 'knowledge-based approach' that might inform future policy about how to reduce smoking prevalence in a rational and transparent way (Reddy et al.). Therefore, the SYMPLE approach was designed to bring together a range of opinions which should be used to present a range of policy options to each borough's Director of Public Health (DPH).

Seven steps are listed in Table 10.3 based on the ISPOR task force—Emerging good practices guidelines (Thokala et al. 2016). The original guidelines used eight steps, but in our study, measuring and scoring had to be carried out at the same time and so were merged in the table. The sequence of stages allowed the views of the general public, expert opinion and other stakeholders to be incorporated at various stages. The findings were ultimately used as a basis for prioritisation between the options under consideration. The entire process is perhaps best seen as a framework for investigating and discussing the objectives and issues rather than a rigid formula.

10.4.1 *Defining the Decision Problem*

The decision problem and corresponding decision goal should be understood and defined as a point of departure for any MCDA; this, of course, includes the identification of appropriate stakeholders, alternatives to be considered and output required (Thokala et al. 2016).

In this case study in order to demonstrate the legitimacy of the prioritisation process, an expert steering group comprising of about 30 stakeholders from a broad range of relevant settings in tobacco consumption reduction were identified by the TCCs (such as stop smoking providers, midwifery, elected councillors, the fire service and a local chamber of commerce).

Table 10.3 Involvement by relevant groups in each of the tobacco prevalence project's stages and phases using ISPOR task force value measurement guidelines

Steps from ISPOR task force	Project phases and stages	General public	Stakeholder expert group	Tobacco Control Commissioners	Lead researcher	Local decision makers
Defining the decision problem	Establish the decision context; identify relevant stakeholder expert steering group; identify intervention alternatives			✓	✓	
Selecting and structuring criteria	Identify relevant criteria to the decision problem	✓	✓	✓	✓	
Weighting criteria	'Weighting', reflecting relative importance of each criterion to the decision	✓	✓	✓		
Measuring performance and scoring alternatives	Estimate performance of the interventions on the criteria by gathering evidence or expert opinion		✓			
Calculating aggregate scores	Estimate the overall score of each intervention, which can be used for prioritisation	✓	✓	✓		
Dealing with uncertainty	Examine the results, sensitivity analyses			✓	✓	
Reporting and examination of findings	Implementing findings			✓		✓

Fifteen interventions were examined and chosen to represent a broad range of potential techniques. There are potentially a limitless number of interventions available given various levels of investment, but MCDA techniques could not investigate every such intervention in practice. Given the subsequent findings would still ultimately be subject to political factors; the list was intended to be broad and representative rather than comprehensive. Through deliberation with the TCCs, a final list that met these requirements was developed, and three to four page business cases for each intervention were prepared, giving a broad outline of how the intervention would likely be implemented in practice and written in language accessible to all stakeholders.

10.4.2 Selecting and Structuring Criteria

After a decision problem is identified, criteria for evaluating the alternatives should be agreed; there are a number of methods for determining the criteria, for example, using facilitated workshops and focus groups. Certain requirements need to be met if an additive model is used (Marsh et al. 2016). Having identified the criteria, they should then be structured using an appropriate method, for example, a value tree (Marsh et al. 2016), which can be used to highlight the uncertainties inherent in the decision and the possible outcomes in each scenario.

For all prioritisation setting methods, identifying relevant criteria for comparison of interventions 'requires considering the underlying reasons for the organisation's existence, and the core values that the organisation serves' (Dodgson et al. 2009) and is potentially the most important part of the process. All the prioritisation setting methods presented in Sect. 10.2 use stakeholders to identify the criteria.

For this case study, the first attempts to identify suitable criteria were carried out through public consultation. Workshops were set up to engage with volunteers from the public to discuss a series of potential interventions and describe why they would prefer investment in one rather than another. These criteria were ranked according to participants' views. They were sent out to the expert group for comment and ranking and were subsequently revised. These steps were nonbinding but were used to inform the subsequent debate on which criteria and weightings to use.

In order to attain a final workable set of criteria, a number of iterations were necessary. So as not to bias the results, a number of criteria which may have been highly related were removed or revised (to avoid double counting). This was achieved by consensus between the TCCs (who attempted to ensure that the findings from the expert group were taken into appropriate account), and six headline criteria were identified (Table 10.4). The first stages of these iterations were realised through correspondence so as to have some points (broad criteria) to discuss during the decision conference. The lack of clear, quantitative data made the identification of suitable proxy variables difficult. The results of the MCDA model were to be indicative to the DPH, rather than conclusive. The DPH could subsequently incorporate other aspects such as synergies between programmes and political considerations. The themes presented in Table 10.4 instead ensured that a roadmap could be followed to ensure that all major, relevant issues would be addressed in the discussion at the decision conference through expert judgement, though in an ideal world, it would have been better to define them more clearly.

10.4.3 Weighting Criteria

Weighting allows for trade-off between an alternative's performance on criteria and is used to group the scores of individual criteria into a total value measure. It is normally done by eliciting stakeholders' preferences, and as the scores given for each criterion all have a representative value and are not commensurate, weights must be given (Dodgson et al. 2009).

Choices concerning the preferences that are relevant to a decision problem are normative; the outcomes of which may be sensitive to the scoring and weighting used. However, it is unclear if any human prioritisation decisions can be characterised as value-free, and a key advantage of MCDA techniques is in making explicit these weights, allowing for the management of and analyses of these subjective aspects (Belton and Stewart 2002). Such analyses are impossible with deliberative processes that instead use implicit weights.

Table 10.4 presents the preference weights for criteria; these criteria were elicited using swing weighting and synthesised the viewpoints of the expert panel, the TCCs and the level of difference between the best and worst performing intervention on each criterion. The importance of each criterion was determined by gathering correspondence before the meeting of the expert group because of expected time constraints on the day. Stakeholders expressed a view that equity aspects were considered from the outset than after cost-effectiveness analysis. There was also a preference stated by many stakeholders for interventions with higher impacts to individuals rather than lower impacts to larger groups. On the other hand, the TCCs were more concerned about the prevalence rates given in the national priorities. After some deliberation with the TCCs, the prevalence rates were converted into swing weights from the best to worst performing intervention in each criterion.

10.4.4 Measuring Performance

Upon agreeing the criteria, a performance matrix, for example, can be used to report or measure the performance of each alternative as applied to each criterion. There are a range of data gathering tools from standard evidence synthesis techniques to elicitation of expert opinion (Thokala et al. 2016).

Due to lack of evidence, for this case study, expert opinion was elicited based on the performance of different interventions which converted as scores (see section below; 10.4.5 Scoring alternatives). In practice, this meant scoring (shown

Table 10.4 Inputs to the MCDA process developed prior to the decision conference—the criteria and their weightings

Criterion definition	Considerations	Weight
How well does it meet our priorities on the national indicators to		50 %
	Reduce smoking amongst adults	*(20 %)*
	Reduce smoking amongst young people	*(15 %)*
	Reduce smoking amongst pregnant women	*(15 %)*
How much will this improve a person's health or quality of life?	*Will it improve their heath or help them to live longer?* *Are there other aspects of a person's life that will improve money, better environment, lower crime, etc.?*	15 %
Will it help the difference in health or length of life between our communities?	*Can the people who need this intervention get to it?* *Will it reach our high-risk groups and communities?* *Will people use the service or intervention?*	15 %
Value for money	*Does it work?* *How many people will benefit—both directly and indirectly?* *Can we afford to do it?*	10 %
Ease of implementation	*Will it contribute to and enhance services/pathways?* *Can we get the right staff, buildings, equipment, etc.?*	5 %
Sustainability	*Is it sustainable?* *Are there any risks associated with this intervention?*	5 %

below) and measuring were carried out at the same time, as there was no intermediate step of carrying out a literature search or specifying the key metrics for each criterion.

10.4.5 Scoring Alternatives

Stakeholders' preferences within criteria are collected after an analysis of each alternative performance. Performance measurements are then converted into scores based on predefined rules or functions—scores are used to transform performance measures into a common scale or to incorporate priorities within the criteria.

Therefore, the next part of the process necessitated scores be given to each intervention on each criterion. For this particular case study, there was not enough data on the interventions, and, hence, to elicit the scores, subjective opinion from key experts was sought during a decision conference setting. An impartial facilitator worked iteratively with stakeholders to generate an explicit model in order to help those present to think clearly about the more important issues (Phillips and Bana e Costa 2007). A broad range of potential stakeholders were included in the process—the same group who had weighted criteria by correspondence. This allowed for a fuller spectrum of views to be included and potentially increased the legitimacy of the findings, as practically all relevant parties were represented in the process.

So as to guarantee that all participants had the opportunity to express a view at each stage, they were initially divided into four groups. Participants were asked to consider how an intervention might perform on each criterion using a score from 0 to 10, where 0 indicates having the least imaginable impact for that criterion and 10 indicated the biggest imaginable impact. Batches of four interventions at a time were presented and debated between groups to ensure an overall consensus score for each intervention on each criterion. Due to time pressure towards the end of the day, two larger groups were formed to score the final interventions in parallel.

10.4.6 Calculating Aggregate Scores

When calculating aggregate scores in the Portsmouth approach, VFM analysis is used, Star uses the same analytical approach but with extensive stakeholder engagement through decision conferencing, PBMA evaluates the possible outcomes against their opportunity costs using a deliberative process and HELP utilises DCE-calculated value.

For this case study, an additive model was used, in this instance a weighted sum approach. Scores elicited from participants on each intervention were combined with the weight on each criterion to calculate total scores for each intervention under consideration. This was performed as shown below:

$$v_j = \sum_{0}^{i} s_{ij} . w_i$$

where

v_j is the overall value for intervention j estimated from MCDA model
S_{ij} is the score for intervention j on criterion i
w_i is the weight attached to criterion i

Interventions were subsequently ranked based on the total scores as shown in Table 10.5.

10.4.7 Dealing with Uncertainty

Uncertainty can have a major impact on an assessment, influencing both the design and nature of the evidence and when evaluating the robustness of the decision outcomes. Uncertainty in MCDA has not been explored extensively. In an MCDA, the selected criteria, performance against those criteria and stakeholders' perspectives are subject to uncertainty. Probabilistic sensitivity analysis techniques can be used to combat parameter uncertainty, whilst scenario analyses can address structural uncertainty.

Table 10.5 Consensus scores generated for each anti-tobacco intervention on each criterion and total scores for each

Intervention	Reduce smoking amongst adults	Reduce smoking amongst young people	Reduce smoking amongst pregnant women	How much will this improve a person's health or quality of life?	Will it help the difference in health between our communities?	Value for money	Ease of implementation	Sustainability	Total score
Weighting	*20*	*15*	*15*	*15*	*15*	*10*	*5*	*5*	*100*
Enforcement	7	8	7	7	6	7	8	8	**71**
Maternity SSS	3	5	8	8	7	9	9	9	**66**
Communications and markcting	8	6	7	5	5	8	7	4	**64**
Training for brief interventions	7	5	5	5	7	7	4	7	**59.5**
Social norms to influence behaviour change	6	8	5	6	6	5	4	5	**59**
Young people education programme	5	6	4	7	6	5	5	6	**55**
R&M SSS	5	4	4	6	6	6	8	8	**54**
Long-term conditions SSS	5	3	3	7	6	7	8	7	**53**
Parents SSS	4	6	6	6	4	5	5	6	**51.5**
BME SSS—high VfM	4	3	2	4	6	**8**	6	5	**44**
Smoke-free spaces—only open spaces	3	4	4	3	3	7	**7**	7	**41**

(continued)

Table 10.5 (continued)

Intervention	Reduce smoking amongst adults	Reduce smoking amongst young people	Reduce smoking amongst pregnant women	How much will this improve a person's health or quality of life?	Will it help the difference in health between our communities?	Value for money	Ease of implementation	Sustainability	Total score
BME SSS—low VfM	3	4	4	3	3	**3**	7	7	**37**
Smoke-free spaces—private spaces	3	4	4	3	3	3	**2**	7	**34.5**
Mental health SSS—high VfM	2	2	2	5	4	**6**	5	5	**34.5**
Preoperative SSS	2	1	1	7	3	8	4	5	**34.5**
Mental health SSS—low VfM	2	1	1	7	3	**2**	4	5	**28.5**
Hospital SSS	3	1	1	5	3	5	2	4	**29**
Replication of A Stop Smoking in School Trial (ASSIST) programme	2	4	1	2	2	2	1	1	**20.5**

It is important to note that MCDA can only be considered as a decision support tool, and therefore there is no correct answer. Subsequently, sensitivity analyses were performed to investigate the robustness of the findings including on the fluctuations in weighting scores for each criterion. This required investigating by how much the weighting on each criterion would have to change in order to alter the final ordering of interventions. These are difficult to illustrate here for 15 alternatives on 8 criteria. However, it was found that the magnitude of change required implied the results were stable. After the sensitivity analyses, it was found that interventions with equal scores performed relatively poorly and were unlikely to be funded. Moreover, the interventions that performed particularly well (and were likely to be funded) continued to perform well throughout the analyses. The smallest change required to alter rankings, for example, related to the weighting on reducing prevalence amongst adults—if this was reduced from 20 % of weighting to 18.75 %, maternity SSS would instead receive the highest score overall. But given these were the highest two performing interventions, they were likely to be funded regardless.

The findings show that MCDA techniques are typically robust (Von Winterfeldt and Edwards 1986) as there was little overall impact when the attributed scores were changed, but this stage is vital in such circumstances where there is the risk of confusion or disagreement.

10.4.8 Reporting and Examination of Findings

The results of an MCDA can be shown in either tabular or graphic forms. Aggregate value scores can help rank the alternatives in order of importance or give a measure of value to each alternative. It is important to recognise that MCDA is a tool to help decision-makers come to a satisfactory decision rather than making a definitive or conclusive decision, allowing them to explore a range of results in differing scenarios.

In this case study, ranking was used to allocate the different budgets for smoking cessation interventions. The South Yorkshire area acted on the results of the study and has redistributed their spending in accordance with the recommendations. For instance, prevention and education activity with young people has been prioritised, and they have also increased spending on smoke-free spaces.

10.4.9 Reflections

The SYMPLE approach used subjective scores and weighted criteria based upon value judgements—as such it cannot offer an objective, 'correct' ranking of results. Nonetheless, the results still make clear which interventions may be considered useful (or otherwise) in future, and they were found to be robust to changes in weights. The approach used an open, deliberative process bringing together experts and stakeholders to rank interventions and make explicit any assumptions made.

Final investment decisions are made in a political context— this must be borne in mind—and the findings appear to have ultimately provided suitable leverage to empower decision-makers to make more sweeping and relevant changes than might otherwise have been possible, as well as giving clarity in renegotiating the services offered by providers.

There are well-established tensions possible between evidence and policy (Dowie 1996), and this is likely to equally be the case at local government level. However, as previously explained, such concerns are likely to reflect real value judgements and may in fact be useful in situations such as this. The results were intended to point decision-makers in the right direction, and it is appropriate that final decisions can be adjusted to address shortcomings in the model's assumptions and to ensure they conform to common sense and public preferences.

The steps taken through were paired directly with the nature of the problem and the constraints of the real-life problem, such as the need to incorporate large numbers of stakeholders, but the impossibility of getting everyone together over a number of days. This context dependency makes it difficult to draw conclusions about how successful it would have been had a different MCDA approach been used. This project was nonetheless successful in terms of establishing whether an MCDA framework would be suitable for enabling prioritisation in such circumstances. This is not to say that the exact approach used here should be adopted for all local government decisions lacking definitive evidence. At practically all stages, compromises were required to incorporate the views of as many stakeholders as possible; the public and the TCCs to ensure the prioritisation progress could be progressed from its starting point. A key issue that this chapter highlights is that in the real world, such compromises are often necessary, and researchers undertaking similar issues in future must use their own judgement to match such issues with the local context of the decision (Craig et al. 2008). The results indicate that there may be further challenges ahead given the increased local discretion now encouraged. Given that public health is no longer the responsibility of the NHS, it is unclear whether public health guidance will carry the same weight as previously. Local decision-makers (and previously the public workshop participants) did not believe ASSIST, for example, would be suitable in a South Yorkshire context as it was felt it might lead to issues around bullying. This is despite the fact that it is recommended as cost-effective by NICE. Public health interventions can prove highly cost-effective (Owen et al. 2012), but this is only demonstrable where there is a way to measure their effectiveness. There is a lack of clear evidence for most other interventions under consideration in this study, and hence they could not be recommended in the same way.

Variation in effectiveness is also possible across the country for interventions depending on a number of local factors such as demography, providers, the manner in which it is implemented and so on, and such issues can be more prominent in public health decisions. This project was driven by the counterintuitive realisation that such an evidence-driven approach in public health had led to perverse and suboptimal outcomes in smoking prevalence in South Yorkshire. In future, consideration needs to be given about how best to manage such variation across the country given the increased powers available to local authorities over their public health budgets. One potential approach is to work with local government using formal approaches such as the one outlined in this paper in future to aid decision-making and increase comparability between council decisions. The approach outlined in this paper has the added advantages of increased transparency and meaningful engagement with stakeholders.

The opportunity to collaborate directly with the TCCs may have increased the likelihood of implementation and generated further insights (Innvær et al. 2002; Lavis et al. 2003). The TCCs knew the realities of the prior decision-making system and could ensure that technical issues are dealt with appropriately as are institutional factors (Williams and Bryan 2007). These institutional and structural factors tend to be particularly pronounced at local level (Duthie et al. 1999). Local governments must also take responsibility for their own decisions at the coal face with their own electorate (more directly than more technocratic bodies such as NICE), which may face further possible constraints on their possible actions. Policy development may not necessarily be wholly evidence based in practice (Lindblom 1959). Understanding how to navigate such issues is vital.

A recent systematic review of the use of economics in health-care decision-making, for example, found its use to be 'small and patchy' (Niessen et al. 2012). As has been noted, acceptance of economic perspectives in public health has been slow, and this has been in part influenced by the complex and multifactorial nature of public health problems, and the prevalence of a range of national, local political and contextual influences which impact on decision-making. In supporting the use and development of MCDA tools in the prioritisation of public health interventions, the study carried out by NICE (Morgan et al. 2011) showed the importance of developing methods perceived as useful by commissioners in ways that were transparent and easy to grasp. Most tools can, however, involve stakeholders and the public in the selection and valuing of criteria. Partnership working and well-developed stakeholder relationships are key to the successful use of prioritisation techniques.

10.5 Limitations of This Study

This chapter does not attempt to take a systematic approach to identifying the list of areas where MCDA approaches have been used in local government settings. Instead, it seeks only to demonstrate the kinds of areas in which they have been used in the past and, through the case study, to highlight the kinds of approaches (and compromises) needed to ensure that models (even imperfect ones) are fit for purpose. Because the approach was not systematic, however, it is possible that some inadvertent bias may exist in reporting the results.

The case study describes a specific project which took place in England. Case studies are valuable where broad, complex questions have to be addressed in complex circumstances (Keen and Packwood 1995). By incorporating the context of the decision, practical concerns are highlighted (Eckstein 2000) and provide rich, contextual information (Flyvbjerg 2006). Such contextual factors can make it difficult to draw clear, generalisable conclusions. However, many of the lessons may be applicable in any such policymaking setting, which compromises are inevitable (Lomas et al. 2005).

Within the case study itself, there were a number of stages to the process, each of which helped inform decision-makers. But the approach is not without limitations, and it would be inappropriate to use the findings of the MCDA stages in isolation and without further reflection. The supplementary steps examining the results better inform decision-makers on the outcomes of the decisions in the real world and help to reduce the risk of bias, increasing the chances of achieving successful policy outcomes. The political context and oversight likely helped to ensure results aligned with perceived 'common sense'.

The length of time available at the decision conference was an issue, most obviously in the fact that scores for the final interventions were decided by two parallel subgroups rather than by all participants simultaneously. However, it is worth emphasising that this was only part of one stage of the overall project. Scores generated at the meeting were not intended to be the final piece in the jigsaw puzzle but the next step on a ladder towards the decision. They serve to highlight potentially new avenues for decision-makers, but no ranking could be said to be the final word, as the model is by necessity limited, and subsequent decisions could not be made in a political vacuum.

Issues such as synergies between interventions and how to manage the timings of disinvestment for previous interventions were also not considered in the model. The approach was meant to offer a tool by which to examine and understand, rather than the final, ideal ranking of interventions. These ultimately require the judgement of DPHs, particularly in the new, more openly political setting. The approaches outlined in this study could only inform these decisions, and the criteria used are not necessarily exhaustive.

10.6 Conclusions

The ability of MCDA techniques to incorporate data and both qualitative and quantitative judgements in a formal manner means that they are well suited to support public health decision-making, where evidence is often only partially available and many policies are value driven. A number of MCDA methods exist for local resource allocation, ranging from quick and simple methods (e.g. Portsmouth scorecard) to more sophisticated methods such as PBMA/DCEs. The local decision-makers need to choose the appropriate method based on their resource/ time constraints, scientific validity and the significance and broader context of the decision problem.

References

Aberdeen City CHP (2010) Final option appraisal for health service redesign for children with complex needs

Airoldi M (2013) Disinvestments in practice: overcoming resistance to change through a sociotechnical approach with local stakeholders. J Health Polit Policy Law 38(6):1149–1171

Airoldi M et al (2011) Healthcare prioritisation at the local level: a socio-technical approach. Priority-setting for Population Health Working Paper Series, Working Paper (7)

Airoldi M et al (2014) STAR—people-powered prioritization a 21st-century solution to allocation headaches. Med Decis Making 34(8):965–975

Ashton, Leigh and Wigan PCT (2005) Options appraisal for the management, organisation and delivery of mental health services

Austin D, Edmundson-Jones P, Sidhu K (2007) Priority setting and the Portsmouth scorecard: prioritising public health services: threats and opportunities. 7/10/09. Available from: http://www.publichealthconferences.org.uk/health_services_2007/presentations.php

Baltussen R et al (2010) Multi-criteria decision analysis to prioritize health interventions: capitalizing on first experiences. Health Policy 96(3):262–264

Belton V, Stewart T (2002) Multiple criteria decision analysis: an integrated approach. Kluwer, Boston

Bohmer P et al (2001) Maximising health gain within available resources in the New Zealand public health system. Health Policy 55(1):37–50

Bridges J (2003) Stated preference methods in health care evaluation: an emerging methodological paradigm in health economics. Appl Health Econ Health Policy 2(4):213–224

Craig P et al (2008) Developing and evaluating complex interventions: the new Medical Research Council guidance. BMJ 337:a1655

Dodgson J et al (2009) Multi-criteria analysis: a manual. Department for Communities and Local Government, London

Donaldson C, Mitton C (2009) Priority setting toolkit: guide to the use of economics in healthcare decision making. John Wiley & Sons, New York

Donaldson C et al (2010) Rational disinvestment. QJM 103(10):801–807

Dowie J (1996) 'Evidence-based', 'cost-Effective' and 'preference-Driven' Medicine: decision analysis based medical decision making is the pre-requisite. J Health Serv Res 1(2):104–113

Duthie T et al (1999) Research into the use of health economics in decision making in the United Kingdom—Phase II: Is health economics 'for good or evil'? Health Policy 46(2):143–157

Eckstein H (2000) Case study and theory in political science. London. Case study method, Sage Publications:119–164

Flyvbjerg B (2006) Five misunderstandings about case-study research. Qual Inq 12(2):219–245

Health England (2009) Matrix Insight, Prioritising investments in preventative health

Health Foundation (2012) Looking for value in hard times. Health Foundation, London

HM Treasury (2003) The green book: appraisal and evaluation in central government: treasury guidance. Stationery Office, London

Innvær S et al (2002) Health policy-makers' perceptions of their use of evidence: a systematic review. J Health Serv Res Policy 7(4):239–244

Keen J, Packwood T (1995) Case study evaluation. BMJ Br Med J 311(7002):444

Keeney RL, Raiffa H (1993) Decisions with multiple objectives: preferences and value trade-offs. New York: Wiley, 1976

Lavis JN et al (2003) How can research organizations more effectively transfer research knowledge to decision makers? Milbank Q 81(2):221–248

Lindblom CE (1959) The science of "muddling through". Public administration review. 19(2): 79–88. DOI 10.2307/973677

Lomas J et al (2005) Final report-conceptualizing and combining evidence for health system guidance. Canadian Health Services Research Foundation, Ottawa

Marsh K et al (2014) Assessing the value of healthcare interventions using multi-criteria decision analysis: a review of the literature. Pharmacoeconomics 32(4):345–365

Marsh K, IJzerman M, Thokala P, Baltussen R, Boysen M, Kalo Z, Lönngren T, Mussen F, Peacock S, Watkins J, Devlin N (2016) MCDA for Health Care Decisions – Emerging Good Practices: Report 2 of the ISPOR MCDA Task Force. Value Health 19:125–137

Morgan A, Ellis S, Field J, Owen L, Jones D, Minchin M, McArthur C, Doohan E, Hodgson G, Pickard L (2011) NICE* Supporting investment in public health: review of methods for assessing cost effectiveness, cost impact and return on investment. NICE, London

Niessen LW et al (2012) Assessing the impact of economic evidence on policymakers in health care—a systematic review

Owen L et al (2012) The cost-effectiveness of public health interventions. J Public Health 34(1):37–45

Peacock S et al (2009) Overcoming barriers to priority setting using interdisciplinary methods. Health Policy 92(2):124–132

Perry A et al (2000) Measuring the costs and benefits of heart disease monitoring. Heart 83(6):651–656

Phillips LD, Bana e Costa CA (2007) Transparent prioritisation, budgeting and resource allocation with multi-criteria decision analysis and decision conferencing. Ann Oper Res 154(1):51–68

Reddy B et al (2016) Using MCDA to generate and interpret evidence to inform local government investment in public health. EURO Journal on Decision Processes. 27:1–21

Reed Johnson F et al (2013) Constructing experimental designs for discrete-choice experiments: report of the ISPOR conjoint analysis experimental design good research practices task force. Value Health 16(1):3–13

Robinson S (2011) Setting priorities in health: a study of English primary care trusts. Nuffield Trust, London, Lulu.com

Robinson S, Dickinson H, Williams I (2009) Evaluation of the prioritisation process at South Staffordshire PCT. Health Services Management Centre, Birmingham

Robinson S et al (2011) Disinvestment in health—the challenges facing general practitioner (GP) commissioners. Public Money Manag 31(2):145–148

Ruta D et al (2005) Programme budgeting and marginal analysis: bridging the divide between doctors and managers. BMJ Br Med J 330(7506):1501

Thokala P et al (2016) Multiple criteria decision analysis for health care decision making—an introduction: report 1 of the ISPOR MCDA Emerging Good Practices Task Force. Value Health 19(1):1–13

UK Government (2011) Option appraisal: making informed decisions in government. National Audit Office, Editor

Von Winterfeldt D, Edwards W (1986) Decision analysis and behavioral research, vol 604. Cambridge University Press, Cambridge

Williams I, Bryan S (2007) Understanding the limited impact of economic evaluation in health care resource allocation: a conceptual framework. Health Policy 80(1):135–143

Williams I, Robinson S, Dickinson H (2011) Rationing in health care: the theory and practice of priority setting. Bristol: Policy Press

Chapter 11
Shared Decision-Making

James G. Dolan and Liana Fraenkel

Abstract Shared decision-making is a collaborative process whereby patients and their providers make healthcare decisions together, taking into account both the best scientific evidence available and the patient's values and preferences. Effective implementation of shared decision-making therefore requires ready access to current evidence comparing expected outcomes of decision alternatives, assessment of decision-related values and preferences, and integration of this information to identify the most suitable course of action. Multi-criteria decision analysis (MCDA) is designed to help people make better choices when faced with complex decisions that involve trade-offs between competing objectives. MCDA methods fulfill all of the required elements of shared decision-making. This similarity suggests that MCDA methods could be used effectively to facilitate shared decision-making in practice.

The evidence currently available supports this hypothesis. This chapter will illustrate how two MCDA methods – the conjoint analysis and analytic hierarchy process (AHP) – have been used to foster shared decision-making in clinical settings.

Conjoint analysis refers to methods that derive an individual's decision-related preferences by examining how they make a series of hypothetical decisions that involve alternatives that differ in how well they achieve a set of decision objectives. We illustrate the use of conjoint analysis to foster shared decision-making by discussing how it has successfully been used to facilitate osteoarthritis treatment choices in real time and improve physician understanding of patient preferences for treatment of lupus nephritis.

The analytic hierarchy process (AHP) is an example of a value-based multi-criteria method. Value-based methods provide a framework for structuring a decision, comparing alternatives relative to specific criteria, defining the relative priorities of criteria in achieving the decision goal, and synthesizing this information to create scores that summarize how well the alternatives are judged to meet the

J.G. Dolan, MD (✉)
Department of Public Health Sciences, University of Rochester,
Rochester, NY, USA
e-mail: james_dolan@urmc.rochester.edu

L. Fraenkel, MD, MPH (✉)
Department of Medicine, Yale School of Medicine, New Haven, CT, USA
e-mail: Liana.Fraenkel@yale.edu

© Springer International Publishing AG 2017

K. Marsh et al. (eds.), *Multi-Criteria Decision Analysis to Support Healthcare Decisions*, DOI 10.1007/978-3-319-47540-0_11

decision goal. They also allow for sensitivity analyses that allow users to explore the effects of different judgments and perspectives on the relative evaluations of the alternatives. We will illustrate the use of the AHP to foster shared decision-making in practice by describing how it has been used to facilitate decisions regarding colorectal cancer screening.

We conclude with a list of suggestions regarding further research to continue this line of investigation with an emphasis on research needed to effectively implement these methods in routine practice settings.

11.1 Introduction

11.1.1 Medical Decisions Are Frequently Complex and Involve Trade-Offs Among Alternatives

The proliferation of medical treatments and diagnostic modalities has resulted in multiple alternatives for managing numerous healthcare problems. In many cases none of the options is clearly superior to the others. In these situations, management decisions depend on preference-driven trade-offs between the pros and cons of the alternatives available. This growing number of preference-driven healthcare decisions has highlighted the importance of patient-centered care that incorporates patient preferences and perspectives into clinical decisions. This approach is based on the principle that these decisions should reflect individual patient preferences and values since the patients are the ones who will experience the decision outcomes (Wennberg et al. 2002; Veroff et al. 2013; O'Connor et al. 2007; Brownlee et al. 2011).

11.1.2 What Is a Good Decision?

In this context, a good decision is one that reflects current clinical evidence, incorporates patient values and preferences, involves patients to the extent that they wish, and is acceptable to patients and their healthcare providers (Politi and Street 2011). Making high-quality clinical decisions that meet these criteria requires shared decision-making, which can be defined as: "an interpersonal, interdependent process in which the health care provider and the patient relate to and influence each other as they collaborate in making decisions about the patient's health care" (Légaré 2013).

The most common approach to promoting shared decision-making in practice has been through the use of patient decision aids designed to inform patients about the decision they face and help them assess their treatment goals and preferences. Compared to usual care, patient decision aids have been shown to clarify patient values, lower decisional conflict, improve patient-practitioner communication, and increase patients' knowledge, accuracy of risk perceptions, and involvement in decision-making (Stacey et al. 2014). However, it has been difficult to implement shared decision-making in practice settings, and there is considerable evidence that many clinical decisions that should be made using a shared decision-making framework are not being made this way (Joseph-Williams et al. 2014; Mulley et al. 2012). Therefore, discovering and implementing clinically feasible and effective ways to routinely implement patient-centered, shared decision-making into clinical practice is needed to promote high-quality care.

11.1.3 Relationship Between Shared Decision-Making and MCDA

Shared decision-making is a challenging task. It requires a clear definition of the decision at hand, descriptions of the options available, succinct summaries of pertinent clinical evidence, assessment of the decision-maker(s) preferences and priorities, and successful integration of this information to identify a sound choice.

Situations like these are not unique to healthcare; they occur frequently in many areas of human endeavor. The techniques of multi-criteria decision analysis (MCDA) were developed to help people make judicious choices when faced with complex decisions like these. The similarity between MCDA and the required elements of shared decision-making suggests that it could serve as the foundation for new methods to implement shared decision-making in practice. The goal of this chapter is to illustrate how two types of MCDA have been used to facilitate shared decision-making in practice and suggest areas for future research.

The chapter is organized as follows. First, to illustrate how MCDA can support patient-centered decision-making by providing information that can be integrated into a wide range of decision-making methods, we will review studies that have used conjoint analysis to derive patient priorities regarding treatment of lupus nephritis and osteoarthritis. Then, to illustrate how MCDA could be used to directly support shared clinical decisions, we will review studies that have used the analytic hierarchy process (AHP) to study patient decision-making regarding colorectal cancer screening. Finally, we will discuss the current state of the art regarding the use of these and other MCDA methods to support clinical decisions and describe directions for future research.

11.2 Conjoint Analysis

Conjoint analysis has long been recognized as a robust method for quantifying preferences for competing options (Bridges 2003; Fraenkel et al. 2001; Ryan and Farrar 2000). In this section, we describe examples of how this method can be used to elicit and explain patient preferences and serve as a tool to support shared decision-making.

When faced with complex decisions, consumers typically evaluate a number of attributes and then make trade-offs among them to arrive at a final choice. Conjoint analysis evaluates these trade-offs to determine which combination of attributes would be most preferred by consumers. Data derived from conjoint analysis studies can also be used to measure the relative importance that respondents assign to specific product characteristics. This feature allows one to observe the influence of specific treatment characteristics on individual patient's treatment choice.

Three major assumptions underlie the ability of conjoint analysis to quantify values.

The first assumption is that each product is a composite of different attributes and that each attribute is specified by a number of levels. For example, in choosing between alternative drug treatments, attributes refer to specific medication characteristics such as route of administration, probability and magnitude of benefit, and risk of toxicity. Levels refer to the range of estimates for each characteristic.

The second assumption underlying conjoint analysis is that respondents have unique values, or utilities, for each attribute level. In this context "utility" is a number that represents the value a respondent associates with a particular characteristic, with higher utilities indicating increased value. The least preferred level of each attribute is arbitrarily given a utility of zero, because conjoint analysis measures utilities on an interval scale. Differences in utilities between alternative levels of an attribute indicate the relative importances that patients assign to changes in specific treatment characteristics. For example, in the limited sample of possible attributes described below, the respondent values decreasing the risk of depression from 40 to 10 % (60 utility units) more than improving the chance of treatment success from 50 to 80 % (40 utility units).

Attribute	Levels	Utility
Chance of treatment success	40 %	0
	50 %	50
	80 %	90
Duration of treatment	12 months	0
	6 months	30
Risk of depression	40 %	0
	25 %	40
	10 %	60

The final assumption underlying conjoint analysis is that utilities can be combined across attributes. That is, if the sum of a patient's utilities for the attributes of Medication A is greater than the sum of utilities for the attributes of Medication B, the patient should prefer Medication A to B. For example, using the utility values shown above, if the researcher defines Medication A as a medication taken over 12 months, with an 80 % chance of success and 25 % risk of depression (total utility = 130), and Medication B as a medication taken over 6 months, with a 40 % chance of success and 10 % risk of depression (total utility = 90), the patient should prefer Medication A over Medication B.

In conjoint analysis, choice simulations are used to convert the raw utilities into preferences for specific options defined by the researcher. Several models are available. One of the most commonly used is the randomized first choice model in which utilities are summed across the levels corresponding to each option and then exponentiated and rescaled so that they sum to 100. This model is based on the assumption that subjects prefer the option with the highest utility. The randomized first choice model accounts for the error in the point estimates of the utilities as well as the variation in each respondent's total utility for each option. This approach has been shown to have better predictive ability than other models (Huber et al. 2007). Simulations also allow the researcher to examine how changing specific medication characteristics (such as lowering the co-pay or changing the route of administration) influences patient preferences.

There are several ways to collect data for conjoint analyses. Adaptive conjoint analysis (ACA) (Sawtooth Software, Inc., Orem, UT (Huber et al. 2007)) collects and analyzes preference data using an interactive computer program. This method is unique in that it uses individual respondent's answers to update and refine the questionnaire through a series of graded-paired comparisons. As a result, each respondent answers a customized set of questions. ACA constructs pairs by examining all the possible ways the levels can be combined and then chooses pairs of options with similar utilities for which it expects respondents to be indifferent (based on previous responses). If one option is clearly superior to the other based on ACA's initial estimate of utilities, no additional information is learned. Because it is interactive, ACA is more efficient than other techniques and allows a large number of attributes to be evaluated without resulting in information overload or respondent fatigue. This is an important advantage, since complex treatment decisions often require multiple trade-offs between competing risks and benefits.

11.2.1 Lupus Nephritis

Lupus nephritis is a serious complication of systemic lupus erythematosus, an autoimmune disorder that can affect multiple joints and internal organs, which may progress to end-stage renal disease requiring dialysis or transplantation. Treatment for lupus nephritis consists of high-dose corticosteroids in combination with one of several possible immunosuppressive agents which differ in their toxicity profiles. We used adaptive conjoint analysis (ACA) to assess patient treatment preferences for lupus nephritis by examining: (i) the relative preferences that patients assign to specific immunosuppressive medication characteristics, (ii) the percentage of women preferring cyclophosphamide over azathioprine (two immunosuppressive drugs) for a given probability of renal survival and risk of adverse effects, and (iii) how changing the probability of renal survival or risk of major toxicity influences preference (Fraenkel et al. 2001). Both cyclophosphamide and azathioprine are equally effective in terms of overall survival. Cyclophosphamide is more effective than azathioprine at preventing end-stage renal disease, but carries a greater risk of

Example of first set of questions

If two medications were acceptable in all other ways, how important would this difference be?

No added risk of hair loss versus **50% risk of hair loss**

1. Not important at all
2. Somewhat important
3. Very important
4. Extremely important

Example of second set of questions

Which would you prefer?

95% have functioning kidneys / 5% need dialysis after 10 years + 50% chance of infertility	OR	60% have functioning kidneys / 40% need dialysis after 10 years + No added risk of infertility

Strongly prefer left **No Preference** **Strongly prefer right**
1 2 3 4 5 6 7 8 9 10

Fig. 11.1 Examples of conjoint analysis questions

infection and a unique risk of infertility and premature ovarian failure. We hypothesized that women of childbearing age wanting to have more children would be more likely to reject cyclophosphamide.

The ACA survey contained nine attributes: efficacy (prevention of dialysis) and the risks of infection, cancer, hair loss, shingles, nausea and vomiting, bleeding from the bladder, oral ulcers, premature ovarian failure, and infertility. Respondents first rated the importance of the difference between the best and worst estimates of each characteristic on a four-point scale ranging from not important at all to extremely important. Second, to refine respondents' utilities, respondents evaluated a series of paired comparisons involving a trade-off between two attributes. Examples of these tasks are provided in Fig. 11.1.

The relative importances of the attributes studied were similar across the two groups of women except for the risk of premature ovarian failure (Table 11.1). Variation in efficacy and risk of infection had the greatest impact on choice, each accounting for approximately 20 % of the total relative importance. Of note, a 50 % increase in the risk of reversible hair loss had a similar impact on patient preference as the much rarer risk of cancer.

Similar to sensitivity analyses conducted for decision analytic models, we conducted simulations to examine preferences under different assumptions. For the base-case scenario, which modeled preferences for the maximum renal survival advantage of cyclophosphamide reported in the literature and a low probability of adverse effects, 56 % of premenopausal women wanting more children preferred cyclophosphamide over azathioprine. In contrast, the majority of premenopausal

Table 11.1 Importance of attributes regarding treatment of lupus nephritis based on adaptive conjoint analysis

Attribute	Premenopausal women wanting more children ($N=25$)	Premenopausal women not wanting more children ($N=40$)
Efficacy	19 ± 4	22 ± 5
Infection	19 ± 4	18 ± 5
Cancer	12 ± 5	12 ± 5
Alopecia	11 ± 4	11 ± 5
Ovarian failure	14 ± 7	9 ± 5
Zoster	9 ± 3	9 ± 4
Nausea	8 ± 4	9 ± 4
Cystitis	5 ± 3	6 ± 4
Oral ulcers	4 ± 2	4 ± 3

women not wanting more children (80 %) preferred cyclophosphamide. A decrease in the risk of premature ovarian failure to 12.5 % (the risk associated with short-term therapy) increased the percentage of respondents preferring cyclophosphamide by only 8 %. Only in the hypothetical situation where cyclophosphamide carries no additional risk of infertility were women wanting more children as likely to choose this drug as those who do not (88 % versus 90 %).

This study suggests that a significant number of premenopausal women wanting more children are unwilling to accept even the smallest risk of infertility associated with cyclophosphamide, no matter how much better it is at preventing renal failure than azathioprine. While newer treatment options are now available for lupus nephritis, cyclophosphamide remains an option for many serious inflammatory diseases. The results of this study underscore the importance of including patients' values for the trade-offs involved in these difficult decisions.

11.2.2 Knee Osteoarthritis

Knee osteoarthritis (OA), also known as degenerative arthritis, is associated with loss of cartilage and bone spur formation. It is the most common form of arthritis and leads to pain and stiffness (Osteoarthritis 2015). Knee OA is currently the most common cause of lower extremity disability. Explicit elicitation of patient preferences is of particular importance in the treatment of patients with knee OA, because pharmacologic options have relatively modest efficacy and differ significantly with respect to their risk of drug toxicity and cost. Given the extant data documenting relative risk aversion among older adults, we hypothesized that current practices for the treatment of knee OA, in which the majority of subjects are treated with nonselective nonsteroidal anti-inflammatory drugs (NSAIDs), are not concordant with patient preferences.

We composed an ACA survey to quantify patient preferences for available treatment options. The ACA task was composed to ascertain patients' preferences for five options: nonselective nonsteroidal anti-inflammatory drugs (NSAIDs), cyclooxygenase inhibitors (COX-2 inhibitors), opioids, glucosamine and chondroitin sulfate, and capsaicin. We measured patient utilities for seven medication characteristics including label, route of administration, time to benefit, response rate, common adverse effects, risk of ulcer, and monthly co-pays. Levels for benefits and harms were drawn from published studies (Fraenkel et al. 2004).

As shown in Table 11.2 below, we found that topical capsaicin (the safest but least effective medication) was the most preferred option. In contrast, nonsteroidal anti-inflammatory drugs (NSAIDs), the most widely prescribed medications for patients with arthritis, are the least preferred therapeutic options when patients are responsible for the full cost of their medications. Decreasing the risk of ulcers associated with NSAIDs or increasing their efficacy did not change to rank ordering of preferences. However, Cox-2 inhibitors became the preferred choice when they were assumed to cost $10.00 per month (reflecting the typical co-pay in an insured patient).

In this study, as shown in Table 11.3 below, the risk of adverse effects had the strongest impact on patient decision-making which explains why patients with knee OA strongly preferred capsaicin and rejected NSAIDs. Preferences for capsaicin were unlikely to be due to a dislike for taking pills, since route of administration was one of the least influential medication characteristics. Despite the widespread use of complementary therapies among patients with arthritis, the label "natural supplement" also had little influence on treatment preferences when rated in comparison to other medication characteristics. The magnitude of the discrepancy between patient preferences in this study and the widespread use of nonselective NSAIDs raise important questions about how patient preferences are elicited and how treatment decisions for OA are made in clinical practice.

Table 11.2 Osteoarthritis treatment preferences assuming patients are paying the full cost of their medications

	Patients preferring each treatment option		
		Change from base case	
Option	Base case	Risk of ulcer decreased[a]	Efficacy of anti-inflammatory drugs increased[b]
	Percent ± SD		
Nonselective NSAIDs	2.0 ± 1.4	9.0 ± 2.9	5 ± 2.2
COX-2 inhibitors	7.0 ± 2.6	7.0 ± 2.6	17 ± 3.8
Opioids	23.0 ± 4.2	20.0 ± 4.0	18 ± 3.8
Glucosamine and/or chondroitin sulfate	24.0 ± 4.3	21.0 ± 4.1	19 ± 3.9
Capsaicin	44.0 ± 5.0	43.0 ± 4.9	41 ± 4.9

Abbreviations: *COX* cyclooxygenase, *NSAID* nonsteroidal anti-inflammatory drug

[a]Risk of ulcer associated with nonselective NSAIDs, 1 %; COX-2 inhibitors, 0.5 %

[b]Efficacy of nonselective NSAIDs and COX-2 inhibitors, 75 % of patients' benefit; opioids and glucosamine and/or chondroitin sulfate, 50 %; and capsaicin, 25 %

Table 11.3 Utilities for osteoarthritis medication characteristics derived from conjoint analysis

Medication characteristic	Relative importances Mean ± standard deviation
Label	9.7 ± 4.9
Route of administration	11.9 ± 4.6
Time to benefit	13.6 ± 4.7
Chance of benefit	15.1 ± 4.6
Common adverse effects	18.5 ± 3.3
Gastrointestinal ulcer	19.2 ± 3.4
Out-of-pocket monthly cost	12.2 ± 4.5

Given these findings, we sought to determine whether conjoint analysis could be used as a decision support tool for decisions regarding treatment of OA in the clinical practice setting. We performed an experiment in which all patients with knee OA were randomized to receive a conjoint analysis-based decision support tool or to a control arm at the time of their appointment.

Subjects in the control arm were given an information pamphlet on OA by the research assistant that they could read while waiting for their appointment.

Those in the intervention arm were asked to complete the ACA task on a laptop computer with the help of a research assistant before seeing their physicians. The ACA survey was similar to that described in the first study which included the following treatment characteristics: route of administration (pills, cream, injection, exercise), likelihood of expected benefit (decrease in pain and improvement in strength and endurance), and risk of adverse effects (dyspepsia and ulcer). After answering the ACA questions, the tool calculated patient-specific relative importances and estimated treatment preferences in real time, thus enabling us to provide patients with a handout illustrating the relative influence of each characteristic on their treatment preferences and a graph demonstrating the relative ranking of the options on a scale ranging from 0 (worst choice) to 100 (best choice) (see Figs. 11.2 and 11.3) (Fraenkel et al. 2007).

We found that subjects who were randomized to the ACA decision support tool had greater self-confidence in their ability to participate in shared decision-making, felt better prepared to participate in decision-making, and reported greater arthritis self-efficacy compared to those receiving the information pamphlet. Most (74 %) of the participants felt that the ACA task was "very easy" to do, and 86 % would recommend the ACA task for other knee pain patients. These results support the use of conjoint analysis as a potential approach to elicit patients' preferences in clinical practice.

11.3 The Analytic Hierarchy Process

The analytic hierarchy process (AHP) is a widely used, theory-based multi-criteria decision analysis method developed in the 1980s by Thomas Saaty. It was designed to be both applicable to a wide range of decision problems and simple enough to be

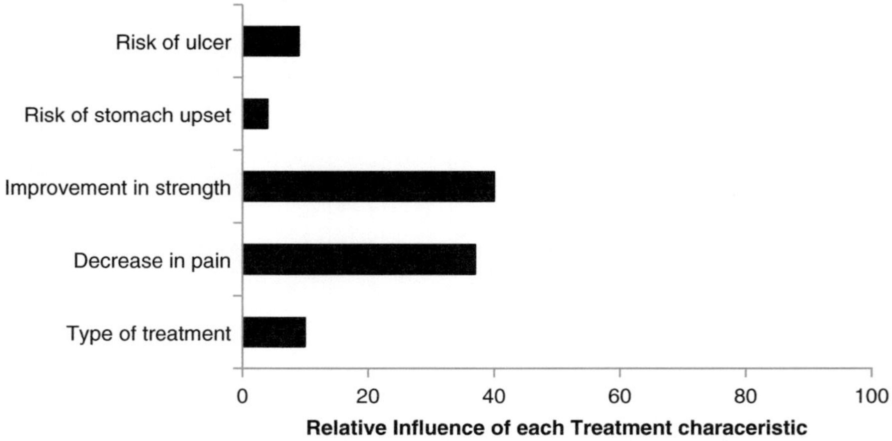

Fig. 11.2 Example of summary of osteoarthritis treatment priorities provided to patients after performing conjoint analysis

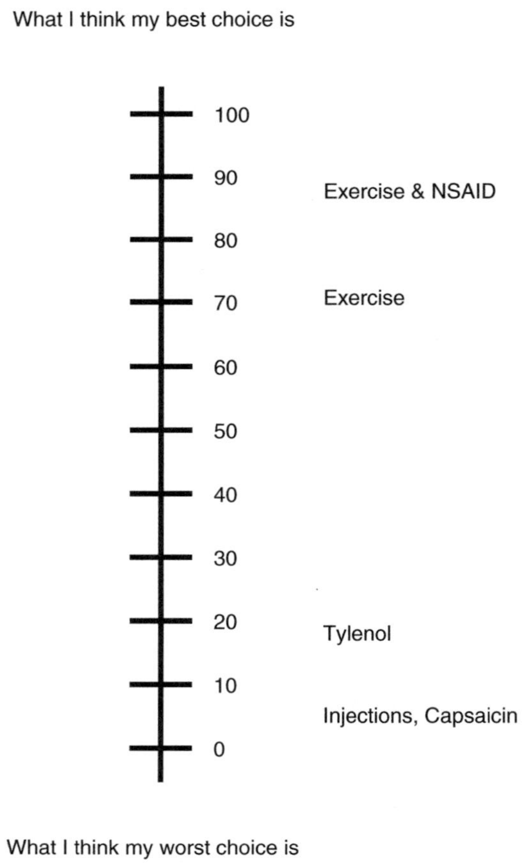

Fig. 11.3 Example of treatment preference summary provided to patients after performing conjoint analysis

readily accessible to a broad range of decision-makers. As a result, the AHP is one of the most widely used multi-criteria methods in the world and has been successfully applied to a wide range of decision problems (Ishizaka and Labib 2011; Ho 2008; Liberatore and Nydick 2008; Subramanian and Ramanathan 2012; Vaidya and Kumar 2006).

An AHP analysis consists of four steps: (1) creating a decision model, (2) gathering pertinent information about the options being considered, (3) performing the analysis, and (4) exploring the results.

The decision model is organized as a series of levels with the goal of the decision at the top, the options being considered at the bottom, and the criteria that will be used to determine how well the options are likely to meet the goal in the middle. The AHP is flexible enough to accommodate criteria that reflect differences among the options based on both objective data and subjective considerations. All criteria should be independent of each other to ensure that all important decision-making considerations are considered equally. They can be divided into one or more levels of sub-criteria if necessary to compare the options more precisely.

Information gathering consists of collecting information that indicates how well the options meet the decision criteria and creating data summaries for objective criteria and descriptions for subjective ones.

The analysis phase uses the structure provided by the decision model to break down the decision into a series of comparison sets consisting of elements (criteria or options) on the same hierarchy level relative to one of the elements on the next higher hierarchy level. Each pair of elements is compared in terms of their importance, likelihood, or preference, depending on the context, using a nine-point scale. When all of these pairwise comparisons are completed, they are combined to derive a ratio-level scale running from 0 to 1. A measure of the consistency of the comparisons called the consistency ratio is also routinely calculated. A perfectly consistent set of comparisons has a consistency ratio of 0. The AHP does not require perfect consistency, but consistency ratios above a certain threshold, 0.1 for technical analyses and 0.15–0.20 for applied analyses, should be reviewed and improved if possible. When all of the comparison sets in the model have been analyzed, they are combined to create an overall score, also reported on a ratio scale running from 0 to 1, which indicates how well the options are likely to meet the decision goal.

The exploration stage of an AHP analysis consists of varying the comparative preferences and priorities contained in the initial analysis to determine the impact on the results. If further analysis is deemed important, the initial model can be adjusted by adding or deleting criteria, options, or information and the analysis is repeated until the decision-makers are satisfied with the analysis and comfortable making a decision. Note that the AHP is not intended to be prescriptive. Rather it should be considered a tool for helping decision-makers gain insight into the problem they face, how the options differ, and their own preferences regarding decision-related trade-offs between competing objectives.

A more complete description of the AHP is beyond the scope of this chapter; several are available in the literature (Dolan et al. 1989; Dolan 2010; Saaty 2008; Saaty 1994).

11.3.1 Colorectal Cancer

Cancer of the colon or rectum, colorectal cancer (CRC), is common. Worldwide, it is the second and third most commonly diagnosed cancer in women and men, respectively, and, in 2012, accounted for almost 700,000 deaths (UK CR 2014). Most colorectal cancers develop over a period of many years from asymptomatic, noncancerous mushroom-shaped growths on the inside wall of the large intestine called adenomatous polyps. Removing these polyps has been shown to prevent cancer (Winawer et al. 1993). This prolonged natural history and proven early intervention makes CRC an ideal target for screening programs that aim to identify people at an early, asymptomatic stage of disease to prevent its progression to a more advanced stage. Because most colorectal cancers occur in people who do not have a family history or medical condition that increases their chances of developing it, population-wide screening of average risk people is recommended in many countries.

Although widely recommended, there is no clearly preferred screening approach to population-based colorectal cancer screening. Several screening tests are available that differ across several dimensions including accuracy, complexity, effectiveness, side effects, and cost. Some countries, such as Australia and Canada, have chosen to implement just one screening option (Australian CRC Screening Guidelines ; Canadian CRC Screening Guidelines). Others, such as the United States, endorse several screening options and rely on clinicians and patients to choose which is most appropriate (USPSTF CRC Screening Guidelines 2008).

Regardless of which approach is taken, selection of a CRC screening strategy involves trade-offs between the advantages and disadvantages of the screening tests available. In other words, it is a multi-criteria decision. At the time the initial US screening guidelines were first issued in 1996, we had already shown that MCDA implemented using the analytic hierarchy process (AHP) could be readily applied to clinical problems and that both patients and clinicians could provide the information needed to conduct an analysis with minimal training. Based on this preliminary work, we conducted a series of studies to explore whether the AHP could be used at the clinical level to help doctors and patients make colorectal cancer screening decisions together in accordance with the guideline recommendations.

11.3.2 The Colorectal Cancer Studies

The first study was a small pilot designed to compare AHP-based decision support with a standard patient information pamphlet. The second was a large-scale survey designed to assess patient priorities for colorectal cancer screening programs, explore the extent to which patients could complete a challenging AHP analysis, and record their impressions of the procedure including the usefulness of the information obtained and willingness to use similar procedures in the future. Both studies were conducted when the CRC screening guidelines endorsed the five screening strategies listed in the table below (Table 11.4).

Table 11.4 Colorectal cancer screening options included in the analytic hierarchy process studies

Screening strategy	Description
Annual stool tests	Checking stool for signs of abnormal bleeding
Flexible sigmoidoscopy every 5 years	Examination of the lower 60 cm of the colon using a flexible fiberoptic scope
Stool tests and flexible sigmoidoscopy	Annual stool tests and flexible sigmoidoscopy every 5 years
Barium enema every 5 years	X-ray examination of the colon
Colonoscopy every 10 years	Examination of the entire colon bowel using a flexible fiberoptic scope

11.3.3 Colorectal Cancer Study 1

The first study was a randomized controlled trial comparing an AHP-based decision aid with educational material describing five recommended screening strategies. The figure below shows the decision model that was used. The goal is at the top: choose the best approach to colorectal cancer screening. The five recommended screening programs are shown at the bottom along with a no screening "wait-and-see" option. In the middle are the decision criteria that were used. They are based on differences among the recommended screening programs that were discussed in both the guidelines and the educational material. Three considerations – screening frequency, preparations needed for the screening tests, and the nature of the test procedure(s) – were combined because criteria on any level of a decision hierarchy need to be comparable using the standard 1–9 scale. In this case, we judged that none of these considerations by itself was of the same order of magnitude as the other major criteria but that, when considered together, they would be (Fig. 11.4).

The study population consisted of patients at average risk of colorectal cancer recruited from two internal medicine practices in Rochester, New York, who were due for a screening test according to the guideline recommendations. Eligible patients were randomly assigned to either the control group or the intervention group and interviewed just prior to a regularly scheduled appointment with their primary care physician. People assigned to the control group were asked to review a short written document that described colorectal cancer and the rationale for screening along with the recommended screening tests. Those assigned to the intervention group, with the assistance of a research assistant, completed a full AHP analysis of the screening decision, as described above, using a dedicated commercial AHP software program running on a laptop computer. Both groups were encouraged to discuss colorectal cancer screening with their physician at the upcoming visit.

The primary study outcomes were patient-reported decisional conflict and the number of screening plans that were carried out. Decisional conflict refers to the amount of uncertainty a person has regarding pursuing a course of action. We assessed decision conflict using the decisional conflict scale that measures overall decisional conflict as well as five contributing factors: uncertainty, feelings of being uninformed, clarity of decision-related values, feelings of being supported

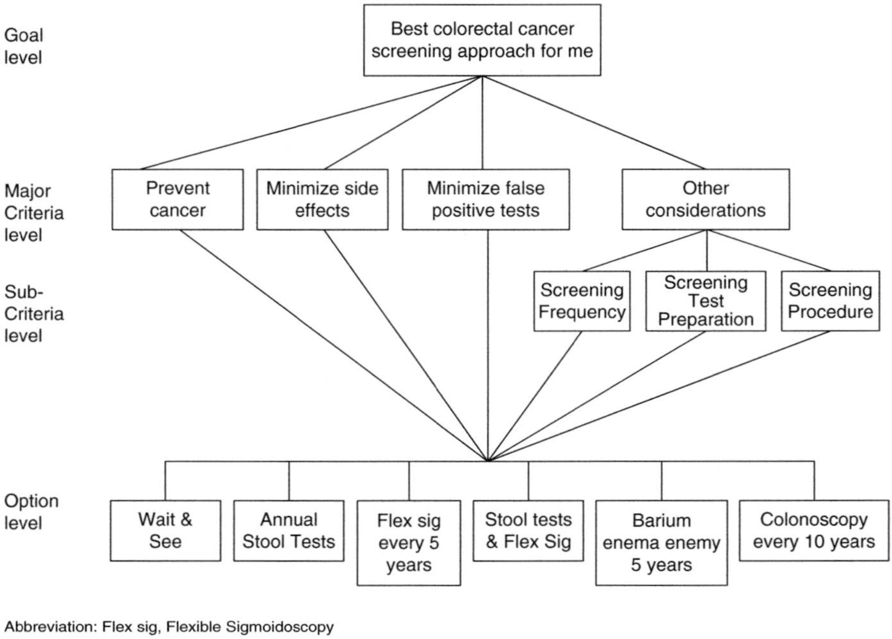

Fig. 11.4 Colorectal cancer screening model

by others, and a personal assessment of the effectiveness of a decision (O'Connor 1995). We hypothesized that patients in the intervention group would have lower decisional conflict and would be more likely to complete screening plans.

Ninety-five patients completed the study, 46 (48 %) in the control group and 49 (52 %) in the experimental group. All but two patients in the experimental group were able to complete the study intervention in the allotted 1 h time. Patients in the experimental group had lower (better) decisional conflict scores and felt more informed, had clearer values, and were more likely to think they had made an effective decision than those in the control group. Patients also assigned widely variable priorities to the decision criteria – the average range was 46 on the 100-point priority scale – and cluster analysis identified six different combinations of priorities for the four major decision criteria (Dolan 2005). The most commonly preferred option was combined fecal occult blood testing and flexible sigmoidoscopy, preferred by 58 % of patients. Fewer patients in the intervention group preferred the no screening "wait-and-see" option. Patients rated both interventions highly and supported their use in routine clinical practice (Dolan and Frisina 2002).

11.3.4 Colorectal Cancer Study 2

The second study was designed to extend the results of the prior study by investigating patient preferences regarding colorectal screening programs and to determine if patients could complete a complex clinical AHP analysis with minimal training in a larger, more representative sample. We surveyed 484 patients at average risk for CRC at internal medicine practice sites in Rochester New York, Birmingham Alabama, and Indianapolis Indiana. All study patients were asked to complete an AHP analysis of the CRC screening decision. We used the same decision model as the first study except that we expanded the range of options to encompass the full range of programs endorsed by guidelines current at the time of the study, a total of ten options. Patients performed their analyses with the assistance of a research assistant using a laptop computer running an AHP software program designed specifically for this study.

Seventy-eight percent of study patients were able to perform a technically adequate AHP analysis which we defined as an overall consistency ratio of less than or equal to 0.15. The primary factor affecting the likelihood of a technically adequate analysis was study site: rates of adequate analyses ranged from 32 % in Indianapolis to 99 % in Birmingham. Patient characteristics including age, race, gender, literacy, numeracy, and household income had little or no effect.

Patient preferences regarding the decision criteria were again heterogeneous. Cluster analysis revealed six distinct preference combinations for the major criteria and four for the logistical sub-criteria. Every decision criterion and sub-criterion was considered most important by at least one cluster group. Major criteria cluster groups were not associated with patient characteristics or study site. However, patients with median household incomes <$35,000 were more likely to be in a cluster where preventing cancer was not the most important consideration.

Patients rated their experience using the AHP highly: 92 % indicated that they understood the decision criteria, 91 % that it was not hard to understand the pairwise comparison process, 85 % that it was not hard to make the comparisons, and 88 % that they were willing to use a similar procedure to make an important decision regarding their healthcare.

11.4 Overall Results and Conclusions

The hallmark of good clinical decision-making is the careful integration of clinical evidence with the preferences and priorities of decision stakeholders. The importance of evidence-based medical decision-making is widely recognized and has been increasingly emphasized. One of the results of increased attention to clinical evidence has been the recognition that many decisions made in contemporary medical practice depend on preference-driven trade-offs among several alternatives. The heterogeneity of patient preferences seen in the studies discussed above clearly demonstrates the importance of identifying individual patient preferences when making clinical decisions that are preference sensitive. This realization has led to efforts to integrate patient preferences and involve patients in decisions regarding their care through a process of shared decision-making.

Both of these key aspects of clinical decision-making are difficult to accomplish in clinical practice. Efforts to increase evidence-based decision-making have largely focused on summarizing the data available through methodologically rigorous systematic literature reviews and the creation of practice guidelines that reflect the strengths and weaknesses of the evidence available. Efforts to increase patient involvement have led to the development of enhanced patient communication formats that help patients become more involved in their care and formal decision aids to help them understand the decision and assess their preferences and priorities. Although great progress has been made in both of these areas, much work remains to be done to develop effective ways to integrate these two tasks.

MCDA tools are well suited to help clinical decision-makers integrate clinical evidence with patient preferences. Taken together, the studies reviewed here provide evidence that patients are able to use powerful MCDA tools with minimal training and that their use leads to an improved decision-making process. These results illustrate the importance and usefulness of addressing clinical decisions from a multi-criteria perspective and warrant additional development and testing of MCDA-based methods to support high-quality, patient-centered clinical decision-making.

However, despite promising results so far, a number of significant issues need to be addressed before MCDA-based clinical decision-making tools can be implemented in practice settings. Perhaps the most important is the need to demonstrate that they provide tangible benefits for both patients and providers. Related issues include the creation of tools that are readily adaptable for clinical use and the development of efficient methods to maintain the currency of the evidence included in them.

Although these concerns are far from trivial, the close match between the needs of clinical decision-makers and the functionalities of MCDA tools, the ready acceptance by minimally trained patients, and the rapid advances in computer and communication technology all suggest that they are not insurmountable. We therefore believe that MCDA-based tools will play a major role in promoting high-quality, evidence-based clinical decision-making in the years to come.

References

Australian CRC Screening Guidelines [Internet]. [cited 4–30/15]. Available from: http://www.cancerscreening.gov.au/internet/screening/publishing.nsf/Content/bowel-screening-1

Bridges JFP (2003) Stated preference methods in health care evaluation: an emerging methodological paradigm in health economics. Appl Health Econ Health Policy 2(4):213–224

Brownlee S, Wennberg JE, Barry M, Fisher ES, Goodman DC, Byrum JPW. Improving patient decision-making in health care: a 2011 Dartmouth Atlas report highlighting Minnesota

Canadian CRC Screening Guidelines [Internet]. [cited 4–20/15]. Available from: http://www.cancer.ca/en/prevention-and-screening/early-detection-and-screening/screening/screening-for-colorectal-cancer/?region=bc

Dolan JG (2005) Patient priorities in colorectal cancer screening decisions. Health Expect 8(4):334–344

Dolan JG (2010) Multi-criteria clinical decision support. Patient: Patient-Centered Outcom Res Springer, 3(4):229–248

Dolan JG, Frisina S (2002) Randomized controlled trial of a patient decision aid for colorectal cancer screening. Med Decis Making 22(2):125–139

Dolan JG, Isselhardt BJ, Cappuccio JD (1989) The analytic hierarchy process in medical decision making a tutorial. Med Decis Making 9(1):40–50

Fraenkel L, Bodardus S, Wittink DR (2001) Understanding patient preferences for the treatment of lupus nephritis with adaptive conjoint analysis. Med Care 39(11):1203–1216

Fraenkel L, Bogardus ST, Concato J, Wittink DR (2004) Treatment options in knee osteoarthritis: the patient's perspective. Arch Intern Med 164(12):1299–1304

Fraenkel L, Rabidou N, Wittink D, Fried T (2007) Improving informed decision-making for patients with knee pain. J Rheumatol 34(9):1894–1898

Ho W (2008) Integrated analytic hierarchy process and its applications-A literature review. Eur J Oper Res 186(1):211–228

Huber J, Orme B, Miller R (2007) The value of choice simulators. In: Gustafsson A, Herrman AF (eds) Conjoint measurement. Springer, New York, pp 347–362

Ishizaka A, Labib A (2011) Review of the main developments in the analytic hierarchy process. Exp Syst Applic 38(11):14336–14345

Joseph-Williams N, Elwyn G, Edwards A (2014) Knowledge is not power for patients: a systematic review and thematic synthesis of patient-reported barriers and facilitators to shared decision making. Patient Educ Couns 94(3):291–309

Légaré F (2013) Shared decision making: moving from theorization to applied research and hopefully to clinical practice. Patient Educ Couns 91(2):129

Liberatore MJ, Nydick RL (2008) The analytic hierarchy process in medical and health care decision making: a literature review. Eur J Operat Res 189(1):194–207

Mulley AG, Trimble C, Elwyn G (2012) Stop the silent misdiagnosis: patients' preferences matter. BMJ 345:e6572

O'Connor AM (1995) Validation of a decisional conflict scale. Med Decis Making 15(1):25–30

O'Connor AM, Wennberg JE, Legare F, Llewellyn-Thomas HA, Moulton BW, Sepucha KR et al (2007) Toward the "tipping point": decision aids and informed patient choice. Health Aff 26(3):716–725

Osteoarthritis [Internet]. [cited 2015]. Available from: http://www.cdc.gov/arthritis/basics/osteoarthritis.htm

Politi MC, Street RL (2011) The importance of communication in collaborative decision making: facilitating shared mind and the management of uncertainty. J Eval Clin Pract 17(4):579–584

Ryan M, Farrar S (2000) Using conjoint analysis to elicit preferences for health care. BMJ 320:1530–1533

Saaty TL (1994) How to make a decision: the analytic hierarchy process. Interfaces 48(24):19–43

Saaty TL (2008) Decision making with the analytic hierarchy process. Int J Serv Sci 1(1):83–98

Stacey D et al (2014) Decision aids for people facing health treatment or screening decisions. Cochrane Database Syst Rev (1):CD001431

Subramanian N, Ramanathan R (2012) A review of applications of analytic hierarchy process in operations management. Int J Produc Econ 138(2):215–241

UK CR. Worldwide cancer mortality statistics [Internet]. 2014 [cited 23 Apr 2015]. Available from: http://www.cancerresearchuk.org/cancer-info/cancerstats/world/mortality/

USPSTF crc screening guidelines 2008 [Internet]. [cited 4–30/15]. Available from: https://www.uspreventiveservicestaskforce.org/Page/Document/UpdateSummaryFinal/colorectal-cancer-screening2

Vaidya OS, Kumar S (2006) Analytic hierarchy process: an overview of applications. Eur J Operat Res 169(1):1–29

Veroff D, Marr A, Wennberg DE (2013) Enhanced support for shared decision making reduced costs of care for patients with preference-sensitive conditions. Health Aff 32(2):285–293

Wennberg JE, Fisher ES, Skinner JS et al (2002) Geography and the debate over Medicare reform. Health Aff 21(2):10

Winawer SJ, Zauber AG, Ho MN, O'Brien MJ, Gottlieb LS, Sternberg SS et al (1993) Prevention of colorectal cancer by colonoscopic polypectomy. N Engl J Med 329(27):1977–1981

Chapter 12
The Role of MCDA in Health Research Priority Setting

Roderik F. Viergever, Dimitrios Gouglas, and Noor Tromp

Abstract Health research priority-setting exercises aim to maximize the impact of investments in health research. An increasing number of priority-setting exercises for health research have taken place in the past two decades. These exercises have been conducted for various areas of health research and at various levels (global, regional, national, local and institutional). In this chapter, we discuss the similarities and differences between health research priority setting and health intervention priority setting, and we describe the current methodologies used in health research priority setting and the role of multi-criteria decision analysis (MCDA) therein. We provide three concrete suggestions for future methodological development in the field of health research priority setting: (1) recognize that many of the methodologies used to set health research priorities apply MCDA, (2) make use of well-established approaches or best practices for health research priority setting and (3) study in more detail the differences between health intervention and health research priority setting.

R.F. Viergever (✉)
Department for Health Evidence, Radboud University Medical Center, P.O. Box 9101, 6500 HB, Nijmegen, Netherlands

Research4health, Utrecht, The Netherlands
e-mail: rviergever@research4health.org

D. Gouglas
CEPI – Coalition for Epidemic Preparedness Innovations, Norwegian Institute of Public Health, Oslo, Norway

N. Tromp
Department for Health Evidence, Radboud University Medical Center, P.O. Box 9101, 6500 HB, Nijmegen, Netherlands

Royal Tropical Institute (KIT), Mauritskade 63, 1092 AD, Amsterdam, Netherlands

© Springer International Publishing AG 2017
K. Marsh et al. (eds.), *Multi-Criteria Decision Analysis to Support Healthcare Decisions*, DOI 10.1007/978-3-319-47540-0_12

12.1 Introduction

Health research[1] provides us with opportunities to mount a better response to health problems. There are different types of health research, and each type offers different opportunities for improving our responses to health problems. Research might measure the magnitude and distribution of a health problem; help to understand the causes of the problem; elaborate solutions; help to translate the solutions or evidence into policy, practice and products; or evaluate the impact of solutions (WHA document A63/22: WHO's role and responsibilities in health research: Draft WHO strategy on research for health 2010). Some research takes place on an individual level (i.e. biomedical research or clinical research); other research takes place on a population level (i.e. epidemiological research or health systems research) (Frenk 1993). Research that focuses on developing products can aim to develop a variety of different products, such as devices, medicines, vaccines, procedures or systems (Health technologies: Report by the Secretariat. World Health Organization Executive Board document EB 121/11 2007). Every year, approximately 240 billion US dollars are spent globally on health research (Røttingen et al. 2013). The challenges associated with distributing these funds in an optimal way have given rise to the growing field of health research priority setting.

Health research priority-setting exercises are used by researchers and policymakers to help them make choices about what health research to conduct or to invest in. These exercises range widely in coverage (global, regional, national, local and institutional) (Viergever et al. 2010a; McGregor et al. 2014), in scope (generalized vs. context specific) (Baltussen et al. 2010) and in their aims (e.g. setting a 'road map' for health research needs vs. prioritizing optimal investment options for funders of health research) (McGregor et al. 2014). A large number of health research priority-setting exercises have been conducted globally in recent years. Two reviews from 2006 to 2008 identified 344 and 258 reports of health research priorities, respectively (Oliver and Gray 2006; Stewart and Oliver 2008); a review of WHO-based health research priority setting from 2009 found 230 reports of health research priorities that were organized or coordinated through WHO headquarters in roughly 5 years before (Viergever et al. 2010a), and a review from 2014 by McGregor identified 91 health research priority-setting exercises from low- and middle-income countries (McGregor et al. 2014).

This chapter reviews the methodologies that have been developed to guide such priority setting, with a specific focus on the role of multi-criteria decision analysis (MCDA) in these methodologies. The chapter has three sections. First, to introduce the chapter, we discuss the similarities and differences between health research

[1] Research is defined here as in the *Frascati Manual* by the Organisation for Economic Co-operation and Development (OECD): 'Creative work undertaken on a systematic base in order to increase the stock of knowledge, including knowledge about man, culture and society, and the use of this knowledge to devise new applications' (Frascati manual: proposed standard practice for surveys on research and experimental development 2002). Health research is defined as in the *Revised field of science and technology (FOS) classification* in the *Frascati Manual* and includes the fields of basic medicine, clinical medicine, health sciences, medical biotechnology and other medical sciences (Working Party of National Experts on Science and Technology Indicators 2007).

priority setting and health intervention priority setting. Second, we describe the types of methodologies that are being used to set health research priorities and to what degree these apply MCDA. From this, several suggestions follow for future methodological development in the field of health research priority setting that we discuss in the final section of the chapter.

12.2 What Are the Similarities and Differences Between Health Research and Intervention Priority Setting?

12.2.1 Similarities

Health research priority setting and intervention priority setting are similar in many ways. Both fields know a large variety of priority-setting methodologies and contexts for which priorities can be set, for example, ranging from deliberative to quantitative methodologies (IJzerman et al. 2014) and from generalized to context-specific contexts (Baltussen et al. 2010). Exercises in the two fields also share many considerations around aspects of the priority-setting process, such as the theories that underlie the methods for priority setting (e.g. multi-attribute utility theory), stakeholder mapping and selection, identifying and choosing criteria, assigning weights to criteria, scoring options, aggregating scores, reaching agreement on the final list of priorities (e.g. consensus approaches or majority rules approaches), presenting the priorities and implementing the priorities (IJzerman et al. 2014; Viergever et al. 2010b; Okello and Chongtrakul 2000).

12.2.2 Differences

However, there are also differences between these two areas of priority setting. The main conceptual difference between the two is that the problem that needs to be solved differs: prioritizing research is not the same as prioritizing interventions. In considering the value of various research options against a set of criteria, there is inherently more uncertainty about these values than in health intervention priority setting, because making decisions about which research will pay off requires an amount of future foresight. As Callahan has noted, ‘While priority setting for health-care delivery is concerned only with meeting present needs, research aims at future as well as present needs’ (Callahan 1999).

This conceptual difference has several practical consequences. First, the criteria that are used to appraise the various options differ between the two fields. There is certainly an overlap between the criteria used in both fields: both might take into account, for example, the (expected) health impact, cost or equity of the research or intervention options. However, other criteria differ: the expected feasibility of development of a health technology does not apply to interventions, because they have already been developed. The criteria that are used in both fields are listed in reviews of health intervention (Tromp and Baltussen 2012) and health research (McGregor et al. 2014; Noorani et al. 2007) priority-setting exercises.

Second, because of the uncertainty associated with health research priority setting, the manner in which options are scored against criteria is often more subjective in health research priority setting, i.e. less directly based on data and more on stakeholder opinion. While subjectivity is inherent to both settings to some degree (e.g. in eliciting preferences for weights of criteria), many exercises that use MCDA to establish intervention priorities make use of objective data to populate the performance matrix.[2] Examples of such objective data about interventions are the effectiveness of the interventions and their cost (Baltussen et al. 2006; 2007). These data are commonly derived from the literature and may be used in mathematical modelling estimations. When such data are not available, which might be the case for criteria for which data are sparser and/or more difficult to quantify (such as equity), subjective judgements are used to score the intervention options based on the various criteria. Conversely, in health research priority setting, where objective data to populate a performance matrix are often not available, stakeholders are commonly presented with evidence collected prior to the exercise, but the dominant method for scoring research options against criteria is through stakeholder opinion (Viergever et al. 2010b).

There are several additional reasons for the use of stakeholder opinion, rather than objective data, in health research priority-setting exercises. First, while in health intervention priority-setting exercises, the number of intervention options that are prioritized (e.g. interventions to combat HIV/AIDS (Youngkong et al. 2012)) is often limited; in health research, the number of options that can be identified and prioritized is virtually unlimited. Even when the health research priority-setting exercise is limited to one health area (e.g. HIV), and even when it is limited to one area of research (e.g. biomedical research, clinical research, epidemiological research or health systems research (Frenk 1993)), the options are endless. Moreover, the level of granularity in defined research options can vary greatly per exercise, ranging from precise research questions to broad research areas (McGregor et al. 2014). In the aforementioned review of health research priority-setting exercises in low- and middle-income countries by McGregor, 35 % prioritized broad research areas, 42 % research topics and 23 % specific research questions (McGregor et al. 2014). Additionally, in health research priority setting, the research options are almost always identified by stakeholders during the priority-setting exercise, while in intervention priority setting, existing options are more often evaluated in advance (we reviewed the priority-setting studies compiled by McGregor (McGregor et al. 2014) and found that only one used a list of predetermined research options). The large amount of possible research options, combined with the fact that their level of granularity is often not yet determined prior to the exercise and that the options are mostly identified by stakeholders during the exercise, makes it difficult to collect objective data on the various research

[2] The population matrix describes the performance of the options against each criterion (Baltussen and Niessen 2006).

options in advance to support populating the performance matrix with objective data. It is noteworthy that while these are common aspects of many health research priority-setting exercises, that there are also health research priority-setting exercises where the number of options is more limited (e.g. (very) early HTAs can help to prioritize various research options and often only have a limited amount of options (Highlights in Early Health Technology Assessment 2011)). For these priority-setting exercises, the use of objective data might be more feasible.

To provide some insight into the workings of health research priority-setting exercises, we describe a case study of the development of a national health research agenda in Papua New Guinea (Box 12.1).

Box 12.1

A case study of health research priority setting in Papua New Guinea

To exemplify the methods used in health research priority-setting exercises, we provide a case study here of a recent exercise that developed a national health research agenda for Papua New Guinea for the years 2013–2018 (Viergever et al. 2014). The purpose of the agenda was to inform the priorities for a planned national health research grants programme, funded by both the Papua New Guinea government and development partners. The development of the agenda was led by a steering committee that was assembled by the National Department of Health. Methodologically, the development of the priority-setting exercise was based mainly on the 'checklist for health research priority setting' and the essential national health research (ENHR) strategy. The exercise involved two stages. In the first, four workshops were held that each focused on a different research domain: reproductive, maternal and child health research, communicable disease research, research on healthy lifestyles and health systems research. For each domain, technical experts, including policymakers, practitioners and researchers, discussed the appropriate values underlying the exercise, decided on criteria that should be used in the priority-setting exercise, decided on the relevant more specific research areas under each research domain and identified 10–15 research topics for each research domain. In stage two, during one workshop, senior policymakers, practitioners and researchers further refined these topics. They also divided 100 points over the three criteria decided upon by the groups in the first stage to reflect their relative importance and then scored the research options against these criteria. In addition, they were asked to provide a score for the overall importance of each research option. Criteria-based scores and overall scores were then combined to form a final ranking of research topics. That final ranking was discussed and modified by the stakeholders in the meeting until a final consensus on the research topics was achieved. After this, participants in the meeting discussed the next steps, including the implementation of the agenda and plans for revision.

12.3 Health Research Priority Setting and MCDA

So, health research priority setting is similar in many ways to health intervention priority setting, but there are also differences. In this section, we review the various *methodologies* that are used to set health research priorities. To assess the degree to which MCDA is being applied in the field of health research priority setting, we compare these methodologies with MCDA. After that, we present an analysis of the degree to which MCDA has been applied in a sample of health research priority-setting *exercises*. In the final part of this section, we describe what the implications are from these analyses for the links between health research priority setting and MCDA.

12.3.1 Methodologies to Health Research Priority Setting (And Their Link with MCDA)

12.3.1.1 Three Types of Methodologies

Table 12.1 presents an overview of the three types of priority-setting methodologies that have been used to establish health research priorities in the past.

The first set of methodologies in Table 12.1 consists of methodologies that use multiple criteria in their decision-making processes but that have not been labelled as MCDA explicitly. These are all approaches that have been developed specifically for prioritizing health research. This set contains most[3] of the dominant approaches to health research priority setting: the essential national health research (ENHR) strategy, the Child Health and Nutrition Research Initiative (CHNRI) and the combined approach matrix (CAM) (Okello and Chongtrakul 2000; Rudan et al. 2006; The 3D combined approach matrix: an improved tool for setting priorities in research for health 2009). These approaches are 'comprehensive' in that they provide step-by-step guidance for the whole health research priority-setting process from planning to implementation, including, for example, preparatory activities (e.g. guidance for which stakeholders to include) and activities that come after priorities have been established (e.g. guidance for reporting of established priorities) (more detailed descriptions of these three approaches are provide in Table 12.1) (Viergever et al. 2010b).

The second set of methodologies in Table 12.1 consists of several MCDA methods that have been used to set health research priorities. The MCDA methods that have been applied in health research priority-setting exercises are, according to the classification of MCDA methods by Belton and Stewart (2002):

[3]Another is the Priority Setting Partnerships approach, which is mentioned under the third set of approaches, because it does not make use of multiple criteria.

- Qualitative MCDA methods (Owlia et al. 2011; Smith et al. 2009; Hummel et al. 2000)
- Value measurement methods, which can be further subcategorized as:
  - Scoring, weighted sum and linear additive models (Phelps et al. 2014; Doble et al. 2013; Research priorities for the environment, agriculture and infectious diseases of poverty: technical report of the TDR thematic reference group on environment, agriculture and infectious diseases of poverty 2013; Bahadori et al. 2011)
  - Analytic hierarchy process (AHP), analytic network process (ANP) and fuzzy AHP methods (Velmurugan and Selvamuthukumar 2012; Kahraman et al. 2014; Husereau et al. 2010; Ijzerman and Steuten 2011)
  - Multi-attribute utility methods (Phillips and Bana e Costa 2007)

Table 12.1 Three types of methodologies that are used to set health research priorities

	Context in which priority setting methodologies are applied	Examples of specific methodologies
1. Methodologies that use multiple criteria (not explicitly classified as MCDA)	National and global health research policy	*Essential National Health Research (ENHR) strategy*: the ENHR approach provides an approach for national-level health research priority setting with a strong focus on context specificity. It is flexible and at various steps of the priority-setting process, such as for the selection and weighting of criteria, offers options rather than prescriptive guidance. The ENHR strategy is commonly used for developing national health research agendas (Okello and Chongtrakul 2000) *Child Health and Nutrition Research Initiative (CHNRI)*: CHNRI provides a method for conducting pairwise comparisons and elimination of options that are dominated by direct comparison, followed by scoring and weighted sum methods for valuing and ranking the competing options based on the relative importance of five predefined criteria: answerability, effectiveness, deliverability, equity and impact on disease burden. The method is commonly used in setting priorities for specific health areas at both the national and global level (Rudan et al. 2006) *Combined approach matrix (CAM)/CAM3D*: the combined approach matrix (CAM) mainly offers a structured framework for the collection of information according to several preselected criteria, including disease burden, current level of knowledge, cost-effectiveness and current resource flows. The method is commonly used to set priorities for specific health areas at both the national and global level (The 3D combined approach matrix: an improved tool for setting priorities in research for health 2009; Ghaffar 2009). These approaches are reviewed in the 'checklist for health research priority setting' (Viergever et al. 2010b)

(Continued)

Table 12.1 (Continued)

	Context in which priority setting methodologies are applied	Examples of specific methodologies
2. Methodologies that use multiple criteria (classified as MCDA)	National and global health research policy, pharmaceutical R&D portfolio management, health-care organization specific priority setting, early HTA	*Qualitative MCDA methods*, such as *listing/checklist* methods and *group decision/team expert choice* methods: deliberative processes that use multiple criteria to inform decisions in the presence of few discrete options and often in the absence of clearly defined contexts or sufficient data. Such methods have been applied in priority setting for health research in low- and middle-income countries, in health-care organizations and for new product development (Owlia et al. 2011; Smith et al. 2009; Hummel et al. 2000) *Value measurement methods*, such as Scoring, weighted sum, linear additive models: variety of simple additive models that combine option values on multiple criteria into aggregate values, multiplying the value scores on each criterion by the weight of that criterion, then adding all weighted scores together. Such models have been applied in priority setting for new product development, health-care organizational contexts and research for infectious diseases of poverty (Phelps et al. 2014; Doble et al. 2013; Research priorities for the environment, agriculture and infectious diseases of poverty: technical report of the TDR thematic reference group on environment, agriculture and infectious diseases of poverty 2013; Bahadori et al. 2011) Analytic hierarchy process (AHP), analytic network process (ANP) and fuzzy AHP methods: AHP structure options into a hierarchy of an overall objective with multiple criteria through pairwise comparisons between options and consistency checks of stakeholder preferences. ANP is an advanced version of AHP which uses a network structure to value and rank options. Fuzzy set theory can be combined with AHP for priority ranking when data is incomplete. AHP, ANP and fuzzy AHP have been applied in priority setting for pharmaceutical R&D portfolio management, health research investments, health-care organizational contexts and early HTAs (Velmurugan and Selvamuthukumar 2012; Kahraman et al. 2014; Husereau et al. 2010; Ijzerman and Steuten 2011) Multi-attribute utility methods: multi-attribute utility theory (MAUT), multi-attribute value theory (MAVT) or multi-criteria portfolio analysis (MCPA) models aim to rank options through use of value functions of options against a set of multiple criteria in light of uncertainty. MAUT has been applied in budget planning and resource allocation in the pharmaceutical sector (Phillips and Bana e Costa 2007)

Table 12.1 (Continued)

	Context in which priority setting methodologies are applied	Examples of specific methodologies
		Outranking methods: direct comparison models and cross-examining option performances, followed by elimination of outperformed options across a set of multiple criteria. Outranking methods have been applied in the prioritization of contract research organizations in the pharmaceutical industry (Varlan and Le Paillier 1999) *Goal, aspiration or reference-level methods*: range of mathematical models which focus on deriving maximum/minimum values of options against a set of multiple objectives or constraints (criteria). Examples of such models include integer, multi-objective programming, multi-objective optimization and heuristics. Their application in health research priority setting concerns predominantly the domain of pharmaceutical R&D portfolio management (Hassanzadeh et al. 2014; Patel et al. 2013; Subramanian et al. 2000; Sonntag and Grossman 1999; Grossman 1975)
3. Methodologies that do not use multiple criteria	National and global health research policy, pharmaceutical R&D portfolio management, health-care organization specific priority setting, early Health Technology Assessment (HTA), priority setting for health services and health outcomes research, national health research policy	*Patient priority-setting partnerships*: collaborative methods bringing patients, carers and clinicians together to establish priorities for health research, particularly for health service and health outcome research (Cowan and Oliver 2013). Used often in the United Kingdom for establishing national research priorities for specific areas of health *Payback analysis*: family of return on investment methods, commonly used in setting priorities as part of early HTA and pharmaceutical R&D portfolio management (Chilcott et al. 2003; Fleurence 2007) *Value of information*: willingness-to-pay method for information guiding decision-making, commonly used in setting priorities for pharmaceutical R&D portfolio management, health services research and health outcomes research (Claxton and Sculpher 2006; Myers et al. 2011; 2012; Eckermann et al. 2010; Meltzer et al. 2011; Hassan et al. 2009; Schmidt 2010) *Real options*: option valuation methods for capital budgeting decisions under uncertainty, commonly used for setting priorities in pharmaceutical R&D portfolio management (Lo Nigro et al. 2014; Zapata and Reklaitis 2010; Johal et al. 2008; Hartmann and Hassan 2006; Kolisch et al. 2005; Jacob and Kwak 2003; Rogers et al. 2002; Rosati 2002) *Various clinical trial simulation, investment appraisal and threshold analyses*: wide range of methods spanning from trial design optimization techniques to horizon scanning of trends and unexpected issues and health economic modelling, commonly used in setting priorities as part of early HTA and for health services and health outcomes research (Miller 2005)

- Outranking methods (Varlan and Le Paillier 1999)
- Goal, aspiration or reference-level methods (Hassanzadeh et al. 2014; Patel et al. 2013; Subramanian et al. 2000; Sonntag and Grossman 1999; Grossman 1975)

In contrast with the methodologies in the first set, none of these methods are specific to health research priority setting: all are generic MCDA methods that have been applied to establish health research priorities. Moreover, these methods are not 'comprehensive' priority-setting approaches: they often only provide guidance for the decision-making process itself, while comprehensive priority-setting approaches provide broader guidance for all steps of the priority-setting process (Viergever et al. 2010b).

Finally, the third set of methodologies in Table 12.1 consists of methodologies that do not make use of multiple criteria. For example, an approach that is frequently used in priority-setting exercises for health research in the United Kingdom, the Priority Setting Partnerships approach, only uses one, prespecified criterion (overall importance) to appraise research options (Cowan and Oliver 2013). This set consists of methodologies that are only used in health research priority setting (the Priority Setting Partnerships approach) as well as generic methods for prioritizing various options (most others).

12.3.1.2 An Implicit Link Between Health Research Priority Setting and MCDA

As noted above, this first set of approaches – consisting of many of the dominant approaches to health research priority setting – makes use of multiple criteria, but the explicit links between these approaches and MCDA are minimal: none of them make any mention of MCDA. To consider whether these approaches do apply MCDA (just without explicitly mentioning it), we have taken the key principles of MCDA as recently proposed by the International Society for Pharmacoeconomics and Outcomes Research (ISPOR) MCDA Task Force (IJzerman et al. 2014) and compared these with the characteristics of these three approaches (Okello and Chongtrakul 2000; Rudan et al. 2006; The 3D combined approach matrix: an improved tool for setting priorities in research for health 2009) and with 'the checklist for health research priority setting' (see Box 12.2), a checklist that was developed based on a review of the dominant approaches in health research priority setting and that describes nine 'things to think about' when doing health research priority setting (the checklist also makes no explicit mention of MCDA) (Viergever et al. 2010b). The results of this comparison are described in Table 12.2, which make clear that many of the 'things to think about' that the checklist for health research priority setting describes as important are aimed at promoting the use of criteria, structure, explicitness and transparency – the key principles of MCDA (Viergever et al. 2010b). Many of the specific, comprehensive approaches to health research priority setting (ENHR, CHRNI, CAM) also note to aim to enhance systematicness, explicitness and transparency (Okello and Chongtrakul 2000;

Rudan et al. 2006; The 3D combined approach matrix: an improved tool for setting priorities in research for health 2009) Moreover, the common steps undertaken in these approaches are similar to the steps taken in MCDA. In health research priority setting, a stepwise approach is usually followed that includes (1) the identification of health research options, (2) the (pre-)specification of criteria and their relative weights against which the research options are appraised and (3) the assessment, comparison and prioritization of options based on their performance against the criteria (Viergever et al. 2010b; Okello and Chongtrakul 2000; Rudan et al. 2006; The 3D combined approach matrix: an improved tool for setting priorities in research for health 2009). MCDA approaches generally also follow a series of steps: (1) the identification of options to be appraised, (2) the specification of criteria and their relative weights against which the options are appraised and (3) the assessment, comparison and prioritization of the options based on their performance against the criteria (Devlin and Sussex 2011).

Therefore, while the dominant approaches in health research priority setting do not mention to use MCDA, they do appear to adhere to the principles of MCDA and generally follow similar steps as in MCDA.

Box 12.2

The checklist for health research priority setting

The checklist for health research priority setting (Viergever et al. 2010b) provides guidance for planning and organizing health research prioritization exercises and recommends that there are at least nine things to think about when setting health research priorities:

1. Context: defining the contextual factors that underpin the priority-setting exercise
2. Use of a comprehensive approach: deciding whether a 'comprehensive' approach to priority setting is appropriate
3. Inclusiveness: deciding which stakeholders should be involved and why
4. Information gathering: considering what information should be collected in preparing the priority-setting exercise
5. Planning for implementation: establishing plans for translation of the priorities to actual research (via funding and policies) as soon as possible
6. Criteria: selecting the right criteria for setting priorities
7. Methods for deciding on priorities: deciding what methods to use for identifying research options and for arriving at priorities from a list of research options
8. Evaluation: planning how and when to re-evaluate the established priorities
9. Transparency: making sure to transparently report both the priorities and the priority-setting process

Table 12.2 The characteristics of several 'comprehensive' approaches for health research priority setting and the 'checklist for health research priority setting' (see Box 12.2), assessed against the key principles of multi-criteria decision analysis (MCDA)

According to the ISPOR MCDA Task Force (IJzerman et al. 2014), MCDA, as generally understood…	In health research priority setting …
… comprises a broad set of methodological approaches, stemming from operations research	… a broad set of approaches is used. The 'checklist for health research priority setting' explicitly recommends using a 'comprehensive' approach, which are approaches that provide step-by-step guidance for the entire priority-setting process. Examples of such approaches include The essential national health research (ENHR) strategy (Okello and Chongtrakul 2000), the Child Health and Nutrition Research Initiative (CHNRI) (Rudan et al. 2006), the combined approach matrix (CAM) (The 3D combined approach matrix: an improved tool for setting priorities in research for health 2009) and Priority Setting Partnerships (Petit-Zeman et al. 2010)
… decomposes complex decision problems, where there are many factors to be taken into account ('multiple criteria') by using a set of relevant criteria	… criteria are recommended in many of these approaches, as well as by the checklist for health research priority setting (the exception is the Priority Setting Partnerships which does not recommend the use of multiple criteria but uses one criterion for overall importance). There are ten larger groups of criteria that are typically used in health research priority-setting exercises (McGregor et al. 2014). Different criteria can be used in priority-setting exercises for specific types of research, such as health technology assessments (Noorani et al. 2007) However, priority-setting exercises only rarely use one of the comprehensive approaches listed above – most develop their own methods (Viergever et al. 2010a; McGregor et al. 2014). A review from 2014 of priority-setting exercises in low- and middle-income countries showed that 67 % of these exercises used criteria (McGregor et al. 2014). Amongst research priority-setting exercises organized or coordinated through WHO headquarters, this percentage is lower (10–31 %) (Viergever et al. 2010a)
… provides a way of structuring such decisions and aims to help the decision-maker be clear about what criteria are relevant and the relative importance of each in their decisions	… when criteria are used, emphasis is commonly placed on the judgement of the decision-maker in establishing the values or objectives of the exercise and, to a variable extent, in identifying relevant criteria, in determining their relative importance and in assessing the contribution of each option to each performance criterion Structure is provided by most comprehensive health research priority-setting approaches by providing guidance on Identifying the options (or alternatives) to be appraised Identifying the criteria (or attributes) against which the options are appraised Considering the relative importance between the different criteria Assessing the performance of options against a number of criteria

Table 12.1 (Continued)

According to the ISPOR MCDA Task Force (IJzerman et al. 2014), MCDA, as generally understood…	In health research priority setting …
	Moreover, if the approaches recommend a quantified process, rather than a deliberative process (IJzerman et al. 2014), the approaches also provide guidance on Eliciting weights that reflect the relative importance between the different criteria based on some sort of preference assessment or modelling Using a certain valuation metric to estimate values that reflect the performance of options against a number of criteria Calculating the overall (weight-adjusted or unadjusted) value of options against all the relevant criteria in a performance matrix, supported by some sort of trade-off analysis in order to list, rank, select or sort the various options
… generally entails being explicit about both the criteria and the weights	… explicitness is a key aspect of health research priority setting. This includes explicitness about criteria and the weights that are used but also about the context (because it determines aspects of the priority-setting process); which approach is used (and why); which stakeholders are included as decision-makers (and why); which information needs to be collected; how the priorities will be implemented; how to reach final agreement on priorities, such as via consensus, pooled ranking or both (and why); and when the priorities will be evaluated and revisited (Viergever et al. 2010b)
… facilitates transparent and consistent decisions	… transparent reporting of both the methods (see points under explicitness above), and the results of a health research priority-setting exercise is considered important in most methodologies for health research priority setting. The checklist for health research priority setting, for example, argues that transparency, amongst others, allows for consistent revision of the priorities when they are evaluated (Viergever et al. 2010b)

12.3.2 Health Research Priority Exercises and MCDA

In the previous section, we described the types of methodologies that are being used to set health research priorities. In this section, we present an analysis of a sample of health research priority-setting *exercises*. Specifically, we assessed the degree to which MCDA methods were applied in these exercises. To do so, we assessed the methodologies applied in the 118 studies relating to a total of 91 health research priority exercises listed in a review by McGregor et al. (2014) for health research priority setting in low- and middle-income countries (McGregor et al. 2014). The large majority of these exercises did not explicitly mention to have used an MCDA approach: only one noted to have used MCDA. A minority of studies used a specific, comprehensive health research priority-setting approach (24 used CHNRI, 7 used ENHR and 3 used CAM). As we established in the previous section, these approaches do not explicitly mention MCDA but do adhere to the principles of MCDA and generally follow the same steps as MCDA. Therefore, in this analysis of exercises, we have considered the exercises using these approaches as applying MCDA, only implicitly so (except in the case of two exercises that used the ENHR method but did not describe the explicit use of criteria).

Our analysis of the 118 studies compiled by McGregor et al. showed that:

- While only one of the 118 studies is explicitly mentioned to have used MCDA, more than 60 % of the 118 studies applied some sort of qualitative (23 %) or quantitative (39 %) form of MCDA:
  - Amongst the 27 studies that applied qualitative MCDA, 15 studies applied some sort of listing/sorting model, 5 studies applied ENHR (with use of explicit criteria), 4 studies applied a consensus-based approach and 3 studies applied CAM for the prioritization of research options. All studies listed the prioritized options as their final output, without generating any values or scores for the listed options.
  - Amongst the 46 studies deploying quantitative MCDA, 31 studies deployed a scoring, weighted sum, linear additive model (of which 7 studies used their own scoring, weighted sum, linear additive model and 24 used a specific model (CHNRI)). In addition, 14 studies used a scoring model but not weighted. Finally, one study used the nominal group technique (not weighted), making explicit use of well-defined, multiple criteria. Almost all studies ranked the prioritized options as their final output, using Likert and/or visual analogue scales to measure their performance. Only one study provided a rating without ranking the options (Lawn et al. 2007), and one additional study sorted the prioritized options in a list without further ranking (Chapman et al. 2014).
  - The remaining 45 studies (that did not apply MCDA methods) applied a wide range of formal or less formal methods, including consultative group processes (12 %); priority listing/sorting approaches (8 %); informal consensus-based methods (7 %); ENHR with no use of explicit criteria (2 %); stepwise approaches, i.e. combinations of literature reviews, key informant interviews and consultative group processes (4 %); formal consensus-based methods (e.g. the nominal group technique with no use of explicit criteria) (3 %); survey-based methods (2 %); and concept-mapping approaches (1 %).
- As it becomes clear from the previous points, in this analysis, we did not consider the assignment of weights to criteria a condition for MCDA. Although in all of the studies that applied quantitative MCDA weights could have been assigned to criteria through a simple, weighted sum approach, in order to reflect their relative importance, 31 studies assigned weights to criteria and 15 did not. We looked in more detail at the seven non-CHNRI studies that assigned weights to criteria: five of these assigned equal weights to all criteria and two studies assigned unequal weights.

- In terms of option identification, only one study used a list of predetermined research options (Technical workshop on setting research priorities for reproductive health in crisis settings: Summary of Proceedings 2011). All other studies constructed the options through similar techniques including Delphi/Hanlon methods, consultative group processes, surveys or combinations of literature reviews, key informant interviews and group discussions. Studies deploying the CHNRI methodology used an outranking approach of direct pairwise comparisons and elimination of options.
- In contrast, the majority of the studies applied predefined criteria, using either a previously established framework (Viergever et al. 2010b; Rudan et al. 2006; Varkevisser et al. 2003) or without specifying further. The few studies that determined criteria as part of the priority-setting process employed a mix of consultative group processes.
- Only one study included some form of deterministic sensitivity analysis to address uncertainty in the priority-setting process (Madi et al. 2007). In addition, a few studies calculated mean scores and standard deviations for the ranked options.

12.3.3 Implications: Health Research Priority Setting and MCDA

In our view, three conclusions follow from the two sections above that assess the role of MCDA in health research priority-setting methodologies and exercises:

1. Many health research priority-setting methodologies and exercises adhere to the principles of MCDA and follow the same steps as in MCDA.
2. However, many of these methodologies and exercises do not explicitly make reference to MCDA. Particularly, many of the dominant approaches for health research priority setting, such as ENHR, CHNRI and CAM, do not make any mention of MCDA, while they all adhere to MCDA's principles and propose multi-criteria decision models for establishing health research priorities that emphasize structure, explicitness and transparency. Moreover, in the review by McGregor, only one health research priority-setting exercise in low- and middle-income countries noted to have applied MCDA, while, according to our analysis and interpretation of methods deployed, more than 60 % in fact appears to have applied some form of qualitative or quantitative MCDA.
3. There are issues with the quality of priority-setting exercises in the area of health research. Several reviews in health research priority setting have shown that amongst the exercises that use multiple criteria, the degree of explicitness, systematicness and transparency varies on a grey scale from non-existent to highly explicit, systematic and transparent (McGregor et al. 2014; Viergever et al. 2010b; Reveiz et al. 2013). In our own review of the 118 health research priority-setting studies in low- and middle-income countries compiled by

McGregor, we found that research options were not always independent, the criteria against which options were prioritized were not always preference independent or mutually exclusive, scoring options based on Likert and/or visual analogue scales masked the frequent lack of objective data and validated measurement instruments for some of the criteria considered and priority-setting outcomes are generally not certain but the scoring models applied only rarely dealt with that uncertainty. In the next section, we provide suggestions for how the quality of these exercises might be improved.

12.4 Methodological Development in Health Research Priority Setting: The Way Forward

This chapter shows that there is a wide range of health research priority-setting methodologies and approaches that all take a different view on how health research priorities should be set. Because of the different contexts for which health research priorities are set (in terms of coverage, scope and aims), one best practice or gold standard for health research priority setting is not appropriate (Viergever et al. 2010b). However, there is consensus that health research priority-setting exercises can benefit from process guidance and that there are at least nine aspects to any health research priority-setting process on which such guidance is needed (see Box 12.2) (Viergever et al. 2010b). Several recommendations follow from this chapter with regard to next steps for guidance development in the area of health research priority setting.

First, while MCDA has become a well-recognized methodology for health *intervention* priority setting (IJzerman et al. 2014), as we have shown above, explicit reference to MCDA is almost completely absent from the methodological literature on health *research* priority setting. The large majority of the health research priority-setting exercises that have been conducted in recent years and the dominant approaches to health research priority setting (Viergever et al. 2010b; Okello and Chongtrakul 2000; Rudan et al. 2006; The 3D combined approach matrix: an improved tool for setting priorities in research for health 2009; Cowan and Oliver 2013) do not make any mention of MCDA. As we have shown in this chapter, while not all methodologies for setting health research priority setting can be classified as MCDA, most do adhere to the principles of MCDA and follow the same steps as in MCDA, even when they do not explicitly make mention of MCDA. The methodological development in health research priority setting appears to have taken place largely separately from development in the area of MCDA for health intervention priority setting in the past two decades. This lack of explicit use of MCDA in health research priority-setting exercises may reflect a lack of awareness by health research priority-setting experts on the body of literature around MCDA. In our view, it would be advantageous to bring these two bodies of literature together. By recognizing that the dominant approaches to health research priority setting apply MCDA, the field of health research priority setting could benefit from the experience that has been developed with the application of MCDA, both in health and in other areas.

This could, for example, expand the number of methodologies and approaches that decision-makers in health research can choose from to set health research priorities. Moreover, more explicit use of MCDA in health research priority setting would allow decision-makers to benefit from the guidance that has been developed in the field of MCDA for more specific aspects of the priority-setting process, such as on the theories that underlie MCDA (e.g. multi-attribute utility theory), stakeholder mapping and selection, identifying and choosing criteria, eliciting weights to address the relative importance of criteria, selecting the most appropriate technique for scoring the options, aggregating these scores, reaching agreement on the final list of priorities (e.g. consensus methods or majority rules methods), presenting the priorities and implementing the priorities (IJzerman et al. 2014).

Second, in order for health research priority-setting exercises to benefit from such methodological developments, it is important that these exercises apply standard approaches to priority setting. Yet, several reviews, and our own analysis for this chapter, have shown that the use of standard approaches to priority setting is rare in health research priority-setting exercises (Viergever et al. 2010a; McGregor et al. 2014). Following best practices, such as the checklist for health research priority setting (Viergever et al. 2010b) or one of the specific, comprehensive approaches to health research priority setting (ENHR, CHNRI, CAM) (Okello and Chongtrakul 2000; Rudan et al. 2006; The 3D combined approach matrix: an improved tool for setting priorities in research for health 2009), can help health research priority-setting exercises to adhere to the MCDA principles of structure, explicitness and transparency. As noted by McGregor, in her review of health research priority-setting exercises in low- and middle-income countries, 'While not consistently used, the application of established methods provides a means of identifying health research priorities in a repeatable and transparent manner' (McGregor et al. 2014).

Third, lessons might be learned from comparisons between the fields of health intervention priority setting and health research priority setting, for example, by comparing the preparatory activities that are generally conducted in these two fields, by comparing how priority-setting methods are generally applied and by comparing how established priorities are implemented and reported. Studying any differences in these areas in more depth and creating further clarity on what the two fields might learn from each other might help both fields to advance methodologically. Particularly, the field of health research priority setting might be able to learn from the experience that has been acquired in health intervention priority setting with using objective data to populate performance matrices. Although, as we have argued above, the different conceptual nature of research priority setting necessitates a more subjective approach, there might be middle ground that deserves to be explored more than it has been to date. In many health research priority-setting exercises, research options are scored against criteria by stakeholders while for some criteria, such as the burden of a particular health problem, more objective judgements might be feasible. Vice versa, the field of health research priority setting has developed extensive experience with the inclusion of a wide range of stakeholders, including patients, service providers, researchers, policymakers and others in the priority-setting process and with soliciting subjective judgements about the value of research options against criteria (Viergever et al. 2010b). In areas of health intervention priority setting where objective data are not available and which are based more on stakeholder opinion, this experience may prove useful.

References

Bahadori M, Teimourzadeh E, Farzaneh A, Nejati M (2011) Prioritizing research needs: insights from a healthcare organization in Iran. Arch Pharm Pract 2(3):135–140

Baltussen R, Niessen L (2006) Priority setting of health interventions: the need for multi-criteria decision analysis. Cost Eff Resour Alloc 4(1):14. doi:10.1186/1478-7547-4-14

Baltussen R, Stolk E, Chisholm D, Aikins M (2006) Towards a multi-criteria approach for priority setting: an application to Ghana. Health Econ 15(7):689–696. doi:10.1002/hec.1092

Baltussen R, ten Asbroek AHA, Koolman X, Shrestha N, Bhattarai P, Niessen LW (2007) Priority setting using multiple criteria: should a lung health programme be implemented in Nepal? Health Policy Plan 22(3):178–185. doi:10.1093/heapol/czm010

Baltussen R, Youngkong S, Paolucci F, Niessen L (2010) Multi-criteria decision analysis to prioritize health interventions: capitalizing on first experiences. Health Policy 96(3):262–264. doi:10.1016/j.healthpol.2010.01.009

Belton V, Stewart T (2002) Multiple criteria decision analysis: an integrated approach. Springer, Boston

Callahan D (1999) Shaping biomedical research priorities: the case of the National Institutes of Health. Health Care Anal 7(2):115–129. doi:10.1023/A:1009401507982

Chapman E, Reveiz L, Sangalang S et al (2014) A survey study identified global research priorities for decreasing maternal mortality. J Clin Epidemiol 67(3):314–324. doi:10.1016/j.jclinepi.2013.10.007

Chilcott J, Brennan A, Booth A, Karnon J, Tappenden P (2003) The role of modelling in prioritising and planning clinical trials. Health Technol Assess 7(23):iii, 1–125. Available at: http://www.ncbi.nlm.nih.gov/pubmed/14499052. Accessed 21 Jan 2015

Claxton KP, Sculpher MJ (2006) Using value of information analysis to prioritise health research: some lessons from recent UK experience. Pharmacoeconomics 24(11):1055–1068. Available at: http://www.ncbi.nlm.nih.gov/pubmed/17067191. Accessed 21 Jan 2015

Cowan K, Oliver S (2013) The James lind alliance guidebook: Version 5. James Lind Alliance, London. Available at: http://www.lindalliance.org/pdfs/JLA_Oliver and Gray report 07_01_20.pdf

Devlin N, Sussex J (2011) Incorporating multiple criteria in HTA: methods and processes. Office of Health Economics, London. Available at: https://www.ohe.org/publications/incorporating-multiple-criteria-hta-methods-and-processes

Doble B, Harris A, Thomas DM, Fox S, Lorgelly P (2013) Multiomics medicine in oncology: assessing effectiveness, cost-effectiveness and future research priorities for the molecularly unique individual. Pharmacogenomics 14(12):1405–1417. doi:10.2217/pgs.13.142

Eckermann S, Karnon J, Willan AR (2010) The value of value of information: best informing research design and prioritization using current methods. Pharmacoeconomics 28(9):699–709. doi:10.2165/11537370-000000000-00000

Fleurence RL (2007) Setting priorities for research: a practical application of "payback" and expected value of information. Health Econ 16(12):1345–1357. doi:10.1002/hec.1225

Frascati manual: proposed standard practice for surveys on research and experimental development, 6th edn. Organisation for Economic Co-operation and Development (OECD), paris (2002)

Frenk J (1993) The new public health. Annu Rev Public Health 14:469–490. doi:10.1146/annurev.pu.14.050193.002345

Ghaffar A (2009) Setting research priorities by applying the combined approach matrix. Indian J Med Res 129(4):368–375. Available at: http://www.ncbi.nlm.nih.gov/pubmed/19535830. Accessed 20 Mar 2015

Grossman D (1975) Dynamic time-staged model for R&D portfolio planning—a real world case. R D Manag 5(S1):81–87. doi:10.1111/j.1467-9310.1975.tb01358.x

Hartmann M, Hassan A (2006) Application of real options analysis for pharmaceutical R&D project valuation—Empirical results from a survey. Res Policy 35(3):343–354. doi:10.1016/j.respol.2005.12.005

Hassan C, Hunink MGM, Laghi A et al (2009) Value-of-information analysis to guide future research in colorectal cancer screening. Radiology 253(3):745–752. doi:10.1148/radiol.2533090234

Hassanzadeh F, Modarres M, Nemati HR, Amoako-Gyampah K (2014) A robust R&D project portfolio optimization model for pharmaceutical contract research organizations. Int J Prod Econ 158:18–27. doi:10.1016/j.ijpe.2014.07.001

Health technologies: report by the secretariat. World Health Organization Executive Board document EB 121/11. (2007). Available at: http://apps.who.int/iris/bitstream/10665/22966/1/B121_11-en.pdf

Highlights in early health technology assessment (2011) Department Health Technology & Services Research MIRA institute for Biomedical Technology & Technical Medicine, Enschede

Hummel JM, Rossum W van, Verkerke GJ, Rakhorst G (2000) The effects of team expert choice on group decision-making in collaborative new product development: a pilot study. J Multi-Criteria Decis Anal 9(1–3):90–98. Available at: http://doc.utwente.nl/71575/1/Hummel00effects.pdf. Accessed 13 Feb 2015

Husereau D, Boucher M, Noorani H (2010) Priority setting for health technology assessment at CADTH. Int J Technol Assess Health Care 26(3):341–347. doi:10.1017/S0266462310000383

Ijzerman MJ, Steuten LMG (2011) Early assessment of medical technologies to inform product development and market access. Appl Health Econ Health Policy 9(5):331–347

IJzerman M, Devlin N, Thokala P, Marsh K, on behalf of the ISPOR MCDA Task Force (2014) "Multi-criteria decision analysis for healthcare decision making", presented at the ISPOR 17th Annual European Congress Amsterdam, The Netherlands 8–12 November 2014. Available at: http://www.slideshare.net/OHENews/mcda-devlin-nov14

Jacob WF, Kwak YH (2003) In search of innovative techniques to evaluate pharmaceutical R&D projects. Technovation 23(4):291–296. doi:10.1016/S0166-4972(01)00116-X

Johal SS, Oliver P, Williams HC (2008) Better decision making for evaluating new medical device projects: a real options approach. J Med Mark 8(2):101–112. Available at: http://www.rti.org/publications/abstract.cfm?pubid=17672

Kahraman C, Süder A, Kaya İ (2014) Fuzzy multicriteria evaluation of health research investments. Technol Econ Dev Econ 20(2):210–226. doi:10.3846/20294913.2013.876560

Kolisch R, Meyer K, Mohr R (2005) Maximizing R&D Portfolio Value. Res Manag 48(3):33–39. Available at: http://www.ingentaconnect.com/content/iri/rtm/2005/00000048/00000003/art00006?crawler=true. Accessed 13 Feb 2015

Lawn JE, Manandhar A, Haws RA, Darmstadt GL (2007) Reducing one million child deaths from birth asphyxia–a survey of health systems gaps and priorities. Health Res Policy Syst 5:4. doi:10.1186/1478-4505-5-4

Lo Nigro G, Morreale A, Enea G (2014) Open innovation: a real option to restore value to the biopharmaceutical R&D. Int J Prod Econ 149:183–193. doi:10.1016/j.ijpe.2013.02.004

Madi BC, Hussein J, Hounton S, D'Ambruoso L, Achadi E, Arhinful DK (2007) Setting priorities for safe motherhood programme evaluation: a participatory process in three developing countries. Health Policy 83(1):94–104. doi:10.1016/j.healthpol.2007.01.006

McGregor S, Henderson KJ, Kaldor JM (2014) How are health research priorities set in low and middle income countries? A systematic review of published reports. Molyneux S (ed). PLoS One 9(9):e108787. doi:10.1371/journal.pone.0108787

Meltzer DO, Hoomans T, Chung JW, Basu A (2011) Minimal modeling approaches to value of information analysis for health research. Med Decis Making 31(6):E1–E22. doi:10.1177/0272989X11412975

Miller P (2005) Role of pharmacoeconomic analysis in R&D decision making: when, where, how? Pharmacoeconomics 23(1):1–12. Available at: http://www.ncbi.nlm.nih.gov/pubmed/15693724. Accessed 13 Feb 2015

Myers E, Sanders GD, Ravi D et al (2011) Evaluating the potential use of modeling and value-of-information analysis for future research prioritization within the evidence-based practice center program. Agency for Healthcare Research and Quality (US), Rockville. Available at: http://www.ncbi.nlm.nih.gov/books/NBK62134/

Myers E, McBroom AJ, Shen L, Posey RE, Gray R, Sanders GD (2012) Value-of-information analysis for patient-centered outcomes research prioritization. Duke Evidence-based Practice Center, Durham

Noorani HZ, Husereau DR, Boudreau R, Skidmore B (2007) Priority setting for health technology assessments: a systematic review of current practical approaches. Int J Technol Assess Health Care 23(3):310–315. doi:10.1017/S026646230707050X

Okello D, Chongtrakul P; The COHRED Working Group on Priority Setting (2000) A manual for research priority setting using the ENHR strategy. The Council on Health Research for Development (COHRED), Lausanne

Oliver S, Gray J (2006) A bibliography of research reports about patients', clinicians' and researchers' priorities for new research. James Lind Alliance, London

Owlia P, Eftekhari MB, Forouzan AS, Bahreini F, Farahani M, Ghanei M (2011) Health research priority setting in Iran: introduction to a bottom up approach. J Res Med Sci 16(5):691–698. Available at: http://www.pubmedcentral.nih.gov/articlerender.fcgi?artid=3214383&tool=pmcentrez&rendertype=abstract. Accessed 13 Feb 2015

Patel NR, Ankolekar S, Antonijevic Z, Rajicic N (2013) A mathematical model for maximizing the value of phase 3 drug development portfolios incorporating budget constraints and risk. Stat Med 32(10):1763–1777. doi:10.1002/sim.5731

Petit-Zeman S, Firkins L, Scadding JW (2010) The James Lind Alliance: tackling research mismatches. Lancet 376(9742):667–669. doi:10.1016/S0140-6736(10)60712-X

Phelps C, Madhavan G, Sangha K et al (2014) A priority-setting aid for new vaccine candidates. Proc Natl Acad Sci U S A 111(9):3199–3200. doi:10.1073/pnas.1400945111

Phillips LD, Bana e Costa CA (2007) Transparent prioritisation, budgeting and resource allocation with multi-criteria decision analysis and decision conferencing. Ann Oper Res 154:51–68

Research priorities for the environment, agriculture and infectious diseases of poverty: technical report of the TDR thematic reference group on environment, agriculture and infectious diseases of poverty (2013) World Health Organization, Geneva

Reveiz L, Elias V, Terry RF, Alger J, Becerra-Posada F (2013) Comparison of national health research priority-setting methods and characteristics in Latin America and the Caribbean, 2002–2012. Rev Panam Salud Publica 34(1):1–13. Available at: http://www.ncbi.nlm.nih.gov/pubmed/24006014. Accessed 20 Nov 2013

Rogers MJ, Gupta A, Maranas CD (2002) Real options based analysis of optimal pharmaceutical research and development portfolios. Ind Eng Chem Res 41(25):6607–6620

Rosati N (2002) Decision analysis and drug development portfolio management: uncovering the real options value of your projects. Expert Rev Pharmacoecon Outcomes Res 2(2):179–187. doi:10.1586/14737167.2.2.179

Røttingen J-A, Regmi S, Eide M et al (2013) Mapping available health R&D data: what's there, what's missing and what role for a Global Observatory. Lancet 382(9900):1286–1307

Rudan I, El Arifeen S, Black RE (2006) A new approach for systematic priority setting in child health research investment. Published by Child Health and Nutrition Research Initiative (CHNRI), Dhaka

Schmidt C (2010) Researchers consider value-of-information theory for selecting trials. J Natl Cancer Inst 102(3):144–146. doi:10.1093/jnci/djq015

Smith N, Mitton C, Peacock S, Cornelissen E, MacLeod S (2009) Identifying research priorities for health care priority setting: a collaborative effort between managers and researchers. BMC Health Serv Res 9:165. doi:10.1186/1472-6963-9-165

Sonntag C, Grossman TA (1999) End-user modeling improves R&D management at AgrEvo Canada, Inc. Interfaces (Providence) 29(5):132–142. Available at: http://pubsonline.informs.org/doi/abs/10.1287/inte.29.5.132?journalCode=inte. Accessed 13 Feb 2015

Stewart R, Oliver S (2008) A systematic map of studies of patients' and clinicians' research priorities. James Lind Alliance, London. Available at: http://www.lindalliance.org/pdfs/JLA Internal Reports/090712_JLAreport_RS_map_studies_PPI & Clinicians_research priorities_with appendices.pdf

Subramanian D, Pekny JF, Reklaitis GV (2000) A simulation—optimization framework for addressing combinatorial and stochastic aspects of an R&D pipeline management problem. Comput Chem Eng 24(2–7):1005–1011. doi:10.1016/S0098-1354(00)00535-4

Technical workshop on setting research priorities for reproductive health in crisis settings: Summary of Proceedings (2011) Centers for Disease Control and Prevention International Emergency & Refugee Health Branch, Atlanta

The 3D combined approach matrix: an improved tool for setting priorities in research for health (2009) Global Forum for Health Research, Geneva

Tromp N, Baltussen R (2012) Mapping of multiple criteria for priority setting of health interventions: an aid for decision makers. BMC Health Serv Res 12:454. doi:10.1186/1472-6963-12-454

Varkevisser CM, Pathmanathan I, Brownlee A (2003). Module 3: identifying and prioritising problems for research. In: Designing and conducting health systems research projects: volume I: Proposal development and fieldwork. KIT publishers and the International Development Research Centre (IDRC), Amsterdam. Available at: http://www.idrc.ca/EN/Resources/Publications/openebooks/069-1/index.html#page_27

Varlan E, Le Paillier R (1999) Multicriteria decision making for contract research organisation choice in the pharmaceutical industry. J Oper Res Soc 50(9):943–948

Velmurugan R, Selvamuthukumar S (2012) The analytic network process for the pharmaceutical sector: multi criteria decision making to select the suitable method for the preparation of nanoparticles. Daru 20(1):59. doi:10.1186/2008-2231-20-59

Viergever RF, Terry R, Matsoso MP (2010) Health research prioritization at WHO: an overview of methodology and high level analysis of WHO led health research priority setting exercises. Geneva. Available at: http://www.who.int/rpc/publications/Health_research_prioritization_at_WHO.pdf

Viergever RF, Olifson S, Ghaffar A, Terry RF (2010b) A checklist for health research priority setting: nine common themes of good practice. Health Res Policy Syst 8(1):36. doi:10.1186/1478-4505-8-36

Viergever RF, Kitur IU, Chan G et al (2014) The Papua New Guinea national health and HIV research agenda. Lancet Glob Health 2(2):e74–e75. doi:10.1016/S2214-109X(13)70165-7

WHA document A63/22: WHO's role and responsibilities in health research: draft WHO strategy on research for health (2010)

Working Party of National Experts on Science and Technology Indicators (2007) Revised field of science and technology (FOS) classification in the Frascati manual (DSTI/EAS/STP/NESTI(2006)19/FINAL). Organisation for Economic Co-operation and Development (OECD), Paris

Youngkong S, Teerawattananon Y, Tantivess S, Baltussen R (2012) Multi-criteria decision analysis for setting priorities on HIV/AIDS interventions in Thailand. Health Res Policy Syst 10:6. doi:10.1186/1478-4505-10-6

Zapata JC, Reklaitis GV (2010) Valuation of project portfolios: an endogenously discounted method. Eur J Oper Res 206(3):653–665. doi:10.1016/j.ejor.2010.03.015

Chapter 13
MCDA for the Development of Clinical Practice Guidelines and for the Prioritization Clinical Research Questions

Cheri Deal, Michele Tony, Hanane Khoury, Gihad Nesrallah, Ahmed A. Al-Jaishi, and Mireille Goetghebeur

Abstract The current challenges facing clinicians today include the integration of the best available evidence into their clinical care of patients and into their prioritization of research questions still requiring answers. Multicriteria decision analysis (MCDA) is an application of decision analytics that can provide a method to clarify available evidence, prioritize these research questions, and support decision-making regarding how to address most critical research needs. In this chapter, two case studies illustrate the use of MCDA to support decision-making in clinical research.

The first case study illustrates application of the structuring aspect of a comprehensive MCDA framework to organize data and questions relevant to the development of clinical practice guidelines (CPG) for a rare genetic condition, Prader-Willi syndrome (PWS), and its complementarity with the Appraisal of

C. Deal, MD, PhD (✉)
Endocrinology and Diabetes Service, CHU Sainte-Justine and Faculty of Medicine, University of Montreal, Montreal, QC, Canada
e-mail: cheri.l.deal@umontreal.ca

M. Tony, MSc, PhD Cand
School of Public health, University of Montreal, Montreal, QC, Canada

H. Khoury, PhD
LASER Analytica, Montreal, QC, Canada

G. Nesrallah, MD, MSc
Li Ka Shing Knowledge Institute, St. Michael's Hospital, Toronto, ON, Canada

A.A. Al-Jaishi, MSc, PhD Cand
London Health Sciences Centre, London, ON, Canada

M. Goetghebeur, PhD, MEng
School of Public Health, University of Montreal
and LASER Analytica, Montréal, Québec, Canada
e-mail: mm.goetghebeur@umontreal.ca

© Springer International Publishing AG 2017
K. Marsh et al. (eds.), *Multi-Criteria Decision Analysis to Support Healthcare Decisions*, DOI 10.1007/978-3-319-47540-0_13

Guidelines Research and Evaluation (AGREE) Collaboration recommendations for CPGs.

In the second case study, application of MCDA to prioritize clinical research questions involving dialysis for kidney failure is illustrated by two examples. The first details a methodology to rank comparative effectiveness of research hypotheses likely to generate most useful data for clinical practice improvement, and the second shows its application to the identification of priorities to conduct registry-based trials.

These case studies illustrate that MCDA provides a method to structure clinical practice guidelines and to prioritize clinical research questions, and to support identification of the most critical needs from a holistic perspective, in order to advance patient care. MCDA participants of the case studies presented here reported that MCDA provided a valid, transparent, and pragmatic process to prioritize clinical research and identify best practices to improve patient management in the midst of scarce research and healthcare resources. Further research is warranted to develop and integrate MCDA in clinical research and practice to contribute to better health and sustainable healthcare.

13.1 Introduction

Clinical practice guideline (CPG) development is now viewed as generally desirable by dispensers, users, and payers of healthcare; their principal goal is to improve quality of care (Cecamore et al. 2011). One of the major drawbacks to the CPG paradigm, however, is its still limited use by healthcare providers. This reticence is based on innumerable criticisms, including an "over-rationalist model implicit in evidence-based health care" (Gabbay and le 2004) as well as concerns for methodological difficulties encountered during the knowledge synthesis process, generalizability, ease of application for both practitioner and patient, inherent conflicts of interest, and the as yet identified or unidentified gaps in our knowledge that can make us wonder if we are missing a bigger question (Doherty 2005). Factors influencing guideline development, such as the stakeholders involved (patients, physicians, allied healthcare professionals, industry, government) and the cultural, social, and political context in which they will be applied, may make a seemingly scientifically and statistically robust document less useful (Woolf et al. 1999).

Evidence-based medicine (EBM) is the cornerstone of the CPG, and as very succinctly put by Saarni and Gylling (2004) in their thoughtful essay, EBM guidelines exert a "fundamental influence on certain key aspects of medical professionalism." This professionalism is called into question daily, for example, when the clinician is faced with the human being sitting in her examining room with a rare disease and a guideline putting a cost on her expensive medical intervention plan, for which a (less than perfect) medical literature supports it as useful, as does her clinical experience.

On a more philosophical level, does she, or should she, "rank" the implications of her decision for this patient with those for her interventions for the other five patients in the waiting room with the more common problems that will require short-term, inexpensive solutions with proven good outcomes? Or should the clinician try to explain the concept of "number needed to treat (NNT)" to the family whose critically ill child may, but probably will not, benefit from a life-prolonging or quality of life-improving drug? Given that the side effect profile is acceptable to the physician and family, and that there are those for whom the drug has worked, is NNT relevant to this patient-physician interaction? These and other ethical challenges are becoming more prevalent as medical diagnostics and interventions become more costly, and it appears to many clinicians that the CPG does not always address them. And even if the professional and ethical challenges to following an evidence-based medical practice are hopefully surmountable as EBM evolves, at the very least, as one editorial on the subject stated, "doing EBM well—like most worthwhile endeavors—is hard" (Smith 2004).

Over the last 12 years, in part stimulated by the EBM movement, the social sciences have begun to study the way in which clinicians obtain knowledge and develop their clinical method, and the term mindline has come to refer to the "internalized and collectively reinforced tacit guidelines" that clinicians (and patients) use in daily practice, far more than CPGs. Consider the common occurrence of patients with several chronic illnesses, when following the three or more CPG recommendations for each condition would become prohibitive to the patient and likely result in vastly reduced adherence to treatments (Buffel du Vaure et al. 2016). How are clinicians using their experience and knowledge base to come up with a pragmatic approach to treating these complex patients? To the EBM community, mindlines may seem akin to heresy, but they are better understood in terms of the philosophical and theoretical framework behind the concept. The concept speaks to the clinician, however, in that it clearly supports a need for a more *holistic* view of how to approach best practice (Wieringa and Greenhalgh 2015).

The final stage of the CPG process is their dissemination and their implementation in routine clinical practice. Much has been written about the reasons limiting CPG use, including (but not limited to) their sometimes cumbersome use, their perceived oversimplification of the clinical problem at hand, their potential use in litigation and an inability to reconcile patient preferences with the guidelines (Cabana et al. 1999). Attempts have been made to improve their use, including not only how guidelines are derived from available data but also how the message is packaged and presented to intended users (Kastner et al. 2015). The identification of barriers to guideline implementation is one of the key elements of a good CPG that is discussed in frameworks proposed to evaluate and improve CPG development such as the Appraisal of Guidelines Research and Evaluation (AGREE) Collaboration (http://www.agreetrust.org/). This often includes the transparent identification and ranking of the unanswered research questions that may, in fact, be hampering a wider acceptance of a particular clinical guideline. It is generally felt that the quality and importance of the original research hypotheses are also a sine qua non of good clinical research and, hence, good clinical practice guidelines.

With these shortcomings to EBM-driven CPGs in mind, multicriteria decision analysis (MCDA) offers much to the clinician including a means (1) to reflect on their intervention and to the epistemological underpinnings, (2) to consider all aspects of the decision-making process that are important when weighing evidence and nonevidence (i.e., the absence of evidence), (3) to structure guideline development, and most importantly (4) to make CPGs as transparent as possible. MCDA structures complex decision problems into a set of criteria (Chapter 4). Each criterion of decision is weighted—a step that allows decision-makers to clarify their perspective and values, and the performance of the intervention for each criterion is scored, allowing an objective identification of its weaknesses and strengths. Although MCDA may be perceived as not intuitive and potentially usurping decision-making authority, if kept simple, it facilitates an important dialogue between end users (patients and clinicians), clinical investigators, researchers, and payers. It also forces decision-makers to think hard about what they value, why they value it, and in what context they value it.

In this chapter, applications of holistic MCDA to support decision-making for guideline development as well as to support prioritization of clinical research are illustrated with two case studies. For the illustration of MCDA application to CPG development, we selected *EVIDEM* (*E*vidence and *V*alues: *I*mpact on *DE*cision*M*aking) comprehensive and adaptable framework developed collaboratively with an open source philosophy designed to stimulate reflection on all aspects of decision and on the evidence available. *EVIDEM* (https://www.evidem.org/) is an innovative, multipurpose, and pragmatic instrument which allows the synthesis of evidence according to Health Technology Assessment (HTA) principles (Chapter 8) and enables clarification of the different perspectives of decision-makers. EVIDEM includes a comprehensive set of decision criteria (Table 13.1) and a step-by-step process to synthesize and validate evidence for each criterion. Criteria of the framework were defined based on an extensive analysis of the literature and decision processes around the world as well as discussions with a wide range of healthcare stakeholders. They were designed to fulfill MCDA methodological requirements and are rooted in the ethical foundations of healthcare (providing care that matters to the individual patient, best serving the population, sustainability). The open-source EVIDEM tools are developed by the EVIDEM Collaboration, a not-for-profit collaborative with members from 40 countries, translated into 11 languages and run by an international board of directors. The generic tools are meant to be adapted to the context of applications and are used to support policy and clinical decision-making in several regions of the world, including by the WHO.

We have purposely chosen one of the most difficult clinical challenges for this case study: the use of growth hormone (GH) in Prader-Willi syndrome. The CPG example we use examines an expensive treatment with potentially serious side effects, given to children by daily injections, it involves a rare genetic condition which limits sample sizes for clinical trials, it must recognize that the goals of treatment differ among clinicians and among families, its levels of evidence are

Table 13.1 List of criteria of the EVIDEM framework, definitions, and methodology used during the preparation of the clinical practice guidelines for GH therapy in Prader-Willi syndrome (Growth Hormone Research Society Workshop on Adult Growth Hormone Deficiency 1998; Atkins et al. 2005; Busse et al. 2002; Centre for Evidence Based Medicine 2010; Daniels 1999, 2001; Evers et al. 2005; Gerkens et al. 2008; Goetghebeur et al. 2008, 2010; Gruskin and Daniels 2008; Ho 2007; Jadad et al. 1996; Jehu-Appiah et al. 2008; Persad et al. 2009; The STROBE group 2007; World Health Organization 2004)

Criteria	Definition	Methodology used to synthesize evidence
Disease impact		
D1—disease severity	Severity of the health condition of patients treated with the proposed intervention (or severity of the health condition that is to be prevented) with respect to mortality, disability, impact on quality of life, clinical course (i.e., acuteness, clinical stages)	Essential information needed to understand the targeted health condition and its consequences will be provided including a description of the condition (e.g., definition, symptoms, etiology, comorbidities, and associated risks) and its progression; impact of the condition on mortality, morbidity, and quality of life; and stages or subtypes of the condition that differentiate interventions and target populations. Medical literature consulted on disease mechanisms, course and prognosis, focusing on high-quality reviews.
D2—size of population	The number of people affected by the condition (treated or prevented by the proposed intervention) among a specified population at a specified time can be expressed as annual number of new cases (annual incidence) and/or proportion of the population affected at a certain point of time (prevalence)	The size of population affected by the condition identified through the annual number of new cases (annual incidence) and/or the proportion of the population affected (prevalence). Data obtained from relevant published epidemiological studies, recent reviews or national statistics and presented in evidence tables to facilitate comparison (Busse et al. 2002)
Therapeutic context of intervention		
C1—clinical guidelines	Concurrence of the proposed intervention (or similar alternatives) with the current consensus of a group of experts on what constitutes state-of-the-art practices in the management of the targeted health condition; guidelines are usually developed via an explicit process and are intended to improve clinical practice	The status of the intervention in the management of the targeted health condition captured from available expert consensus guidelines. Information on the place of the intervention in therapy and levels of recommendation gathered and presented in tables

(continued)

Table 13.1 (continued)

Criteria	Definition	Methodology used to synthesize evidence
C2—comparative interventions limitations *(unmet needs)*	Shortcomings of comparative interventions in their ability to prevent, cure, or ameliorate the condition targeted; also includes shortcomings with respect to safety, patient-reported outcomes, and convenience	Limitations of comparative interventions regarding efficacy, safety, and patient-reported outcomes, as well as populations eligible to these interventions retrieved from recent reviews in prominent journals
Intervention outcomes		
I1—improvement of efficacy/effectiveness	Capacity of the proposed intervention to produce a desired (beneficial) change in signs, symptoms or course of the targeted condition above and beyond beneficial changes produced by alternative interventions. Includes efficacy and effectiveness data, as available	Criterion divided into subcriteria to allow for separate reporting and appraisal of six outcomes of growth hormone treatment measured in patients with PWS (i.e., growth, body composition, metabolic effects, exercise tolerance, motor development, and bone composition). Priority given to peer-reviewed comparative studies (randomized-controlled trials [RCTs] and observational) and meta-analyses (e.g., Cochrane reviews); other types of studies included if evidence for certain outcomes of interest is limited. Data reported by study (not by publication) to avoid reporting duplicate publications (Busse et al. 2002). In a first step, evidence from RCTs and comparative observational trials organized into comprehensive evidence tables, including description of trials (e.g., type of study, setting, intervention, outcomes measured, duration of treatment, number of patients, patient age, patient inclusion/exclusion, type of analysis, patient disposition) and data available for each outcome thus complying with best practices in HTA (Busse et al. 2002). These comprehensive tables used as a basis to synthesize the most critical data for each outcome in the EVIDEM matrix format, i.e., in easy-to-read concise tables providing sufficient information to allow a wide range of healthcare stakeholders to reach an opinion. The standard format included study information (authors, year, design, level of evidence, number of patients and age, treatment, and duration) and data (results for intervention and comparators, difference, and statistical significance). Study limitations (e.g., selection bias, drop-out rates) analyzed and reported in semiquantitative instruments (see Table 13.3, criterion Q2)

I2—improvement of safety and tolerability	Reduction in intervention-related health effects that are harmful or undesired compared to alternative interventions	Possible harms related to the use of the intervention and its comparators investigated and presented in the most informative way. All-cause as well as treatment-related adverse events for the intervention and key comparators reported in registries, clinical studies (RCTs and observational), and product monographs synthesized in evidence tables to allow for comparison among various sources. Data on serious adverse events and deaths, discontinuations due to adverse events, and warnings collected and reported
I3—improvement of patient-reported outcomes	Capacity of the proposed intervention to produce beneficial changes in patient-reported outcomes (PROs) (e.g., quality of life) above and beyond beneficial changes produced by alternative interventions; also includes improvement in convenience to patients and adherence to treatment course	Studies (RCTs and observational) reporting changes in PROs (e.g., quality of life) related to the intervention and its comparator(s) analyzed and reported in evidence tables indicating population, duration of treatment, PRO instruments used (and whether they have been validated), PRO outcomes reported, etc. Data on patient preferences and convenience also reported, when available
Type of benefit		
T1—public health interest (e.g., *prevention, risk reduction)*	Risk reduction provided by the proposed intervention at the population level (e.g., prevention, reduction in disease transmission, reduction in the prevalence of risk factors)	Data to help define the type of benefit that the proposed intervention can provide at the population level (e.g., prevention, risk reduction, reduction in the prevalence of risk factors) identified based on clinical and PRO data, synthesized, and presented in the MCDA matrix
T2—type of medical service (e.g., *cure, symptom relief)*	Nature of the clinical benefit provided by the proposed intervention at the patient level (e.g., symptom relief, prolonging life, cure)	Data to help define the type of benefit that the proposed intervention can provide to individual patients (e.g., cure, prolonging life, symptom relief) identified based on clinical and PRO data, synthesized, and presented in the MCDA matrix

(continued)

Table 13.1 (continued)

Criteria	Definition	Methodology used to synthesize evidence
Economics		
E1—budget impact on health plan *(cost of intervention)*	Net impact of covering the intervention on the budget of the target health plan (excluding other spending; see E3). This represents the differential between expected expenditure for the proposed intervention and potential cost savings that may result from replacement of other intervention(s) currently covered by the health plan. Limited to cost of intervention (e.g., acquisition cost, implementation cost). Includes consideration on affordability	Information on the resources consumed by the use of the intervention (including price of the intervention, frequency/duration of treatment, estimated annual cost per patient, cost of administration) collected from public sources, as available. Studies of the budget impact of the proposed intervention on health plans described, including the type of model used (e.g., claim based, epidemiological), costs included (e.g., dispensing fees, markups, cost of administration), and major assumptions. The projected budget impact(s) presented including the number of patients treated, potential cost of the intervention to the health plan, and incremental budget impact if existing interventions are projected to be replaced. Simple models will be developed as necessary to calculate budget impact estimates per 1,000,000 population and as percentage of gross domestic product (GDP) for representative countries (Jehu-Appiah et al. 2008)
E2—cost-effectiveness of intervention	Ratio of the incremental cost of the proposed intervention to its incremental benefit compared to alternatives. Benefit can be expressed as number of events avoided, life-years gained, quality-adjusted life-years gained, additional pain-free days, etc.	Sufficient information to understand the design and results of published economic evaluations provided (including population, intervention, comparator(s), perspective of analysis, model type and time horizon, efficacy/effectiveness of data used, patient-reported outcomes of data used, costs included, key model features, incremental cost-effectiveness ratios, and sensitivity analyses)
E3—impact on other spending (e.g., *hospitalization, disability)*	Impact of providing coverage for the proposed intervention on other expenditures (excluding intervention cost; see E1) such as for hospitalization, specialist consultations, adverse events, long-term care, disability, lost productivity, caregiver time, equipment maintenance, etc.	Impact of the proposed intervention and its comparators on other expenditures, such as for hospitalization, specialist consultations, adverse events, long-term care, disability, lost productivity, caregiver time, and equipment maintenance, extracted from available economic studies. The absolute cost difference between the intervention and its comparators calculated and reported

Quality/uncertainty of evidence		
Q1—adherence to requirements of decision-making body	Alignment of the intervention with the mandate/scope of the healthcare system. The goal of healthcare is to maintain normal functioning. Mission and scope of healthcare plans/systems derive from this principle	Not applicable for the international practice guidelines
Q2—completeness and consistency of reporting evidence	Extent to which reporting of evidence on the proposed intervention is complete (i.e., meeting scientific standards on reporting) and consistent with the sources cited	For five types of evidence (clinical, patient-reported outcomes, epidemiological, economic, and budget impact), studies most relevant to the international and Canadian setting critically appraised for level and quality of evidence. Level of evidence determined using the classification of the Centre for Evidence-Based Medicine (seven levels) (Centre for Evidence Based Medicine 2010). Quality of evidence assessed using instruments previously described that were developed based on published tools for the assessment of clinical (e.g., GRADE (Atkins et al. 2005), Jadad et al. (1996)), economic (e.g., CHEC (Evers et al. 2005)), and epidemiological studies (e.g., STROBE (2007)). These instruments pose questions on key study dimensions (including target population, intervention, and comparators, outcome measures, study design, adverse events (for clinical data), time horizon, statistical analyses, and results) to promote a systematic and critical analysis and its transparent reporting (Goetghebeur et al. 2008, 2010)
Q3—relevance and validity of evidence	Extent to which evidence on the proposed intervention is relevant to the decision-making body (in terms of population, disease stage, comparator interventions, outcomes, etc.) and valid with respect to scientific standards (i.e., study design, etc.) and conclusions (agreement of results between studies). This includes consideration of uncertainty (e.g., conflicting results across studies, limited number of studies and patients)	Due to the subjective nature of quality assessments (Gerkens et al. 2008), analyses conducted in a three-step process. First, a trained investigator reviewed the study, provided answers to all questions for each dimension contained in the instrument, and wrote a summary critical analysis (for each study or for a group of studies, e.g., all clinical trials). All evaluations then reviewed by a second trained clinical investigator and validated by an expert in the field during face-to-face workshop

(continued)

Table 13.1 (continued)

Criteria	Definition	Methodology used to synthesize evidence
Contextual decision criteria—qualitative tool Concepts and information on six ethical and contextual decision criteria of growth hormone for PWS categorized and synthesized in the qualitative tool, organized in two clusters. Colloquial and scientific evidence researched and synthesized to support reflection and discussion among workshop participants on specific ethical and system-related issues, as well as to ensure that all aspects of the decision have been considered		
Ethical criteria[a] Although ethical principles are implicitly included in some of the criteria of the MCDA matrix, an explicit discussion of how ethical consideration may influence the decision is important and was supported by synthesized information covering the three often conflicting standard ethical principles outlined by the WHO: utility, efficiency, and fairness (World Health Organization 2004)		
Et1—*utility*—goals of healthcare[a]	The goal of healthcare is to maintain normal functioning. Such consideration is aligned with the principle of utility, which considers the act to produce the greatest good or "greatest benefits for the greatest number"	It is generally agreed that the goal of healthcare is to maintain normal functioning (Daniels 2001). Such consideration is aligned with the principle of utility, which considers the act to produce the greatest good or "greatest benefits for the greatest number" (World Health Organization 2004). To stimulate reflection on whether the intervention is actually producing a good that is a health benefit and falls under the mission and scope of the health plan/healthcare system, information to support a discussion on this topic was synthesized. Information derived from peer-reviewed and gray literature on the proposed (or related) intervention, as well as from rules, laws, and regulations publicly defining the mission and scope of relevant health plans/healthcare systems, as available
Et2—*efficiency*—opportunity costs	Opportunity costs include resources or interventions that may be forgone if the proposed intervention is used/reimbursed. Such consideration is aligned with the principle of efficiency, which considers maximizing health for a given level of resources (efficiency can be considered at the patient level and at the society level)	To stimulate reflection by participants on what may be forgone if the proposed intervention were to be used/reimbursed and whether the use of the intervention would maximize available resources (at patient and societal/institutional level), available literature discussing the role and cost of the intervention with regard to other types of interventions to manage/treat the same condition will be synthesized. Data on interventions that may be discontinued to free resources in limited budget settings (disinvestments) will be explored

Et3—*fairness*[a]—population priority and access	Priorities for specific groups of patients are defined by societies/decision-makers and reflect their moral values. Such considerations are aligned with the principle of fairness, which considers treating like cases alike and different cases differently and often gives priority to those who are worst-off (theory of justice)	The objective of this criterion is to stimulate reflection on priorities and whether the proposed intervention targets a group of patients that belong to prioritized populations. Priorities for specific groups of patients are defined by societies/decision-makers and reflect their moral values. Such considerations are aligned with the principle of fairness, which considers treating like cases alike and different cases differently and often gives priority to those who are worst-off (theory of justice) (World Health Organization 2004). Literature discussing priorities in relevant settings as well as information from laws and regulations outlining priorities of health plans/healthcare systems synthesized. Discussion on whether the proposed inervention is targeting a prioritized group. Consideration given to theory of justice based on information on whether patients with PWS can be considered among the worst-off. Other aspects explored, relating to whether the intervention is associated with issues of access to care and whether the intervention is associated with issues of access to care and whether the intervention triggers issues relating to the concept of "treating like cases alike" (World Health Organization 2004)
Overall context		
O1—system capacity and appropriate use of intervention	The capacity of healthcare system to implement the intervention and to ensure its appropriate use depends on its infrastructure, organization, skills, legislation, barriers, and risks of inappropriate use. Such considerations include mapping current systems and estimating whether the use of the intervention under scrutiny requires additional capacities (note: if available, economic estimate would be included in the economic criterion E3 of the MCDA Value Matrix)	The objective of this criterion is to ensure consideration of the capacity of the healthcare system to implement the intervention and to ensure its appropriate use; this depends on infrastructure, organization, skills, legislation, barriers, and risks of inappropriate use. Such considerations include mapping current systems and estimating whether the use of the intervention under scrutiny requires additional capacities. Available literature synthesized concerning risks of inappropriate use of the intervention and its consequences as well as implementation issues other than economic aspects.

(continued)

Table 13.1 (continued)

Criteria	Definition	Methodology used to synthesize evidence
O2—stakeholder pressures	Pressures from groups of stakeholders are often part of the context surrounding healthcare interventions. Such considerations include being aware of pressures and interests at stake and how they may affect values of decision-makers	The objective of this criterion is to ensure consideration of pressures from groups of stakeholders, which are often part of the context surrounding decisions on healthcare interventions. Such considerations include being aware of pressures and interests at stake and how they may impact the decision. Available information on societal pressures and pressures from specific groups of stakeholders (clinicians, patients, industry, etc.) summarized
O3—political/historical context	Political/historical context may influence the value of an intervention in consideration of specific political situations and priorities (e.g., priority to innovation) as well as habits, traditions, and precedence	Data synthesized on the specific political/historical context that may impact the appraisal of the intervention, scientific literature, disease association web sites, and popular media, addressing such political/historical context or precedence and traditions associated with the intervention or related interventions. As available, data on explicit governmental priorities (e.g., innovation in healthcare, budget constraints in economic recession) beyond healthcare priorities (covered in Et3) reported as well as information on funding decisions for the proposed intervention by relevant jurisdictions

[a]*Ethical criteria* are based on three principles; since these are often conflicting, clearly identify trade-offs and legitimize decision by engaging a broad range of stakeholders and explaining decision (Gruskin and Daniels 2008; Persad et al. 2009); legitimizing decision is key to attaining accountability for reasonableness (Daniels 1999, 2001)

hampered by the difficulty in designing appropriate and robust clinical trials because of the presence of important and strong confounders, and it must face many ethical issues such as treating patients with cognitive disabilities.

For the second application of MCDA, we again use the EVIDEM decision criteria to investigate the identification and prioritization of research projects, explore research design, and facilitate knowledge transfer. The clinical context used for this application was that of hemodialysis. This is another expensive but lifesaving treatment modality for the large and growing numbers of patients with end-stage renal failure; it carries with it significant risk of morbidity and mortality. More recently, CPGs have encouraged the use of intensive hemodialysis, including home intensive hemodialysis, for its cost savings and improved quality of life for patients. However, the transfer of knowledge to clinicians and health professionals in order to encourage and facilitate its use has been limited, in part because of missing evidence. EVIDEM MCDA decision criteria were therefore adapted for the purpose of prioritizing research questions relevant to intensive hemodialysis use and employed by a panel of clinical and methodological experts to prioritize, refine, and improve research in intensive hemodialysis.

13.2 Case Study 1: MCDA for Structuring Evidence and Identifying Most Important Outcomes

The development of evidence-based approaches to clinical decision-making aims at improving medical practice and quality of healthcare services. However, lack of scientific evidence and uncertainties around the robustness of this evidence despite the growing volume of medical literature has hindered clinical decision-making (Alper et al. 2004; Ely et al. 2002). One of the main obstacles that clinicians face is poor access to structured and comprehensive information needed to support patient care (Ely et al. 2002). Clinical practice guidelines (CPGs) are meant to "assist practitioner and patient decisions about appropriate healthcare for specific clinical circumstances" (Committee to Advise the Public Health Service on Clinical Practice Guidelines Institute of Medicine and Medicine 1990). To be more consistent and efficient, the process to generate them needs to be systematic in its assessment of evidence and in the development of questions and recommendations. Development of recommendations to guide clinical practice also requires consideration of a broad range of aspects to ensure optimal care and social responsibility (Brouwers et al. 2010; Dhalla and Laupacis 2008). Potential intellectual or financial conflict of interest compromises CPG credibility and usefulness (Sitges-Serra 2014). The Appraisal of Guidelines Research and Evaluation (AGREE) Collaboration provides an instrument to address the issue of variability in the quality of practice guidelines. Initially developed in 2003 (AGREE Collaboration 2003), it was revised in 2009 as AGREE II, with launching of training tools and a web-based platform to facilitate the work of evidence reviewers (Makarski and Brouwers 2014). The tool, comprising 23 items organized into six quality domains (scope and purpose, stakeholder involvement, rigor of development, clarity of presentation, applicability, and editorial independence), assesses the methodological rigor and transparency in which a guideline is developed; AGREE is used internationally (www.agreetrust.org).

Clinical researchers and decision-makers have used MCDA as an approach to support deliberation and simultaneous consideration of many aspects (scientific, economic, ethical) relevant to research and decision-making (Baltussen and Niessen 2006). EVIDEM is an MCDA-based framework designed to integrate the ethical dilemmas faced by decision-makers in balancing health of patients, health of populations, and health of healthcare systems into a comprehensive range of decision criteria (Goetghebeur et al. 2008, 2010). In this case study, it was selected as a holistic structure to organize evidence for each of the criteria of the framework and thus facilitate reflection and deliberation that took place in the development of CPG for patients with Prader-Willi syndrome that followed the recommendations of the AGREE Collaboration (Table 13.2). It was also selected to explore quantitatively the relative importance of clinical outcomes that can be achieved by this treatment in this patient population.

13.2.1 MCDA to Structure Evidence and Clinical Practice Questions

Decision-making is particularly difficult for interventions targeting patients with rare diseases, owing in part to the difficulties inherent in performing adequately sized clinical trials in limited populations, confusion as to optimal outcomes needed to ascribe efficacy, to the larger periods of time needed to ascertain safety and to the tendency to place a higher value on treating common conditions in order to benefit the largest number of individuals.

Prader-Willi syndrome (PWS) is a rare (1 in 20,000–25,000 births) and heterogeneous genetic condition: it is characterized by hypotonia (decreased muscle tone and mass), poor feeding in infancy, hyperphagia with evolving obesity, hypogonadism (lack of sex hormones), decreased adult height, and cognitive and behavioral disabilities. These serious and long-term health consequences stem in part from hypothalamic dysregulation and may include growth hormone deficiency. Treatment with recombinant human growth hormone (GH) was approved based on short-term data reporting beneficial effects on growth and body composition. However, GH therapy for PWS represents a unique therapeutic challenge which includes treating individuals with cognitive disability, varied therapeutic goals that are not focused exclusively on increased height, and concerns about potential life-threatening adverse events (Burman et al. 2001). In this case study, MCDA was

Table 13.2 Concurrence of EVIDEM and AGREE requirements for development of evidence-based clinical practice guidelines: the example of guidelines for GH treatment in Prader-Willi syndrome (PWS) (Research Trust 2016)

AGREE requirements for scope and purpose	*Consensus guidelines approach using EVIDEM*
Item 1: The overall objective(s) of the guideline is(are) specifically described	Overall objective: to evaluate the effects of GH therapy in pediatric and adult patients with PWS and provide guidelines for its use Goal: reduction of morbidity in patients affected by PWS with the focus on specific endpoints known to be affected by GH including growth, body composition, physical activity, metabolic status, cardiovascular health, bone health, and neurological and motor development
Item 2: The clinical question(s) covered by the guideline is(are) specifically described	Clinical questions identified based on available evidence by experts in relevant fields at the time of content validation Clinical questions/points of discussion will stimulate discussion during presentations and breakout sessions
Item 3: The patients to whom the guideline is meant to apply are specifically described	Available evidence gathered according to the target population, divided in two subcategories: Pediatric patients with PWS Adults patients with PWS
AGREE requirements for stakeholder involvement	*Consensus guidelines approach using EVIDEM*
Item 4: The guideline development group includes individuals from all the relevant professional groups	Stakeholders involved in guidelines development included: Experts in PWS (clinical geneticists, adult and pediatric endocrinologists, nutritionists) Epidemiologists Health economists HTA specialists Ethicists
Item 5: The patients' views and preferences have been sought	An executive member of a Canadian PWS Association (lay organization including parents of patients with PWS) invited to participate in the workshop
Item 6: The target users of the guideline are clearly defined	Physicians treating patient with PWS (pediatricians, internists, endocrinologists, neurologists, orthopedic surgeons, pulmonologists, psychiatrists) Nutritionists, genetic counselors, physiotherapists, occupational therapists, psychologists
Item 7: The guideline has been piloted among target users	The guidelines sent to key professional societies for their comments; access to all validated EVIDEM HTA reports are available online (open source)
AGREE requirements for rigor of development	*Consensus guidelines using EVIDEM*
Item 8: Systematic methods were used to search for evidence	The approach included an algorithm for: Databases and sources to search (Medline, Cochrane, HTA agencies, etc.) Keywords to identify evidence for each decision criterion

(continued)

Table 13.2 (continued)

AGREE requirements for scope and purpose	*Consensus guidelines approach using EVIDEM*
Item 9: The criteria for selecting the evidence are clearly described	The approach included criteria to select evidence (e.g., for clinical data, prioritize randomized-controlled trials and comparative observational studies) The approach included tools for assessment of the quality of selected studies
Item 10: The methods used for formulating the recommendations are clearly described	The results of a systematic analysis of the available scientific evidence for GH and PWS presented to international experts in PWS, epidemiology, health economics, HTA, and ethics in the form of online HTA for validation Key questions identified a priori by workshop organizers Invited presentations by experts at the workshop followed by discussion of key questions and formulation of resulting recommendations Consensus discussions involving all workshop participants used to draft final recommendations (consensus development) The assessment of the extent of agreement (consensus measurement) done using MCDA as per the EVIDEM protocol (Goetghebeur et al. 2008)
Item 11: The health benefits, side effects, and risks have been considered in formulating recommendations	The approach included systematic consideration of 21 decision criteria (see Table 13.1) including clinical criteria such as type of benefit, efficacy/effectiveness, safety, and patient-reported outcomes using the EVIDEM HTA report and expert discussions
AGREE requirements for rigor of development (cont.)	*Consensus guidelines approach using EVIDEM*
Item 12: There is an explicit link between the recommendations and the supporting evidence	The framework aligns evidence available with reflection and discussion to reach recommendations
Item 13: The guideline has been externally reviewed by experts prior to its publication	The guidelines were submitted to a journal requiring external peer review prior to acceptance for publication
Item 14: A procedure for updating the guideline is provided	5–10 year update planned as per guidelines for treatment of adults (not affected by the PWS) with growth hormone deficiency (Growth Hormone Research Society Workshop on Adult Growth Hormone Deficiency 1998; Ho 2007)
AGREE requirements for clarity and presentation	*Consensus guidelines using EVIDEM*
Item 15: The recommendations are specific and unambiguous	Structured HTA report permitted identification of unambiguous and ambiguous risks/benefits of GH therapy in PWS which facilitated the formulation of recommendations Areas of uncertainty clearly identified
Item 16: The different options for management of the condition are clearly presented	The HTA report included alternative therapies (i.e., nutritional, pharmaceutical, behavioral, exercise, anorexigens)

Item 17: Key recommendations are easily identifiable	The final consensus guidelines organized in tables and bullet points Key recommendations highlighted
Item 18: The guideline is supported with tools for application	The guidelines are available through the Internet and publicized through presentations at professional societies
AGREE requirements for applicability	*Consensus guidelines approach using EVIDEM*
Item 19: The potential organizational barriers in applying the recommendations have been discussed	Workshop presentations included discussion of healthcare organization for patients with PWS
Item 20: The potential cost implications of applying the recommendations have been considered	Economic analysis is an integral part of the EVIDEM HTA report and was addressed by a health economist
Item 21: The guideline presents key review criteria for monitoring and/or audit purposes	Treatment clearly defined and key criteria for monitoring treatment established
AGREE requirements for editorial independence	*Consensus guidelines approach using EVIDEM*
Item 22: The guideline is editorially independent form the funding body	Private industry supporters did not participate in the writing of the guidelines
Item 23: Conflicts of interest of guideline development members have been recorded	Conflict of interest statements obtained from all guideline participants including HTA developers and available with the online publication

first applied to facilitate systematic development of evidence-based CPGs for the use of GH in patients with PWS (Deal et al. 2013).

An extensive literature review was performed to identify the most relevant available evidence of GH treatment for PWS for each criterion of the framework covering disease impact, therapeutic context, treatment outcomes (efficacy/effectiveness, safety, and patient-reported outcomes), type of benefits, economic impact, as well as ethical and contextual considerations. Data was organized in evidence tables and synthesized; the level and strength of evidence were assessed using, respectively, the Centre for Evidence-Based Medicine (CEBM) levels of evidence (Centre for Evidence Based Medicine 2010) and EVIDEM data quality instruments. The framework thus developed was adapted into a CPG module in which clinical aspects are the primary focus and used to elicit questions for CPG development. An interactive web information system was developed to facilitate the CPG process.

Based on the analysis of the literature and feedback from experts, CPG questions reflecting current issues in management of patients with PWS were developed and organized using the EVIDEM framework (Table 13.3). The framework was used to organize the program of the workshop and to assign questions to CPG working groups. A face-to-face consensus workshop was held, during which 43 international experts and stakeholders (clinicians, patient representative, ethicist, methodologists, and

Table 13.3 Organization of CPG questions by criteria of the EVIDEM framework (v1.1)

Clinical aspects	
Intervention overview *Indication*: 1. Do patients with PWS need GH testing: In infancy? In childhood? In adulthood? 2. What baseline evaluations need to be performed before GH treatment? *Intervention duration*: 3. For how long should GH therapy be pursued? 4. Should treatment duration be dependent upon response? 5. Should treatment duration be different dependent upon outcome priority? *Administration/description*: 6. What clinical lab tests or imaging studies need to be done to monitor treatment? 7. What doses should be used for GH therapy: In infants? In children and adolescents? In adults? 8. Is there an optimal level of circulating IGF-I to obtain with GH treatment? 9. Should GH dose be titrated to IGF-I, and if so, at what frequency? 10. What is the frequency of follow-up visits necessary to adequately monitor GH therapy? **Comparator(s):** 11. What other therapies/interventions have been tried in PWS?	
Decision criteria	**Proposed questions**
Disease impact	
D1—disease severity	12. What is the frequency of the various genetic subtypes among various populations? 13. How has evolution of our genetic testing methodology changed genetic subtype frequency? 14. Are all patients with PWS equally GH deficient? 15. Are there genotype-phenotype correlations relevant to specific to clinical outcome measures targeted with GH therapy? Other correlations? 16. What are the important comorbidities that need to be considered when considering GH therapy? 17. What is the life expectancy of PWS subjects? 18. What are the major causes of death in PWS subjects?
D2—size of population	19. What is the birth incidence/prevalence of PWS?
Therapeutic context of intervention	
C1—clinical guidelines	20. Why are physicians divided in their belief about the benefits of GH therapy? 21. What role does patient cognitive impairment play in physician attitudes about treatment?
C2—comparative interventions limitations (*unmet needs*)	22. For each of the other therapies/interventions tried in PWS, what were the specific outcomes, the efficacy per outcome, and the safety/tolerability of the therapy/intervention? 23. What specific therapies/interventions have been tried concomitant to GH therapy? 24. What are the nutritional recommendations for infants with PWS, children with PWS, adolescents with PWS, and adults with PWS?

Table 13.3 (continued)

Intervention outcomes		
I1—improvement of efficacy/effectiveness	25. What are the most important clinical outcome priorities when initiating GH therapy in subjects with PWS: In infancy? In childhood? In adolescence? In adulthood?	
	26. What is the best way to measure GH effectiveness on:	
	(a) Growth	(g) Metabolic benefits
	(b) Body composition	(h) Resting energy expenditure
	(c) Motor development (infants and children)	(i) Cardiovascular status
	(d) Neurological status	(j) Bone health
	(e) Physical activity	(k) QoL (specifically in intellectually disabled individuals)
	(f) Muscle strength	
	27. What is the impact of other hormonal deficiencies on GH treatment?	
	28. Does response to GH vary by:	
	(a) Age at start of treatment	(d) Degree of dietary control
	(b) Dose	(e) Level of physical activity
	(c) Body composition at start	
I2—improvement of safety and tolerability	29. What are the major serious adverse events of GH treatment of PWS subjects?	
	30. What is the evidence that GH treatment in PWS increases the risk of:	
	(a) Sleep apnea	(h) Edema
	(b) Sudden death	(i) Breast tenderness/enlargement
	(c) Scoliosis	(j) Risk of infection
	(d) Diabetes	(k) Joint pain
	(e) Intracranial hypertension	(l) Neoplasia
	(f) Epilepsy	(m) Arterial hypertension
	(g) Slipped capital femoral epiphyses	(n) Stroke/intracranial bleeding
	31. What is the tolerability of GH: In published clinical trials (dropout rates)? In patient-reported data? In phase 4 trials? In smaller observational studies?	
	32. What are the main reasons given for patient withdrawal from clinical trials of GH in PWS?	
	33. What is the evidence that adverse events in PWS differ from those in patients with hypothalamic obesity secondary to craniopharyngioma and/or its treatment?	

(continued)

Table 13.3 (continued)

I3—improvement of patient-reported outcomes	34. What are the most significant benefits reported by patients and/or parents after GH treatment?
Type of benefit	
T1—public health interest (e.g., *prevention, risk reduction*)	35. Is there any risk reduction associated with GH treatment in patients with PWS?
T2—type of medical service (e.g., *cure, symptom relief*)	36. What are the least important, but significant, clinical outcomes to GH therapy? 37. What known GH effects have not been adequately studied in PWS?
Quality/uncertainty of evidence	
Q2—completeness and consistency of reporting evidence	38. What are the confounding variables that are difficult to control in PWS GH clinical trials? 39. What is the best way to report efficacy data according to current recommendations and why? 40. Is there a place for a therapeutic trial of GH, and if so, how long before assessing GH effectiveness? 41. When sources of potential study bias are considered (adequate randomization and blinding of patients and health professionals, adequate description of withdrawals and dropouts, provision of intention-to-treat analysis), what proportion of the clinical trials have a high risk of bias (i.e., one or more of the previous criteria not met)?
Q3—relevance and validity of evidence	42. What questions with regard to GH use in PWS require further study? 43. What are the major research areas with regard to PWS that need to be addressed beyond issues of GH use?
Resource allocation and ethical aspects	
Overview *Economic burden of illness* 44. What are the major sources of healthcare costs related to the care of patients with PWS? 45. What are the major costs of treating morbid obesity? 46. What are the major costs of treating diabetes?	
Decision criteria	**Proposed questions**
Economics of intervention	
E1—budget impact on health plan (cost of intervention)	47. What is the cost of GH treatment in patients with PWS? 48. What is the budget impact at the country level?
E2—cost-effectiveness of intervention	49. What is the cost-effectiveness of GH treatment in patients with PWS?
E3—impact on other spending (e.g., hospitalization, disability)	50. What are the economic consequences (beyond drug cost) of GH treatment in patients with PWS?
Ethical criteria	
Et1—utility—goals of healthcare	51. Is the use of GH in patients with PWS aligned with the mission and scope of healthcare systems?
Et2—efficiency—opportunity costs and affordability	52. How do we prioritize resources for PWS care, and how does GH fit into this? 53. What benefits need to be defined to justify an indication for GH therapy?

Et3—fairness—population priority and access	54. Is access to GH therapy available to all PWS patients, and if not, why? 55. Are there issues of fairness in withholding GH treatment or in targeting specific subpopulations of PWS subjects for GH therapy?
Overall context	
O1—system capacity and appropriate use of intervention	56. How do we organize the comprehensive care of the PWS patient, to optimize GH treatment and particularly to decrease/prevent potential side effects? 57. What are the evidence-based steps that are needed to harmonize care of patients with PWS?
O2—stakeholder pressures/barriers	58. Are there any pressures/barriers for the use of GH in patients with PWS?
O3—political/historical context	59. Are there any specific political/historical context impacting the use of GH in patients with PWS?

GH growth hormone, *PWS* Prader-Willi syndrome, *QoL* quality of life

researchers) followed clinical practice guideline development recommendations outlined by the AGREE Collaboration to develop consensus guidelines for GH therapy in PWS (Deal et al. 2013), using a web MCDA interface to facilitate discussion. The web site aided the entire CPG process from its preparatory stages to the practice implementation stages by allowing:

1. Seamless access to highly synthesized evidence, detailed evidence tables and actual publications/reports for each criterion of the framework, as well as quality assessments of evidence
2. Access to CPG questions for each criterion
3. Access to the CPG experts for interactive online validation of evidence and reflection on questions assigned to working groups prior to the consensus workshop
4. Public access to all validated synthesized data on GH for PWS for each criterion used for the CPG process under a Creative Commons license (http://www.evidem.org/tiki/PWGHINConsensusWorkshop (Collaboration 2010))

CPG question elicitation and organization were facilitated by the MCDA framework, providing a pragmatic means to ensure systematic consideration of evidence for a wide range of criteria and associated issues. By structuring the discussions and deliberations and by clearly revealing current knowledge and gaps, the framework facilitated developing evidence-based CPGs and identifying research needed for continued improvement in management of patient with PWS.

13.2.2 MCDA to Identify Most Important Outcomes

In addition to being the most common genetic cause of morbid obesity, PWS is characterized by poor linear growth, hypotonia, delays in developmental milestones, reduced physical activity, and musculoskeletal problems in childhood (Butler et al.

2006). Although GH is indicated to improve growth and body composition in pediatric PWS patients (Australian Government Department of Health and Ageing 2008; electronic Medicines Compendium (eMC) 2011; Pfizer inc 2011), its use and coverage in PWS treatment vary widely, reflecting a need to clarify its clinical benefits. This is one of the most important aspects of CPG development, as discussed in item 1 of the AGREE guidelines (Table 13.2).

The efficacy criteria of the framework were thus expanded to include specific outcome measures of GH treatment in PWS patients, which were transformed into the following subcriteria: growth, body composition, physical activity, metabolic and cardiovascular status, bone health, and motor development (Question 22 in Table 13.3). For each subcriterion, available evidence was synthesized and validated by experts using an interactive web system which provided seamless access to highly synthesized evidence, detailed evidence tables, and actual publications/reports. During the consensus workshop, participants assigned weights to each subcriterion using a point allocation technique (Dolan 2010), reflecting participants' individual perspectives on their relative importance. Then participants assigned scores to each subcriterion on a four-point scale (0–3) to assess the performance of GH for PWS patients relative to each outcome, based on evidence available and presented for each subcriterion. An MCDA value estimate was obtained using a linear model combining normalized weights and scores to identify the most relevant efficacy criteria for value assessment of this treatment.

Analysis of the workshop results revealed that the highest weights were assigned to subcriteria "body composition" (24 % of points) and "physical activity" (18 % of points)

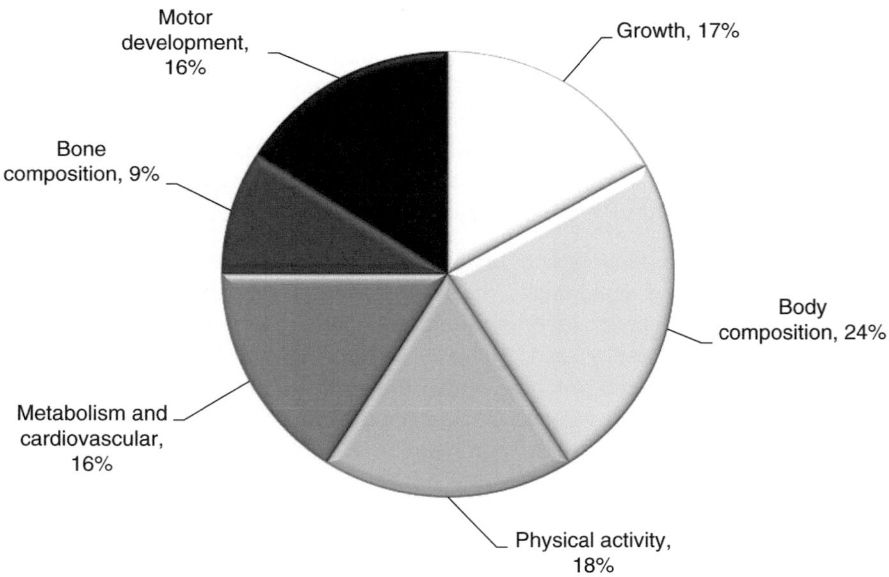

Fig. 13.1 Relative importance of the different outcomes achieved by GH treatment for patients with PWS. Weights elicited by experts using a point allocation technique are reported

(Fig. 13.1). The weight attributed to subcriterion "Growth" received only 17 % of points; 46 % of respondents attributed ≤10 % of points to "Growth." *Score* assignment showed that the highest scores were given to "Body composition" and "Growth" subcriteria (data not shown), suggesting that GH provided the highest benefit on these outcomes. Low scores assigned to subcriteria of "metabolism and cardiovascular," "bone composition," and "motor development" reflected limited GH efficacy and/or limited data on these outcomes. Interestingly, these results are discordant with the indication for which GH was approved for PWS in Europe and North America, namely, mainly to promote growth and secondarily, in Europe only, body composition.

Overall, a majority of participants (70 %) reported an interest in the MCDA exercise, either for stimulating reflection or facilitating discussion and deliberation. This case study showed that holistic and pragmatic MCDA as purported by EVIDEM provides a useful methodology for structuring and prioritizing clinical practice questions and concepts, as well as for identifying most important outcomes for a given pathology using an intuitive approach based on direct clinical experience.

13.3 Case Study 2: MCDA for Clinical Research Prioritization

Health research prioritization is a relatively well-developed field of research with numerous published frameworks that consider both disease/condition-related factors (e.g., burden, unmet need) and research-related factors, including feasibility and impact. Although many of these applications use methodologies that can be related to MCDA, very few have explicitly applied the methodology. Viergever et al. (2010) established a nine-item checklist for health research priority setting. Although they did not provide an explicit set of decision criteria per se, they identified a need to select decision criteria as part of the research prioritization process.

Several research prioritization models have been proposed that are specific to comparative effectiveness research. Comparative effectiveness studies are designed to compare benefits and harms of alternate treatment or diagnostic strategies and are intended to inform individual and population-level decision-making. Consequently, prioritization of comparative effectiveness research (CER) questions requires due consideration of population-level impacts, including the size of the affected population, and opportunities to alleviate disparities in health or health service delivery. Moreover, since CER study designs can include large pragmatic trials, prioritization efforts should consider study size, feasibility, and resource use.

To date, a number of approaches to CER prioritization have been developed in various jurisdictions. The Federal Coordinating Council (FCC) for Comparative Effectiveness Research (Unites States) has established a decision-making framework for CER that includes a number of criteria (appropriateness domains) that are specific to federally funded healthcare programs in the Unites States (Andrews 2013). Dubois and Graff (2011) developed a framework for prioritization of CER that included 8 steps and 11 criteria including conditions-related criteria and research-related criteria. While this framework is comprehensive, it does not explicitly consider the quality of generated evidence (i.e., confidence in treatment effect estimates) or the patient importance of proposed study outcomes (e.g., patient-reported outcomes or outcomes identified as important by patients affected by the target condition). Krishnan et al. (2013) identified and ranked criteria with several groups of stakeholders to define priorities for comparative effectiveness research in chronic obstructive pulmonary disease. The resulting criteria considered outcomes, economic impact, and applicability/feasibility of implementation of research findings, but did not consider feasibility of the CER project or the quality of the resulting evidence.

As described above, the EVIDEM framework provides a holistic, ethical, structured, and transparent process for considering a range of factors relevant to decision-making in healthcare. Moreover, the EVIDEM Collaboration provides (downloadable at https://www.evidem.org/evidem-framework/) customizable tools for weighting and scoring decision criteria using MCDA with a linear model. We therefore adapted the EVIDEM criteria for the purpose of prioritizing research questions related to intensive hemodialysis and dialysis-related registry-based cluster-randomized trials.

13.3.1 MCDA for Clinical Research Prioritization: Case Study of Hemodialysis

Hemodialysis remains the most commonly used treatment for end-stage renal disease; more than 24,000 Canadians received dialysis in 2013 (Canadian Institute for Health Information (CIHI) 2015; Nesrallah et al. 2004; The Kidney Foundation of Canada 2013). This treatment is associated with high morbidity and mortality and a substantial economic burden (Nesrallah et al. 2004). A conventional dialysis prescription is delivered over three to four sessions per week, over a duration of 3.4–5.5 h per session (Nesrallah et al. 2013). Further increasing treatment duration and frequency to provide “intensive” hemodialysis have been shown in observational studies to improve patient survival and other clinical outcomes, including health-related quality of life (Canadian Institute for Health Information (CIHI) 2015; Nesrallah et al. 2004). For logistical reasons, longer and more frequent dialysis is more easily provided in patients’ homes, and most patients receiving home hemodialysis receive some form of intensive hemodialysis (The Kidney Foundation of Canada 2013). Home therapies are also considered cost-effective and afford greater flexibility and ease of scheduling.

Efforts to increase the uptake and improve the practice of home intensive hemodialysis regimens have led to the development of practice guidelines (Nesrallah et al. 2013). These, in turn, have identified significant knowledge gaps in the provision of intensive home hemodialysis, leading to calls for comparative effectiveness studies to identify research needs and priorities (Nesrallah et al. 2013). An international working group—the Scientific Committee of the International

Quotidian Dialysis Registry—identified a number of research questions addressing major knowledge gaps in home intensive hemodialysis prescription. Given the broad range of topics identified by working group members, we developed a transparent and structured approach to research question prioritization. While the EVIDEM framework was originally developed for the purpose of prioritizing candidate clinical interventions, many of the EVIDEM decision criteria are relevant to research design (Goetghebeur et al. 2008) and could be adapted to allow decision-makers to prioritize research projects.

We used an iterative and consultative process with a panel of clinical and methodological experts to adapt and refine the original EVIDEM (Goetghebeur et al. 2012) decision criteria for the purpose of prioritizing research questions relevant to hemodialysis. The objectives were to create a tool that could simultaneously prioritize studies of both observational and experimental designs. The resulting framework included 11 criteria to assess the overall value of CER in improving hemodialysis practice from a holistic standpoint. Criteria pertained to the impact, context, and outcomes of the CER question, CER study feasibility, economics, and implementation of study findings. Quality of evidence generated by a CER question was also included as a criterion, with consideration of 13 subcriteria outlining the risk of bias (the likelihood that due to limitations in execution or design of a study, its findings deviate systematically from the truth) and precision (which typically relates to the adequacy of the study's sample size) (Guyatt and Busse 2011).

The working group, consisting of 28 researchers, then generated 13 candidate CER questions, each question containing information about the population, intervention, comparator, and outcome referred to commonly as PICO. This assumes that a "well-built" question should include four parts that identify the patient problem or population (P), intervention (I), comparison (C), and outcome(s) (O). The questions were refined using a nominal group process (Table 13.4), and the working group recommended a study design most appropriate for the research question, considering the quality of evidence available at the time. For example, for a CER question that had already been adequately explored using observational designs, the working group typically recommended an experimental design as a next step; for largely unexplored areas of inquiry, the working group typically recommended an observational design as a first step. For each CER question, the working group developed a one-page research proposal that included design considerations and other information (e.g., availability of data, reliability of existing data sources, existing funding sources, and others) that would inform the appraisal according to the newly developed decision criteria.

As a first step, participants were asked to weight each criterion in Table 13.5, from their own perspectives and independently from the research questions, according to its importance in rating the CER questions. Weighting scale was 1 (low) to 5 (high). A weight of 0 was allowed if the participant thought the criterion should not be considered. Second, for each of the research questions, participants assigned a score for each criterion of the MCDA matrix, on a scale of 0 (worst) to 3 (best). Average overall value estimates of CER questions were obtained by

Table 13.4 CER questions generated by participant nephrologists using PICO format

#	Questions
1	*Cluster RCT*: Among patients with stage III, IV, or V CKD, does a formal Independent (home HD or home PD) dialysis selection process (e.g., MATCH-D or other decision support tool) increase [intensive dialysis incident rate/utility/mortality] compared with no formal selection procedures/informal modality selection methods? *Secondary objective*: to determine predictors of ID use
2	*Prospective cohort study*: Among patients undergoing home HD, does scheduled re-training/recertification reduce the incidence of complications [access-related infection/technique failure/vascular access failure], as compared with no re-training protocol?
3	*Prospective cohort study*: Among patients undergoing frequent (five or more sessions/week) HD, is vascular access type (CVC vs. other) associated with [*mortality/technique survival/hospitalization*]?
4	*Prospective cohort study*: Among patients undergoing frequent (more than four sessions per week) home hemodialysis with an arteriovenous fistula, is the use of buttonhole cannulation associated with [*bacteremia/mortality/hospitalization/access survival*]?
5	*Factorial (2 × 2) RCT*: Among patients undergoing home HD with an AV fistula, and using buttonhole cannulation, does the use of topical antimicrobial prophylaxis reduce the risk of [*bacteremia/mortality/access survival/hospitalization*]?
6	*Parallel RCT*: Among patients with high levels of comorbidity who are failing to thrive on conventional hemodialysis, is short-daily in-center hemodialysis associated with better outcomes [*quality of life/survival*]?
7	*Registry-based descriptive analysis*: Among developed countries in which more intensive hemodialysis is available, what are incident rates and prevalent rates for patients receiving long hemodialysis, frequent hemodialysis, and long/frequent hemodialysis?
8	*Retrospective cohort study*: Is treatment with longer or more frequent hemodialysis associated with better transplant outcomes [*graft survival/patient survival/acute rejection*] as compared with conventional hemodialysis?
9	*Multinational retrospective cohort study*: Among countries in which longer or more frequent hemodialysis are provided, how do patient characteristics and outcomes compare?
10	*Prospective cohort study*: Among patients who are willing and able to undergo either PD or HD as an initial modality, does the initial modality choice dictate [*survival/hospitalization/technique survival/body access complications*]?
11	*Prospective cohort study*: Among patients undergoing longer and more frequent HD, is a higher dialysate calcium (>1.6 mmol/L) associated with an increase in [coronary artery/peripheral vascular] calcification? *Secondary objective*: Among patients undergoing longer and more frequent HD, which factors are associated with a greater risk of developing coronary artery calcification (e.g., preexisting calcifications, diabetes, C-reactive protein levels, catheter use, etc.)?
12	*Prospective cohort study*: Among patients undergoing home hemodialysis, what are causes of death, compared to a matched cohort on conventional dialysis?
13	*Prospective cohort study*: Among patients undergoing home hemodialysis, what are causes of hospitalization, compared to a matched cohort on conventional dialysis?

RCT randomized-controlled trial, *CKD* chronic kidney disease, *HD* hemodialysis, *PD* peritoneal dialysis

combining weights and scores using a linear additive model. Standard descriptive statistics (mean, min, max) were used to assess variability across participants.

Analyses of the data collected showed that participants assigned highest importance to the following criteria: *impact on patient survival and other major*

Table 13.5 Modified EVIDEM decision criteria definitions and corresponding normalized weights elicited using a five-point scale

Cluster/criteria	Definition	Normalized weights, mean (min, max)
Impact of CER question		
Population size	Relative size of population affected by proposed CER question	8 % (0, 13)
Disease severity	Severity of disease or burden of morbidity or disability addressed by the CER question	10 % (6, 13)
Context of CER question		
Unmet need	CER question addresses unmet need (significant uncertainty, knowledge gap) in an identified priority area, as determined by systematic review, expert panel, clinical practice guideline, consensus statement, healthcare agency mandate, formal information need assessment, or other systematic process	11 % (8, 16)
Outcomes of CER question		
Impact on patient survival and other major clinical outcomes	CER question has potential to impact on patient survival and other major clinical outcomes that are not considered patient-reported outcomes	11 % (9, 16)
Potential to reduce harm or improve safety	CER question has potential to reduce harm or improve safety	9 % (4, 13)
Impact on patient-reported outcomes	CER question has potential impact on patient-reported outcome (QoL, function, well-being)	9 % (5, 12)
Quality of evidence for CER question		
Potential to provide estimates in which we can be confident	The proposed study question allows a CER study design that has the potential to provide estimates in which we can be confident	9 % (3, 13)
Feasibility of CER study		
Feasibility of CER question	CER study is feasible (considering available data sources, data quality, study population size, sample size requirements, enrollment rate if applicable, investigator's interest; cost of study/analysis should not be considered in this criterion)	10 % (3, 16)
Economics of CER study findings		
Potential to result in savings in cost	CER study has potential to result in savings in cost of intervention, other medical costs, nonmedical costs, opportunity costs (consider health system perspective)	8 % (5, 13)
Implementation of CER study findings		
Feasibility of CER study findings implementation	Implementation of the CER study findings is feasible (consider facilitators and barriers to knowledge dissemination and adoption of the recommended practice derived from evidence)	8 % (3, 10)
Potential to reduce unjustified variation in practice	Implementation of CER study findings has potential to reduce unjustified variation in practice	7 % (3, 13)
Total		*100*

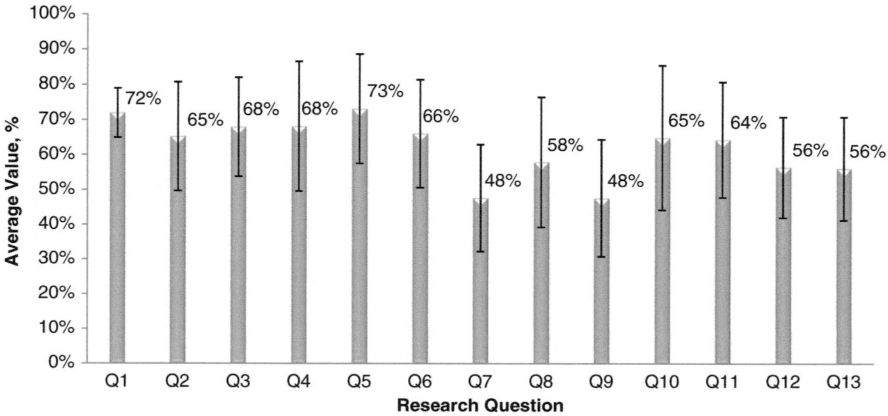

Fig. 13.2 Ranking of CER questions from Table 13.4. Higher average value denotes a higher rank (error bars represent 95 % confidence intervals)

clinical outcomes (mean weight, 4.7; *normalized 11 %*), *unmet needs* (mean weight, 4.5; *normalized 11 %*), and *feasibility of the CER question* (mean weight, 4.3; *normalized 10 %*) (Table 13.5). Wide weight variations across participants were noticed on the remaining criteria.

Value estimates of CER questions, combining weights and scores assigned by participants, varied between 48 and 73 % of maximum value on the MCDA scale (Fig. 13.2). Highest value estimates (>70 %) were obtained for research questions exploring the association between dialysis selection process or vascular access/antimicrobial prophylaxis and mortality/morbidity (Q1 and Q5). Lowest value estimates (48 %) were obtained for CER questions exploring incidence/prevalence rates, baseline characteristics, and outcomes of hemodialysis patients (Q7 and Q9). Ranking had excellent face validity for all criteria.

This application for home-based intensive hemodialysis shows that a holistic MCDA approach provides a useful tool to ensure prioritization of CER questions that provide highest benefits for improving clinical practice. Results of this ranking process were used to prioritize research planning for the international network of nephrologist researchers.

13.3.2 MCDA for Clinical Research Prioritization: Case Study of Registry Trial Prioritization for the Kidney, Dialysis, and Transplantation (KDT) Program

The Kidney, Dialysis, and Transplantation (KDT) program at the Institute for Clinical Evaluative Sciences (ICES, Ontario, Canada) is composed of staff and clinicians that aim to improve health and healthcare of patients with kidney disease. The KDT program was interested in leveraging administrative data to conduct a cluster-randomized trial. The aim was to pursue one of five cluster RCTs in the realm of in-center hemodialysis interventions that would have the highest impact for reducing patient morbidity and burden of dialysis patients on the healthcare system.

The KDT program conducted a prioritization exercise having two goals. Because this was the first cluster-randomized trial for the program, the team wanted to advance the most feasible and scalable trial. Secondly, the researchers wanted to choose the project with the most pragmatic approach so they can leverage the experience gained to conduct future trials in this area.

The team prioritized the five trials using the six criteria developed for the hemodialysis CER case study (Table 13.6). The "impact of the CER question" criteria were excluded in this case study because the patient population and disease process were similar across research proposals; hence, they were not expected to vary across this criterion. Feasibility of implementation of the intervention was added as a separate criterion rather than including it as a feasibility subcriterion, since it was felt to require special consideration in the context of planning cluster-randomized trials.

The analytic hierarchy process (AHP) was used to calculate weights assigned to each criterion. AHP is designed for situations whereby ideas, feelings, and emotions affecting the decision process are quantified to provide a numeric scale for prioritizing alternatives, in this case research projects (Saaty 1982).

Weights were elicited using AHP by which each criterion was ranked relative to every other alternative criterion on a discrete scale of 1 (criteria i and j are of equal importance) to 9 (i is extremely more important than j). A rating of 5 indicated that i is strongly more important than j. This procedure established a 6 × 6 *pairwise comparison matrix* that quantifies the decision-maker's judgment regarding the relative importance of the different criteria (Saaty 1982).

Researchers ($n = 11$) were then asked to assign weights to each criterion. Relative weights were calculated by normalizing the comparison matrix (adapted from Taha 2007; (Taha 2007) results presented in Table 13.6). The highest importance was assigned to the feasibility (*normalized* 30 %), patient impact (*normalized* 27 %), and implementation of intervention (*normalized* 24 %). Economic impact and quality of evidence were judged to be of least importance (lowest weights at *normalized* 4 % and 7 %, respectively). Consistency ratio (CR) of the comparison matrix was then calculated (CR = 0.03), providing a level of coherent judgment on the part of the decision-maker regarding the pairwise comparison. A consistency ratio <0.1 was considered acceptable.[1]

Following the weighting exercise, clinician researchers scored each project based on the a priori selected criteria, on a scale of 0 (worst) to 3 (best). The score for each

[1] A CR ≥ 0.1 means there is high inconsistency and the decision-maker may need to reestimate the importance of the criteria relative to each other. To keep consistency ratio low, some have suggested keeping the number of criteria in a range between 5 and 9 (Saaty 1982). This suggestion is based on our limits for processing information. From Miller's law, it is argued that the number of unique information an average human can hold in working memory is 7 ± 2 (Miller 1956). Thus, if more than nine criteria are necessary, we suggest clustering them in groups of five to nine.

Table 13.6 Criteria definitions and assigned weights

Criteria	Description	Normalized weights
Meets information need	Registry trial addresses *unmet need* (significant uncertainty, knowledge gap) in an identified priority area, as determined by systematic review, expert panel, clinical practice guideline, consensus statement, healthcare agency mandate, formal information need assessment, or other systematic process	8 %
Feasibility	Registry trial is *feasible* (considering available data sources, data quality, study population size, sample size requirements, enrollment rate if applicable, and investigator's interest) Also please consider ethical concerns, regulatory red tape, and consent (patient vs. cluster level vs. Ministry of Health [MOH] guidelines*) **If the MOH is planning on adopting the intervention of interest regardless of the proposed trial, we may not need to consent patients*	30 %
Quality of evidence	The proposed study has the potential to provide *estimates in which we can be confident* (*Consider precision and risk of bias and other factors—see list below adapted from* Guyatt et al. (Guyatt and Busse 2011))*	7 %
Patient impact	The intervention for registry trial has potential to improve: (a) On patient survival and other major clinical outcomes that are not considered patient-reported outcomes (b) Patient *safety* or reduce *harm* *Patient-reported outcomes* (quality of life, function, well-being)	27 %
Economic impact	Registry trial has potential to result in savings in *cost* of intervention, other medical costs, nonmedical costs, opportunity costs (consider health system perspective)	4 %
Implementation of intervention	*Implementation* of intervention into practice is *feasible* considering**:** *Pre-study:* (**a**) Cost of setup (hiring RC, equipment, and training); (**b**) potential of outcome contamination due to switching from intervention to control groups *Post-study:* (**a**) Facilitators and barriers to knowledge dissemination and adoption of the recommended practice derived from evidence generated by registry trial; consider risk of inappropriate information use; (**b**) implementation of registry trial study findings has potential to reduce unjustified *variation in practice*	24 %
Total		*100*

Table 13.7 Criteria scoring and trial ranking

Trial	Mean weighted score	Rank
Trial 1	2.4	1
Trial 2	2.2	2
Trial 3	1.9	3
Trial 4	1.5	5
Trial 5	1.7	4

criterion was multiplied by the predetermined weight to get a weighted score estimate. The sum of the weighted scores was calculated for each alternative project; standard descriptive statistics (sum, mean, median) were used to identify the priority project. As shown in Table 13.7, this prioritization exercise allowed ranking of registry trials according to their weighted scores.

The results revealed that Trials 1, 2, and 3 had the highest priority and were rated as the most feasible projects with the highest likelihood for improving patient outcomes. Because there is little evidence in the literature regarding the efficacy for the intervention of Trials 4 and 5, the team felt these projects would have little patient impact hence were giving a lower rating. Since this priority setting exercise, the top three choices were presented to stakeholders and one of the projects was funded to move forward. Overall, the team considered this MCDA-based prioritization process transparent, valid, and practical.

These case studies demonstrate that MCDA can be used pragmatically to prioritize clinical research questions. It provides a way to ensure a systematic consideration of the relevant aspects of prioritization, with an increased awareness of the feasibility and potential benefits with regard to the triple aim. In the current context of limited resources and the duty to serve patients and populations while maintaining the sustainability of healthcare systems, such approaches are poised to advance patient care in a most meaningful way. This field of research and application is still in its infancy and more research is needed to optimize these approaches.

13.4 Conclusion

In clinical practice, and in the development of CPGs, clinicians have to deal with increasing amounts of evidence while struggling to reconcile their duty to help their patients with population needs and healthcare system sustainability. MCDA, by its very nature, was perceived by clinicians as not only useful for structuring CPGs and CER, since it permits an organized approach to identifying relevant questions and to clarifying evidence, but also as extremely satisfying because of its holistic approach to the patient. Its consideration of all relevant criteria brings the clinician back to the modernized Hippocratic oath emphasizing the moral obligations of physicians to do the best care possible for the patient and includes a pledge to neither subscribe to therapeutic nihilism nor overtreatment, to further share scientific knowledge, to see the patient in the context of his existence, and to not fear, but admit and address, ignorance (Sulmasy 1999). The analyses, reflections, interactions, and discussions that such tools stimulate are a promising avenue to further improving the quality of research that is required to continually advance care delivery.

In clinical research, investigators must consider, and make trade-offs, between multiple and sometimes conflicting criteria that need to be structured to prioritize the most critical research question(s) and to permit more informed funding decisions. MCDA analytics provide the research team with the opportunity to consider the values (or criteria) that each individual perceives as important and provides a unique ability for researchers to consider and discuss complex trade-offs among several options. Last but not least, it ensures that we see the patient and their family as partners in decision-making, and helps to better define issues that matter to patients, by ensuring that decisions, even those taken at the bedside, are rooted in consideration of all relevant criteria (see also Chapter 11 Shared decision-making for bedside applications of MCDA).

In conclusion, MCDA participants in the case studies presented here reported that MCDA provided a valid, transparent, and pragmatic process to identify best clinical practices and prioritize clinical research to improve patient health in a climate of increasingly scarce healthcare resources. The reflective process supported by holistic MCDA includes trade-offs that individuals have to make to tackle ethical dilemmas, awareness of conflicts of interest, and uncertainty implicit in rapidly evolving knowledge. This process, inherent to clinical research and practice, brings us back first and foremost to patient needs, which are, and should be, the ultimate purpose of clinical research and clinical practice guidelines (Sitges-Serra 2014). It also ensures research and practice decision-making is rooted in ethics and a deep awareness of the consequences of choices. As always, further research is compulsory to develop and integrate MCDA in clinical research and practice to contribute to better health and sustainable healthcare.

References

AGREE Collaboration (2003) Development and validation of an international appraisal instrument for assessing the quality of clinical practice guidelines: the AGREE project. Qual Saf Health Care 12(1):18–23

Alper BS, Hand JA, Elliott SG, Kinkade S, Hauan MJ, Onion DK et al (2004) How much effort is needed to keep up with the literature relevant for primary care? J Med Libr Assoc 92(4): 429–437

Andrews J (2013) Prioritization criteria methodology for future research needs proposals within the effective health care program: PiCMe-Prioritization Criteria Methods. PM:23367528

Atkins D, Briss PA, Eccles M, Flottorp S, Guyatt GH, Harbour RT et al (2005) Systems for grading the quality of evidence and the strength of recommendations II: pilot study of a new system. BMC Health Serv Res 5(1):25

Australian Government Department of Health and Ageing (2008) Public summary document for Somatropin. http://www.pbs.gov.au/info/industry/listing/elements/pbac-meetings/psd/2008-03

Baltussen R, Niessen L (2006) Priority setting of health interventions: the need for multi-criteria decision analysis. Cost Eff Resour Alloc 4:14

Brouwers MC, Kho ME, Browman GP, Burgers JS, Cluzeau F, Feder G et al (2010) AGREE II: advancing guideline development, reporting, and evaluation in health care. Prev Med 51(5): 421–424

Buffel du Vaure C, Ravaud P, Baron G, Barnes C, Gilberg S, Boutron I (2016) Potential workload in applying clinical practice guidelines for patients with chronic conditions and multimorbidity: a systematic analysis. BMJ Open 6(3):e010119

Burman P, Ritzen EM, Lindgren AC (2001) Endocrine dysfunction in Prader-Willi syndrome: a review with special reference to GH. Endocr Rev 22(6):787–799

Busse R, Orvain J, Velasco M, Perleth M, Drummond M, Gurtner F et al (2002) Best practice in undertaking and reporting health technology assessments. Working group 4 report. Int J Technol Assess Health Care 18(2):361–422

Butler MG, Lee PDK, Whitman B (2006) Management of Prader-Willi syndrome, 3rd edn. Springer Science Business Media inc., New York

Cabana MD, Rand CS, Powe NR, Wu AW, Wilson MH, Abboud PA et al (1999) Why don't physicians follow clinical practice guidelines? A framework for improvement. JAMA 282(15): 1458–1465

Canadian Institute for Health Information (CIHI) (2015) Canadian organ replacement register annual report: treatment of end-stage organ failure in Canada, 2004 to 2013. https://secure.cihi.ca/estore/productFamily.htm?locale=en&pf=PFC2864&lang=en

Cecamore C, Savino A, Salvatore R, Cafarotti A, Pelliccia P, Mohn A et al (2011) Clinical practice guidelines: what they are, why we need them and how they should be developed through rigorous evaluation. Eur J Pediatr 170(7):831–836

Centre for Evidence Based Medicine (2010) CEBM levels of evidence version #2. http://www.cebm.net/index.aspx?o=5653

Committee to Advise the Public Health Service on Clinical Practice Guidelines Institute of Medicine, Institute of Medicine; Field MJ, Lohr KN (eds) (1990) Clinical practice guidelines: directions for a new program. Washington, D.C.: National Academy Press

Consensus guidelines for the diagnosis and treatment of adults with growth hormone deficiency: summary statement of the Growth Hormone Research Society Workshop on Adult Growth Hormone Deficiency (1998) J Clin Endocrinol Metab 83(2):379–381

Daniels N (1999) Decisions about access to health care and accountability for reasonableness. J Urban Health 76(2):176–191

Daniels N (2001) Justice, health, and healthcare. Am J Bioeth 1(2):2–16

Deal CL, Tony M, Hoybye C, Allen DB, Tauber M, Christiansen JS (2013) Growth Hormone Research Society workshop summary: consensus guidelines for recombinant human growth hormone therapy in Prader-Willi Syndrome. J Clin Endocrinol Metab 98(6):E1072–E1087

Dhalla I, Laupacis A (2008) Moving from opacity to transparency in pharmaceutical policy. CMAJ 178(4):428–431

Doherty S (2005) History of evidence-based medicine. Oranges, chloride of lime and leeches: barriers to teaching old dogs new tricks Emerg Med Australas 17(4):314–321

Dolan JG (2010) Multi-Criteria clinical decision support. A primer on the use of multiple-criteria decision-making methods to promote evidence-based, patient-centered healthcare. Patient 3(4):229–248

Dubois RW, Graff JS. Setting priorities for comparative effectiveness research: from assessing public health benefits to being open with the public. Health Aff (Millwood). 2011;30(12):2235–42.

electronic Medicines Compendium (eMC) (2011) Summary of product characteristics – Genotropin 5.3mg, 12mg. http://www.medicines.org.uk/emc/medicine/13860/SPC/Genotropin+5.3mg,+12mg/

Ely JW, Osheroff JA, Ebell MH, Chambliss ML, Vinson DC, Stevermer JJ et al (2002) Obstacles to answering doctors' questions about patient care with evidence: qualitative study. BMJ 324(7339):710

Evers S, Goossens M, de VH, van TM, Ament A (2005) Criteria list for assessment of methodological quality of economic evaluations: consensus on health economic criteria. Int J Technol Assess Health Care 21(2):240–245

EVIDEM Collaboration (2010) Open access prototypes of the Collaborative registry. https://www.evidem.org/initiatives/collaborative-registry/

Gabbay J, le MA (2004) Evidence based guidelines or collectively constructed "mindlines?" Ethnographic study of knowledge management in primary care. BMJ 329(7473):1013

Gerkens S, Crott R, Cleemput I, Thissen JP, Closon MC, Horsmans Y et al (2008) Comparison of three instruments assessing the quality of economic evaluations: a practical exercise on economic evaluations of the surgical treatment of obesity. Int J Technol Assess Health Care 24(3):318–325

Goetghebeur MM, Wagner M, Khoury H, Levitt RJ, Erickson LJ, Rindress D (2008) Evidence and Value: Impact on DEcisionMaking – the EVIDEM framework and potential applications. BMC Health Serv Res 8(1):270

Goetghebeur MM, Wagner M, Khoury H, Rindress D, Gregoire JP, Deal C (2010) Combining multicriteria decision analysis, ethics and health technology assessment: applying the EVIDEM decisionmaking framework to growth hormone for turner syndrome patients. Cost Eff Resour Alloc 8(1):4

Goetghebeur MM, Wagner M, Khoury H, Levitt RJ, Erickson LJ, Rindress D (2012) Bridging health technology assessment (HTA) and efficient health care decision making with multicriteria decision analysis (MCDA): Applying the EVIDEM framework to medicines appraisal. Med Decis Making 32(2):376–388

Gruskin S, Daniels N (2008) Process is the point: justice and human rights: priority setting and fair deliberative process. Am J Public Health 98(9):1573–1577

Guyatt G, Busse J (2011) Tool to assess risk of bias in cohort studies. http://www.evidencepartners.com/resources/

Ho KK (2007) Consensus guidelines for the diagnosis and treatment of adults with GH deficiency II: a statement of the GH Research Society in association with the European Society for Pediatric Endocrinology, Lawson Wilkins Society, European Society of Endocrinology, Japan Endocrine Society, and Endocrine Society of Australia. Eur J Endocrinol 157(6):695–700

Jadad AR, Moore RA, Carroll D, Jenkinson C, Reynolds DJ, Gavaghan DJ et al (1996) Assessing the quality of reports of randomized clinical trials: is blinding necessary? Control Clin Trials 17(1):1–12

Jehu-Appiah C, Baltussen R, Acquah C, Aikins M, d'Almeida SA, Bosu WK et al (2008) Balancing equity and efficiency in health priorities in Ghana: the use of multicriteria decision analysis. Value Health 11(7):1081–1087

Kastner M, Bhattacharyya O, Hayden L, Makarski J, Estey E, Durocher L et al (2015) Guideline uptake is influenced by six implementability domains for creating and communicating guidelines: a realist review. J Clin Epidemiol 68(5):498–509

Krishnan JA, Lindenauer PK, Au DH, Carson SS, Lee TA, McBurnie MA et al (2013) Stakeholder priorities for comparative effectiveness research in chronic obstructive pulmonary disease: a workshop report. Am J Respir Crit Care Med 187(3):320–326

Makarski J, Brouwers MC (2014) The AGREE Enterprise: a decade of advancing clinical practice guidelines. Implement Sci 9:103

Miller GA (1956) The magical number seven, plus or minus two: some limits on our capacity for processing information. Psychol Rev 63:81–97

Nesrallah GE, Moist LM, Awaraji C, Lindsay RM (2004) An international registry to compare quotidian dialysis regimens with conventional thrice-weekly hemodialysis: why, how, and potential pitfalls. Semin Dial 17(2):131–135

Nesrallah GE, Mustafa RA, MacRae J, Pauly RP, Perkins DN, Gangji A et al (2013) Canadian Society of Nephrology guidelines for the management of patients with ESRD treated with intensive hemodialysis. Am J Kidney Dis 62(1):187–198

Persad G, Wertheimer A, Emanuel EJ (2009) Principles for allocation of scarce medical interventions. Lancet 373(9661):423–431

Pfizer inc (2011) Prescribing info: Genotropin

AGREE Research Trust (2016) Using AGREE II for practice guideline development. http://www.agreetrust.org/resource-centre/agree-ii-as-a-practice-guideline-development-framework

Saarni SI, Gylling HA (2004) Evidence based medicine guidelines: a solution to rationing or politics disguised as science? J Med Ethics 30(2):171–175

Saaty TL (1982) Decision making for leaders: the analytical hierarchy process for decisions in a complex world. California, Belmont

Sitges-Serra A (2014) Clinical guidelines at stake. J Epidemiol Community Health 68(10):906–908

Smith J (2004) Editor's Choice: from optimism to hubris. BMJ 329:0–h

Sulmasy DP (1999) What is an oath and why should a physician swear one? Theor Med Bioeth 20(4):329–346

Taha HA (2007) Operations research. An introduction, 8th edn. Pearson Education Inc, Upper Saddle River

The Kidney Foundation of Canada (2013) Facing the facts. Includes highlights from the Canadian Organ Replacement Register. http://www.kidney.ca/document.doc?id=4083

The STROBE group (2007) The STROBE statement: checklist of items that should be included in reports of observational studies. http://www.strobe-statement.org

Viergever RF, Olifson S, Ghaffar A, Terry RF (2010) A checklist for health research priority setting: nine common themes of good practice. Health Res Policy Syst 8:36

Wieringa S, Greenhalgh T (2015) 10 years of mindlines: a systematic review and commentary. Implement Sci 10:45

Woolf SH, Grol R, Hutchinson A, Eccles M, Grimshaw J (1999) Clinical guidelines: potential benefits, limitations, and harms of clinical guidelines. BMJ 318(7182):527–530

World Health Organization (2004) Guidance on ethics and equitable access to HIV treatment and care. http://www.who.int/ethics/Guidance%20on%20Ethics%20and%20HIV.pdf

Part III
Future Directions

Chapter 14
Using MCDA as a Decision Aid in Health Technology Appraisal for Coverage Decisions: Opportunities, Challenges and Unresolved Questions

Martina Garau and Nancy J. Devlin

Abstract Existing Health Technology Appraisal (HTA) processes almost inevitably require the consideration of multiple criteria which go beyond improvements in patient and population health. MCDA offers a way of structuring these decision processes and making them more transparent and consistent. Its use represents a way of complementing and supporting deliberative processes, rather than supplanting them. This can also assist the accountability of HTA decisions to stakeholders.

MCDA has the potential to address a number of limitations of current HTA systems. However, its application in HTA requires careful consideration of a number of issues, including how the decision criteria are selected and weighted; whose values should be used; how budget constraints and opportunity costs are addressed; and how uncertainty in evidence is handled. The way forward on these fundamental questions will depend on the type of the decision problem and of the objectives of the health-care system within which decisions are being made.

There needs to be a consideration of the balance between additional organisational costs of implementing an MCDA approach and additional benefits of improved decision making process. Even where MCDA cannot follow 'best practise', partial implementation (e.g. use of a performance matrix) may still have the potential to improve the decision making process.

M. Garau (✉) • N.J. Devlin
The Office of Health Economics, London, UK
e-mail: mgarau@ohe.org

© Springer International Publishing AG 2017
K. Marsh et al. (eds.), *Multi-Criteria Decision Analysis to Support Healthcare Decisions*, DOI 10.1007/978-3-319-47540-0_14

14.1 Introduction

Many countries have developed or are in the process of developing collectively funded health-care systems to ensure universal coverage and access to health care for their populations (WHO 2010a). Governments increasingly face budgetary limits on health-care spending, giving rise to a need to make difficult choices about which health interventions should be given priority. This process, usually controlled by third-party payers, aims at maximising the value generated by health interventions given the available budget constraint. Historically, many high-income countries and more recently an increasing set of middle-income countries have established Health Technology Appraisal (HTA) processes to identify and recommend the most valuable health interventions that should be made available within national, or jurisdictional, health-care systems. As pointed out by Batista and Hodge (2009):

> There is no "best" model for HTA but rather different models, which may explain the fragmented picture of HTA in some countries and the successive transformations of HTA organizations witnessed in other countries (Batista and Hodge 2009).

HTA is a broad term that encompasses a variety of approaches: it has been defined as a 'multidisciplinary field of policy analysis. It studies the medical, social, ethical, and economic implications of development, diffusion, and use of health technology' (The International Network of Agencies for Health Technology Assessment, INAHTA).

Although traditionally HTA has been linked to the assessment and appraisal of individual technologies, mainly medicines, it can be more broadly referred to as the assessment and appraisal of any intervention used for the production of health service. Towse et al. (2011) distinguish between:

- Technologies applied within the health-care system – a drug a device, a surgical procedure or other medical interventions (microtechnologies).
- Organisational systems used in health care to organise access, service delivery and payment of providers (Garrido and Rottingen 2010), such as the mix of clinical and related workforce (macro-technologies).
- Groups of individual health interventions which are combined within a delivery system to manage patients efficiently. This is the focus of clinical guidelines which can bring together assessment of microtechnologies, in the way they are used in sequence within a care pathway, and of macro-technologies, when looking at organisational issues such as location of care.

The focus of this chapter is on applications of MCDA in HTA processes for microtechnologies appraised individually or as a group as part of clinical guidelines. However, this does not preclude the use of MCDA in other health-care decision making contexts. On the contrary, we argue that MCDA can help in considering a wider range of criteria, compared to current HTA processes, including health system considerations, which are typically kept separated and considered in macro-technology assessment.

14.2 Why Do We Need MCDA in HTA?

MCDA has the potential to address a number of limitations of current HTA systems, most importantly, being more explicit in the way multiple attributes of value beyond improvements in health are taken into account; reflecting social values; providing more systematic and robust ways of considering evidence from stakeholders; and supporting the way HTA decision makers exercise judgement when making trade-offs between multiple criteria.

HTA processes typically seek to maximise 'value' given limited health-care resources.

However, what is considered to constitute 'value' can vary among jurisdictions. There is general consensus that improvements in health as a result of treatment is the most important benefit: many HTA systems have introduced highly formalised approaches to measure changes in patient health and for choosing interventions that are effective and provide value for money. Those systems, set up in Australia, New Zealand, the UK, European Nordic countries such as Sweden and some Canadian provinces, have primarily relied on the quality-adjusted life year (QALY) for measuring changes in both length and quality of life and focused on its maximisation in their decision making processes.

However, health-care systems face multiple objectives that go beyond improvements in population health. For example, equity considerations, relating to the reduction of inequitable distributions of health across different groups, may be considered relevant. Similarly, an imperative to respond to life-threatening situations may also merit consideration (Baltussen and Niessen 2006). As recently recommended by the WHO, HTA can support countries towards universal health coverage to allocate limited funds efficiently by facilitating uptake of technologies providing good value for money and prevent uptake of less valuable technologies (WHO 2010b).

Golan et al. (2011) report the criteria considered in different countries for health technology prioritisation (Table 14.1). They include considerations of the clinical benefits, efficiency, equality and other social values. The authors note that efficiency-based criteria are common to all health systems. Yet there is a distinction between countries that consider this explicitly – in the form of cost-effectiveness analyses and maximisation of health outcomes given a budget constraint – and countries that consider costs and budgetary impact without directly, or explicitly, comparing them to the benefits accrued (Golan et al. 2011). The latter make decisions based on a two-stage approach where an assessment of therapeutic 'added value' (the relative effectiveness of a new treatment compared to current treatments) feeds into pricing and/or reimbursement decisions taken at either national or local levels.

However, whether cost is explicitly or implicitly or ignored in HTA (e.g. as in the USA), financial factors are ultimately unavoidable in the health-care system's implementation of HTA decisions. These can have a substantial impact on total spending, resource allocation and patients' access to health care.

Table 14.1 Criteria used internationally for prioritising new health technologies

Principles of allocative justice	Criteria	Australia	Canada	Denmark	Finland	France	Israel	New Zealand	Norway	Oregon	Sweden	The Netherlands	UK
Need	General	✓	✓					✓		✓			✓
	Severity of the condition			✓		✓	✓		✓		✓	✓	
	Availability of alternatives		✓			✓	✓	✓					
Appropriateness	Efficacy and safety					✓	✓	✓				✓	✓
	Effectiveness			✓	✓			✓		✓			
Clinical benefits	General	✓	✓	✓			✓	✓			✓		
	Effect on mortality (life-saving)						✓		✓	✓	✓		
	Effect on longevity						✓			✓			
	Effect on health-related quality-of-life	✓	✓				✓			✓			
Efficiency	Cost-effectiveness/benefit	✓		✓		✓		✓	✓	✓	✓	✓	✓
	Budgetary impact		✓		✓		✓	✓					
	Cost		✓				✓						

Equality	General	✓		✓				✓	✓	✓	✓	✓	✓
	Accessibility to the service	✓	✓	✓									
	Affordability to the individual						✓	✓				✓	
Solidarity			✓	✓			✓		✓		✓	✓	
Other ethical or social values	Autonomy	✓		✓							✓		✓
	Public health value					✓							
	Impact on future generations	✓											
'Other' considerations						✓							
Quality of the clinical and economic evidence			✓		✓				✓				✓
Other considerations not elsewhere classified	Strategic issues consistency with previous decisions and precedents		✓					✓					✓

Source: Golan et al. (2011)

There has been growing interest in developing approaches within existing HTA systems that could take into account multiple criteria simultaneously and in a more systematic way (Department of Health 2010; Norheim et al. 2014). In part, this relates to the need for HTA bodies to be accountable for their decisions, which in turn pushes them towards being more explicit about the way competing criteria have been taken into account.

In part, it also relates to policy debates pushing for a departure from a QALY-driven approach (see, e.g. Kind 2015). There is growing recognition of the need to consider outcomes beyond health outcome-related ones and explore alternative methods to measure 'all things that matter to patients' (Brazier and Tsuchiya 2015). The UK government proposal to introduce a value-based pricing system, subsequently renamed 'value-based assessment' because of its potential inclusion in the National Institute for Health and Care Excellence (NICE) process, is an example of an attempt to complement the current system of QALY maximisation with explicit consideration of other factors or attributes of value such as the severity of the disease targeted by interventions (Department of Health 2010).

Similarly, the WHO highlights that current approaches for priority setting in health care in low- and middle-income countries do not address adequately the full range of health system objectives. Current approaches are based mainly on cost-effectiveness analysis. There is a need for explicit recognition and consideration of equity criteria (Norheim et al. 2014).

An example of the use of multiple criteria in a prioritisation process is that of Thailand, where the selection of health topics for the Thai HTA body is conducted by a panel comprising of representatives from four stakeholder groups: health professionals, academics, patient and civic groups. The panel selects at least ten topics yearly for assessment according to prioritisation criteria including size of population, and impact on household expenditure if the intervention was not included in the benefit package. In a pilot to use MCDA in this process, an ad hoc stakeholder panel was created to assign a score from one to five to each of the six selection criteria as shown in Table 14.2 and identified interventions deserving further assessment and appraisal (Youngkong et al. 2012). The impact of the study was deemed positive in terms of improved fairness and transparency of the process, compared to the existing one which was described as 'ad-hoc and driven by stakeholder groups' (Youngkong et al. 2012).

Another factor in HTA policy debate has been the involvement of a range of stakeholders in the decision making process, including the patients who can potentially get access to the interventions. For example, in the case of orphan drugs, it has been recognised that the preferences of people directly affected by these rare and complex conditions are critical to the assessment of relevant treatments. Clinicians who deal with these conditions on a daily basis can also provide valuable insights relating to both health and non-health gains (Sussex et al. 2013a; Paulden et al. 2015).

The inclusion of patient views represents another shift away from the conventional QALY paradigm, which tends to focus on public preferences when

Table 14.2 Example of scores of proposed interventions against selection criteria for the Thai benefit package

Health interventions	Selection criteria					
	Size of population affected by disease	Effectiveness of health intervention	Variation in practice	Economic impact on household expenditure	Equity/ ethical and social implication	Total
1. Anti-immunoglobulin E for severe asthma	4	3	5	5	1	18
2. Treatment for people with chronic hepatitis B	5	4	2	3	3	17
3. System for screening, treatment and rehabilitation of alcoholism	5	5	4	1	1	16
4. Implant dentures for people who have problem with conventional complete dentures	5	2	2	5	1	15
5. Screening for risk factors for leukaemia in people living in the industrial areas	4	3	5	1	2	15
6. Treatment for severe lupus nephritis	2	4	2	5	1	14
7. Smoking cessation programme	5	3	2	1	3	14
8. Treatment for people with chronic hepatitis C	3	5	2	3	1	14
9. Absorbent products for urinary and faecal incontinence among disabled and elderly people	4	2	2	4	1	13
10. Treatment for unfertilised women	5	0	2	5	1	13
11. Renal replacement by dialysis for new final stage renal failure patients	2	1	5	4	1	13
12. Screening and treatment for liver cancer	2	3	2	5	1	13
13. Physical examination package (following the Civil Servant Medical Benefit Scheme)	5	0	5	1	1	12
14. *Cissus quadrangularis* L. for haemorrhoid	5	1	4	1	1	12
15. Biological agents for psoriasis	1	1	2	5	2	11
16. Screening for gall bladder cancer	2	2	2	1	3	10
17. Orbital implant and plastic surgery of orbit and facial bones	1	2	1	1	2	7

Source: Youngkong et al. (2012)

valuing the different health states measuring health-related quality of life.[1] Increased attention to patients' preferences is also arguably consistent with conventional welfare economics aimed at aggregating (and maximising) preferences of affected individuals (Brazier et al. 2005).

Many HTA systems, such as NICE and the Canadian Agency for Drugs and Technologies in Health (CADTH), do involve stakeholders in their decision making through formalised consultation processes and participation in committees meetings (and via the role of the Citizen's Council). Since May 2014, the Scottish HTA body (Scottish Medicines Consortium – SMC) has introduced the option of forming and consulting an external panel of clinicians and patient representatives during the assessment of medicines for rare or end of life conditions (SMC 2015). This further stage in the HTA process allows the main committee to obtain views on the expected benefits of new interventions that are not captured in its standard method of assessment, mainly focused on cost per QALY. However, as noted in Culyer (2009), consultation or commenting is different from participation in decision making. In many HTA systems, it remains unclear how the views of patients, clinicians and other key stakeholders influence the final decisions. MCDA offers a way to improve the transparency and consistency of the extent to which these stakeholders' views are taken into account.

A final reason MCDA could be useful in HTA is that the consideration of complex information, such as decision problems entailing multiple and conflicting criteria, is cognitively demanding and can lead to inconsistent decision making. The decision theory and psychological literature shows that under conditions of complexity and uncertainty, individuals tend to rely on heuristic mental processing. Such processing is mainly based on intuition and fragments of memory which can lead to oversight of relevant information and cognitive biases (Gilovich et al. 2002; Kahneman 2003; Hicks and Kluemper 2011). In the context of HTA, decisions are made not by individuals but by committees, following a 'deliberative process', and this adds a further layer of complexity (Culyer 2009). How information is used and processed to reach a decision will be influenced by a number of factors including group dynamics, unwritten rules and conventions about the way decisions are reached; the chairperson's chairing 'style'; and how many people are on the committee. Committees' members are often required to review and process a large volume of information supporting one or more than one technology, to formulate a judgement and to reach quick decisions within committee meeting discussions. For those reasons, Devlin and Sussex (2011) concluded that 'the preferred options identified by MCDA are likely to out-perform the use of intuitive judgement alone'.

MCDA can facilitate and structure individuals' thinking on specific decision problems and also provide an aid to support group decision making. In particular, it can ensure that all members of decision making committees can input and effectively contribute to the group discussion and development of the final decision. In addition, it can help to minimise the impact of people with dominant personalities

[1] An exception is the Swedish approach to HTA, which stipulates a preference for using patients' 'experience-based' values, rather than those of the general public, in the valuation of quality of life.

or chairing styles who can potentially drive the group discussion and formation of people's preferences.

In summary, MCDA has the potential to improve decision making in HTA by improving its transparency and consistency. It can also address a number of limitations specific to the current HTA decision making processes, such as the consideration of a composite measure of benefit; improving stakeholders' involvement, and supporting individual and group exercise of judgement.

This may be related to recognised frameworks setting out the conditions necessary for a 'legitimate' decision making process. MCDA can help HTA to meet two conditions of the accountability for reasonableness (A4R) framework (Norman and Sabin 2008)[2] as it provides a structure to develop or adapt criteria relevant to stakeholders (the 'reasonableness condition') and could improve clarity on the way evidence and other factors taken into account are presented to outside observers (the 'publicity condition').

In the rest of this chapter, we will explore a number of issues to be considered before introducing MCDA in HTA. They are summarised in Table 14.3 and addressed in the following sections.

14.3 Do the Criteria and Weights Need to Be 'Fixed' in Order to Provide Consistency Between HTA Decisions?

In some types of health-care decisions (e.g. the European Medicines Agency exploratory use of MCDA to assess the benefits and risks of new medicines – see Phillips et al. 2011), it is arguably appropriate to choose both the criteria and the weights to be used on a case-by-case basis. The specific types of benefits and risks will be different in each case, and the key aim of benefit risk assessment (BRA) is to establish the balance of benefits and harms for each technology. In contrast, there is an argument for all HTA decisions to employ a fixed set of criteria, given that each decision affects the same limited budget. Every HTA decision has an opportunity cost – and the metric in which benefits lost are measured needs to be the same as the metric in which benefits obtained are measured, in order to facilitate a weighing up of benefits and costs. If different criteria are used, or the same criteria with a different weight on each, on a case-by-case basis, this could obfuscate a consistent assessment of value for money. In effect, it changes the definition of the maximand at each and every decision point, such that achieving allocative efficiency is difficult.

---

[2] 'The A4R framework consists of four conditions: process must be public (fully transparent) about the grounds for its decisions; the decision must rest on reasons that stakeholders can agree are relevant; decisions should be revisable in light of new evidence and arguments; and there should be assurance through enforcement that these conditions (publicity, relevance, and revisability) are met' (Norman and Sabin 2008).

Table 14.3 Overview of key issues when using MCDA in HTA

	Options	Issues for consideration
Criteria and weights to be fixed?	1. Established in advance; the same across all decisions 2. Chosen on a case-by-case basis and varying across technologies or disease areas	1. Allows using same metric to measure lost and added benefit; consistent consideration of all criteria 2. Flexible approach. However it can hinder systematic consideration of all criteria and predictability of decision making
Whose criteria?	1. Current HTA bodies' criteria 2. Members of an HTA committee on behalf of the health system 3. Reflect views of the general public	1. Assumption is that there is a mandate for those 2. Involvement of health system budget holders can encourage alignment of objectives across various health system decision makers 3. Reflecting taxpayers/potential health system users' views
Whose preferences for weighting the criteria?	1. Any stakeholder as defined by the decision maker 2. Members of an HTA committee 3. Members of the general public	1. In line with extra-welfarist foundation of HTA. However, variations of stakeholders among diseases might require flexible weights 2. Pragmatic approach which can avoid conducting large preference-based studies 3. Consistent with the approach taken to valuing QoL in QALYs
How to factor in opportunity costs?	1. Separate criterion for cost 2. Composite measure of (net) benefits to be weighed-up against (net) costs	1. Risk of overlap with other criteria (e.g. cost and cost-effectiveness) 2. Requires setting an acceptable 'cost per incremental benefit/point score'
How can uncertainty be addressed?	1. A separate, distinct criterion for uncertainty 2. Sensitivity analysis techniques	1. Measuring and valuing such a criterion present challenges. Different criteria can be associated with different types and degrees of uncertainty 2. Ensures that sensitivity to assumptions about key aspects of evidence is taken into account. However, it leaves open the question of how results of sensitivity analyses should affect decisions

Those issues have been recognised by both supporters and critics of MCDA as a guide to health-care decision makers. 'Without a proper assessment of the other attributes of benefit forgone, decisions may reduce both health and the other attributes of benefit that originally motivated the use of MCDA. Therefore, the task of conducting MCDA correctly is considerable and it should not be regarded as a simple alternative to cost effectiveness analysis (CEA) as the same issues and methods apply except that, for MCDA, other attributes of benefit are considered in addition to health outcome (Peacock et al. 2009). If not done properly, instead of making decisions that improve a composite measure of benefit, which better represents society's preferences, it may actually reduce it' (Claxton et al. 2015) (cited in Drummond et al. 2015).

This same argument may not apply with as much force where HTA purposely does not take costs into account. For example, in the USA, the focus of HTA is on establishing the relative effectiveness of new health-care technologies, rather than cost-effectiveness. In these circumstances, each decision is in effect a one-off case, where what constitutes relative effectiveness and how it is measured might plausibly differ from technology to technology. However, even in such cases, the decisions made as a result of these HTA process will inevitably have implications for budget impact, resource allocation and spending on health care. Avoiding the consideration of costs in HTA simplifies the HTA process – but risks extending coverage to technologies which are poor value for money and passing on efficiency issues for decisions for insurers and providers of health care to manage or patients and the public via co-payment and premium insurers.

14.4 Whose Criteria?

One option is to use the criteria which HTA bodies say that they currently use, assuming they have some legitimacy. Alternatively, where an HTA system shifts from a purely deliberative process to an MCDA process and is therefore going to be more explicit about the criteria it uses (such that it will be able to be held to account for decisions), it may wish to revisit its criteria.

Where criteria come from in part relates to the wider question of whose views and opinions are considered relevant in decision making. For example, should the criteria come from the collective expertise of the members of an HTA committee, acting on behalf of the National Health System (NHS)? Should the health-care system whose budgets and health-care delivery mechanisms are affected by HTA decisions be given a say on what criteria to use, so that HTA and health-care system objectives align? Involving health-care budget holders in the selection of criteria to use in HTA could overcome the problem of there being a disjunction between the 'maximands' from the perspective of different parts of the health-care system. For example, Shah et al. (2012) and Karlsberg Schaffer et al. (2015) point out that whilst NICE's process assumes that the principal objective of health care is to maximise QALYs, this is out of keeping both with the objectives of the Department of Health and with the decisions being made in local NHS organisations in England. If HTA bodies are acting as agents (in principal-agent terms) for the health-care system, then there is an argument for the HTA body consulting closely with the health-care system regarding the choice of criteria, rather than selecting them independently of the organisations whose budgets are effected by their recommendations.

A further alternative is to seek input from the general public – as taxpayers and potential patients. For example, the Oregon Health Services Commission undertook an extensive consultation with the public during the establishment of its 'experiment' with prioritisation (Kitzhaber 1993). A similar process could inform the selection of criteria for HTA – which could aid the legitimacy of decisions.

14.5 Whose Preferences Should Be Used in Weighting Criteria?

A related question is whose preferences should count in weighting the criteria. Again, there is no single 'correct' answer to this question: it will depend on the nature of the health-care system in each case, which is in turn a product of the cultural and sociopolitical context. As noted above, in repeated HTA decisions that affect a single, fixed budget, there is an argument to be made for using identical criteria, identically weighted, in order to facilitate the pursuit of allocative efficiency. It is less clear that this same consideration applies where HTA focuses on effects and benefits, rather than addressing cost. Although, as economists, where budgets are fixed, we would argue that thinking about allocative efficiency and opportunity cost should always be the cornerstone of HTA.

The theoretical foundations for HTA have relatively little to say on this matter of whose weights should be used in an MCDA. The use of cost-effectiveness analysis in health care (manifested as cost per QALY) rests on the theory of extra-welfarism, and this arguably also provides the theoretical foundations for extending the formal consideration of other criteria via MCDA. Broadly speaking, extra-welfarism represents a rejection of welfarism, and cost-benefit analysis, as a basis for making public choices, on the grounds that these rely on utility. 'Extra-welfarists' (a.k.a non-welfarists), notably Sen (1977), argue that utility is fundamentally flawed as a basis for social choices. In health care, extra-welfarists argue that things other than utility should therefore be taken into account (Culyer 1991). In practice (rather than as any theoretical requirement of extra-welfarist theory), this has manifested itself as cost per QALY, where the QoL weights in QALYs come from members of the general public. It is important to note that other approaches would be entirely consistent with the extra-welfarist foundations of HTA, as pointed by Morris et al. (2007):

> It is important to note that what has become the orthodox approach to economic evaluation under extra-welfarism has emerged through practice rather than being required by it as a normative framework.

Culyer (2012) notes that in extra-welfarism:

> …any number of stakeholders might be regarded as the appropriate source of different values. (Culyer 2012)

Sources of values might appropriately come from:

> '…an authority (decision makers, wise women, the general public, an elected or appointed committee, a citizen's jury, or some other organ)' and whilst '…economists may be able to derive values from experimental groups or samples of the relevant population through modern methods for eliciting preferences…the choice about which groups to sample are not normally for the analyst to make but for the ultimate decision maker, advised by the analyst'. (Culyer 2012)

This is also a feature of early writings on resource allocation in health care by Alan Williams, which refer to extra-welfarism as 'the decision makers' approach'. Under this pragmatic approach, it is possible for values (such as QoL weights) to come from the decision makers themselves ('postulated values') (Williams 1972, cited by Sugden 2008). This in turn would suggest some legitimacy, in MCDA approaches to HTA decision making, in using the views and preferences of decision makers (i.e. committee members – e.g. via 'decision conferencing' – Phillips 2007) in weighting criteria.

In contrast, Claxton and Devlin (2013) (in a briefing paper commissioned by NICE for its 2013 methodology review) note the parallels between the arguments for using MCDA methods in HTA, the methods used to value the EQ-5D – which comprises multiple criteria of Health-related quality of life (HRQoL) – and methods relating to which are already a standard part of HTA at NICE (NICE 2013). The widespread acceptance and active promulgation of stated preference methods to weigh HRQoL in the EQ-5D, drawing on the preferences of representative samples of the general public, might be considered to set a precedent. The normative position behind the decision to base these weights on the views of the general public is that these are the taxpayers and potential patients, valuing hypothetical health states behind a 'veil of ignorance'.

That same rationale arguably also applies to the weighting of multiple criteria in the HTA decision making process. This would imply that implementing an MCDA approach to HTA in such a situation would make use of information on the relative weights on the criteria derived from the general public (e.g. via a discrete choice experiment).

Where the normative rationale for deciding whose views should count in determining MCDA criteria and weights is not clear, multiple stakeholder perspectives may be indicated (as suggested by the reasonableness condition of the A4R framework). However, this raises two issues. The first relates to the variation in relevant stakeholders, such as patients, among different diseases, which would require flexible weights. Arguably, patients might differ in their willingness to trade off increases in one measure of benefit against the others depending on the disease with which they are affected. For example, patients with rare conditions are likely to assign more importance to criteria relating to the nature of the disease being treated than those concerning the effectiveness of the new medicine (Sussex et al. 2013a).

A related issue is that the weights that may arise from different standpoints – HTA committee members, the general public, clinical experts and patients – may vary substantially or at least to such an extent that the decisions arising from an MCDA process are materially affected. MCDA can help to understand whether using different weights has a significant impact on the aggregate measure of benefit driving the decision or not. In cases where there are widely differing views on the weights – potentially leading to different possible outcomes of the decisions – that information can be taken into account as part of the evidence considered by a decision making committee. This highlights another important feature of MCDA which is to hear and reflect the voice of all participants.

14.6 Can MCDA Incorporate the Concept of Opportunity Cost of New Technologies?

As noted earlier, the remit of HTA bodies varies from jurisdiction to jurisdiction. Depending on the type of health system the HTA body operates in, different types of decision problems are addressed by HTA. For example, some systems involving patient co-payment decisions (such as France and Italy) are primarily focused on defining the level of reimbursement, in which case different MCDA total benefit points might be associated with different degrees of reimbursement.

In other cases (such as Israel), the decision making committee reviews a basket of new technologies at one point in time each year based on the total available budget. The Oregon Health Services Commission looked at all condition/treatment pairs, ranked these in terms of their cost-effectiveness (and later just in terms of their effectiveness) and used that to decide a cut-off point, below which treatments were not funded.

In any resource constrained health system, there is a need to have a value for money benchmark or decision making rule that can ensure efficient resource allocation. In health systems with a fixed budget, the HTA process explicitly recognising the trade-off between costs and benefits and a cost-effectiveness threshold representing the opportunity cost of adoption is often used. It is worth noting that the notion of fixed budget does not always hold and in some cases an increased demand of resources is met, for example, via an increased expenditure in health (Karlsberg Schaffer et al. 2016).

If multiple dimensions of values are considered, the opportunity costs ought to be measured based on the same metrics used to measure those dimensions of value. In other words, there is a need to consider the unit of the attributes of value or MCDA criteria that would be assumed to be foregone elsewhere in the system if a new treatment is implemented. In this way, all the benefits lost and potentially produced as a result of implementing a new intervention can be compared to make a decision.

As explained in Sussex et al. (2013b):

> In the case of the MCDA approach, the weightings applied reflect relative willingness to pay for value, but an 'anchor' is needed to understand the opportunity cost, i.e. what in absolute terms is the hurdle for adoption. (Sussex et al. 2013a, b)

Other dimensions that might be relevant to the use of the threshold and to the budget constraint are the extent to which there is a devolution to local jurisdictions or regions in the management of the health budget and reimbursement decisions (as in Spain and Italy) and the type of financing system (tax funded with a single payer vs insurance-based/Bismarck systems with multiple payers).

Currently, available MCDA frameworks or software only partially address the issue of opportunity cost. For example, EVIDEM (2015) integrates cost as a distinct attribute (or criterion) of value. However, careful definition of such a criterion is needed to avoid overlapping with other criteria (e.g. if the framework includes both cost and cost-effectiveness), and guidance is needed to identify what constitutes good value for money.

In the MCDA framework such as 1000minds® (Golan and Hansen 2012), all incremental benefits are combined into a point score, reflecting the relative importance of each criteria and the degree of achievement of the intervention, compared against the total net costs to the health care system and used to inform resource allocation decision making based on the development of efficiency frontiers. However, in both approaches described, there is a need to identify the 'hurdle for adoption' (e.g. a cost per incremental point score) for repeated HTA decisions affecting a single, fixed budget.

There is substantial controversy, regarding, conceptually:

- What the cost-effectiveness threshold 'means': marginal cost of a QALY foregone, marginal cost of a QALY gained or maybe marginal willingness to pay – or marginal willingness to accept – QALYs gained/lost (Mason et al. 2008; Donaldson 2011; Culyer et al. 2007; Karlsberg Schaffer et al. 2015; Appleby et al. 2009)?
- How to measure the cost-effectiveness threshold. For example, in the UK, Claxton et al. (2015) developed a 'top-down' approach, finding the 'average cost per QALY' in the NHS. Alternatively, 'bottom-up' approaches look at specific cost per QALY of specifically displaced services (Peacock et al. 2009).

Locating the threshold, defined in simple cost per QALY terms, has proved difficult. On one hand, one can argue that extending the attributes of value to consider in resource allocations could make the definition of the threshold even more complicated. This is probably why, in many systems, 'softer' attributes or criteria are not quantified and are incorporated via deliberative processes. On the other hand, the fact that there are so many methodological issues with the definition and the estimation of the cost-effectiveness threshold – and a relatively small evidence base to support the choice of a threshold – suggests MCDA could provide an opportunity to better define the resource allocation decision problem.

14.7 How Can Uncertainty Be Addressed in MCDA Approaches to HTA?

In current HTA systems, the consideration of how robust are expected values of cost and/or effectiveness provided to the decision maker to changes in model parameters generally plays an important role. In particular, decision makers are interested in understanding how confident they can be that the decision they are reaching is the 'right' one. For example, the latest NICE guide to methods states that:

> It is important for the model to quantify the decision uncertainty associated with a technology (that is, the probability that a different decision would be reached if the true cost effectiveness of each technology could be ascertained before making the decision). (NICE 2013)

MCDA approaches generally explore sensitivity analysis at the end of the decision making process to see if variations in criteria, scores or weights affect the decision outcome. There are a number of sensitivity analysis approaches presented and discussed in the literature showing how to explore the magnitude and impact of uncertainty on the final outcome of the MCDA processes (see Thokala and Duenas 2012; Broekhuizen et al. 2015; Chapter 5 of this book). However, there is a lack of guidance or explicit statement on how that should inform decision making. This is because the acceptable level of uncertainty is a matter of judgement and therefore will vary depending on the context of the decision making. As with other criteria, most HTA systems allow considerable discretion to committees to decide on the appropriate level of acceptability which could therefore vary from decision to decision.

As compared to some existing HTA systems, where the focus is on clinical benefits/effectiveness and costs, decision makers using an MCDA approach potentially face higher degrees of uncertainty given the multiple benefit attributes included which all need evidence to determine estimates. In addition, in an MCDA approach, different types of uncertainty (such as parameter uncertainty) might need to be explored for both criteria weights and performance scores (Broekhuizen et al. 2015).

The consideration of uncertainty of performance scores is more similar to some existing HTA systems where uncertainty is quantified, although in MCDA processes there is also an element of preference elicitation scores based on the relevant evidence (presented in the performance matrix, Thokala et al. 2016). The probability that a technology is less effective than expected can be estimated (via probabilistic sensitivity analysis). This can then be compared to a predetermined benchmark value that represents the level of uncertainty tolerated by the decision maker. Alternatively, threshold analysis can show at which score point the decision outcome on an intervention would change (Thokala et al. 2016).

Structural uncertainty which relates to the choice of criteria and the way they are measured and weighed is complex and is not extensively discussed in the literature (Thokala and Duenas 2012; Broekhuizen et al. 2015). Arguably, structural uncertainty is addressed in MCDA processes because there is an explicit discussion at every step (e.g. weighting, scoring, etc.) and a continuous validation and refinement of the criteria used (Broekhuizen et al. 2015). Van Til et al. (2014) explored this issue in the context of the EVIDEM MCDA framework and found that the choice of the elicitation method does not impact the estimated weights when those methods support group decisions. However, more research is needed to compare other approaches and their impact on the weights and on the aggregate measure of value. We note that in many HTA systems, an EQ-5D value set is used for the QALY calculations but uncertainty related to the model and data used to develop the value set is not considered in decision making.

Most importantly, how uncertainty should be factored in depends on the risk attitude of the decision maker. In principle, HTA bodies making a large number of decisions should be risk neutral, as chance of underestimating the overall value of a technology is as much the chance of overestimating it. If this is the case, decision makers should focus on expected values and consider uncertainty around the mean only if investment for additional evidence collection to reduce such uncertainty is required (Barnsley et al. 2016).

However, some HTA bodies, such as IQWiG in Germany, have signalled a preference about certainty of outcome, particularly clinical outcomes, and have tended to reward technologies with more certain estimates of the clinical value over those with less certain estimates (Towse and Barnsley 2013). In cases where the decision maker is explicitly risk averse and a low degree of uncertainty is part of its maximand, there might be an advantage in having a distinct criterion representing uncertainty. First of all, it might help considering the trade-off between the performance score (e.g. the size of the observed clinical benefit) and the strengths of the evidence provided in an explicit and transparent way. Such an approach can also help committees' members to clearly separate the robustness of evidence (which could be captured in an uncertainty/quality of evidence criterion) and the score to assign to specific criteria. There is evidence that people tend to give lower scores when the supporting evidence is not very robust (Marsh et al. 2014).

One challenge of introducing an 'uncertainty' criterion within MCDA is that in principle all criteria require evidence and can have different levels of uncertainty around their estimates. Therefore, there might be a need to have a measure of 'uncertainty' for each criterion. One way to address this could be to develop an aggregate measure to reflect uncertainty of multiple criteria. An attempt in this direction is provided by the EVIDEM framework which includes a quality of evidence criterion considering validity, relevance, completeness of reporting, and type of evidence (EVIDEM 2015). Finally, including an uncertainty criterion would require the elicitation of risk preferences of different stakeholders, which might differ substantially.

Golan and Hansen (2012) suggest that uncertainty should be considered in the context of an assessment of the quality of clinical evidence provided. They propose that this could be represented in a 'bubble chart', as shown in Fig. 14.1, where the size of each bubble is proportional to the strength of the evidence of the technology. The researchers stress that quality of evidence should not be part of the total benefit calculation (represented in the vertical axis) as its relative importance (weight) is likely to change depending on the technology considered. However, this approach does not consider the quality of evidence related to other non-clinical criteria and does not provide guidance on acceptability levels – so decisions ultimately rely on a deliberative process, informed by evidence on the performance of the options presented in this manner.

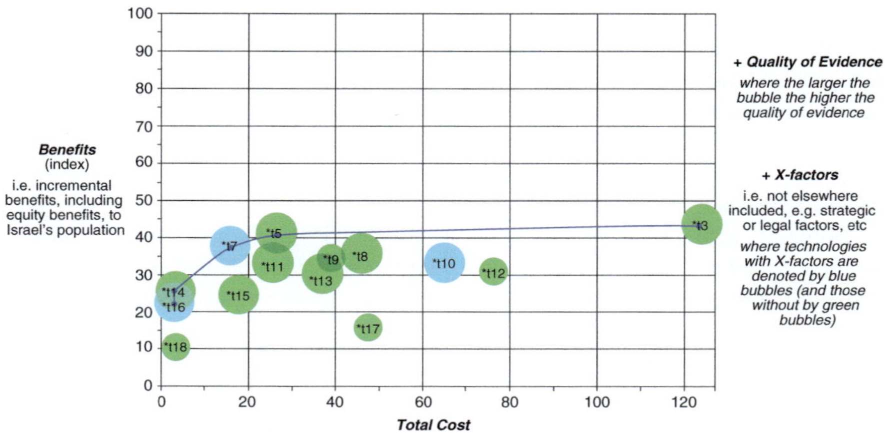

Fig. 14.1 Israel's Health Basket Committee pilot of MCDA. Bubble size = quality of evidence (*Source*: Golan and Hansen (2012))

14.8 Final Issues to Consider

There are a number of concerns that HTA bodies might have about introducing and using MCDA.

The first is that MCDA will attempt to make decision making into a more formulaic approach and, in the more extreme cases, that deliberation will be replaced by an algorithm providing an 'answer' to a decision problem based on a mathematical process (Culyer 2009). Hence, decision makers may fear that MCDA 'locks them in' to a mechanistic approach – or that their judgements may be made redundant. However, as emphasised by many researchers in the field, MCDA instead aims '… to help the decision makers by structuring the information to support their deliberative process' (Thokala et al. 2016). Further, 'MCDA is not simply a technical process. Its successful implementation depends crucially on effective design of social processes by which the analysis is structured and conducted' (Dodgson et al. 2009).

We note that, depending on the specific MCDA approach adopted, the exercise of judgement remains an important part of the process, particularly when weights and criteria are assigned. MCDA provides a structure to guide the decision makers' thinking. As there is a variety of MCDA approaches (even for each MCDA step), the right balance between structure and deliberation will depend on the type of decision problem and on the specific HTA institutional context.

Linked to the previous point is decision makers' potential concerns about being 'too explicit' about decisions, which can open them up to legal or constitutional challenges from external parties, particularly from those with vested commercial interests. However, transparency is an important element of 'fair' processes; therefore, public scrutiny needs to be allowed. In particularly controversial cases, MCDA can help both in identifying the areas of disagreement and explaining how those conflicts were addressed (e.g. if consensus was reached via a group discussion or if the view of the majority was taken).

Ultimately, the overall value added of any new MCDA approach to HTA will need to be tested and clearly demonstrated before implementation. In particular, there is a need to compare its benefits (in terms of 'better' decisions from a resource allocation perspective and in terms of 'better' processes if, for example, it improves acceptability of decisions among those affected) against its implementation costs (e.g. if it requires longer timelines or capability/expertise building).

Finally, there a number of methodological issues that are not solved by using MCDA, such as disagreement on how best to measure certain value criteria (e.g. disease severity), and the possibility of including criteria that overlap or that are not independent when additive models are used. For a discussion on criteria requirements, see the second ISPOR Task Force report on MCDA (Marsh et al. 2016).

14.9 Conclusions

Existing HTA processes almost inevitably require the consideration of multiple criteria. There is growing interest, internationally, in finding ways of systematically considering these other factors. MCDA offers a way of structuring these decision processes. Its use represents a way of complementing and supporting deliberative processes, rather than supplanting them. MCDA does not replace judgement – it is simply a way of ensuring that judgements are exercised in a consistent and transparent way. This can also assist the accountability of HTA decisions to stakeholders.

The use of MCDA creates an opportunity to properly align understanding of the objectives of the NHS with the goals of HTA. MCDA could provide a framework for developing priority setting frameworks for use by local NHS organisations, which in turn can inform the criteria and weights to be applied in HTA. Devlin and Sussex (2011) note a number of examples of the use of MCDA by NHS budget holders.

However, as we have noted, there are non-trivial issues to address in the use of MCDA – in particular, relating to the way budget constraints and opportunity costs are incorporated, and the way uncertainty in evidence is handled. Decisions regarding how criteria are selected and weighted require careful attention.

Further, there needs to be a consideration of the balance between additional organisational costs of implementing an MCDA approach and additional benefits of improved decision making process. Even where MCDA cannot follow 'best practise', 'second best practise' may still have the potential to improve the decision making process. For example, rather than undertaking a 'full' MCDA, simply agreeing the relevant criteria and presenting the evidence on the performance of each technology as a performance matrix – without weighting the criteria – may in itself aid consistency and transparency.

Acknowledgements The authors would like to thank Adrian Towse, Grace Marsden, Hector Castro and the editors for their valuable comments received on an early draft of this chapter.

References

Appleby J, Devlin N, Parkin D, Buxton M, Chalkidou K (2009) Searching for cost-effectiveness thresholds in the NHS. Health Policy 91(Suppl 3):239–245

Baltussen R, Niessen I (2006) Priority setting of health interventions: the need for multi-criteria decision analysis. Cost Eff Resour Alloc 4:14

Batista RN, Hodge MJ (2009) The "natural history" of health technology assessment. Int J Technol Assess Health Care 25(Supplement 1):281–284

Barnsley P, Cubi-Molla P, Fischer A, and Towse A. (2016) "Uncertainty and Risk in HTA Decision Making" OHE research paper. Available at https://www.ohe.org/publications/uncertainty-and-risk-hta-decision-making

Brazier J, Tsuchiya A (2015) Improving cross-sector comparisons: going beyond the health-related QALY. Appl Health Econ Health Policy 13(6):557–565

Brazier J et al (2005) Should patients have a greater role in valuing health states? Appl Health Econ Health Policy 4(4):201–208

Broekhuizen H et al (2015) A review and classification of approaches for dealing with uncertainty in multi-criteria decision analysis for healthcare decisions. Pharmacoeconomics 33:445–455

Claxton K, Devlin N (2013) Report on structured decision making for NICE's 2013 methods review

Claxton K et al (2015) Methods for the estimation of the National Institute for Health and Care Excellence cost-effectiveness threshold. Health Technol Assess 19(14):1–503

Culyer AJ (1991) The normative economics of health care finance and provision. In: McGuire A, Fenn P, Mayhew K (eds) Providing health care: the economics of alternative systems of finance and delivery. Oxford University Press, Oxford

Culyer AJ (2009) Deliberative processes in decisions about health care technologies. OHE Seminar, London, https://www.ohe.org/publications/deliberative-processes-decisions-about-health-care-technologies#sthash.Z4P0eCXU.dpuf

Culyer AJ (2012) Chapter 2. Extra welfarism. In: Cookson R, Claxton K (eds) The humble economist. OHE, London

Culyer AJ, McCabe C, Briggs A, Claxton K, Buxton M, Akehust R, Sculpher M, Brazier J (2007) Searching for a threshold, not setting one: the role of the National Institute for Health and Clinical Excellence. J Health Serv Res Policy 12(Suppl 1):56–58

Department of Health (2010) A new value-based approach to the pricing of branded medicines: a consultation. Department of Health, London

Devlin N, Sussex J (2011) Incorporating multiple criteria in HTA. Methods and processes. OHE research. Available at: https://www.ohe.org/publications/incorporating-multiple-criteria-hta-methods-and-processes

Dodgson JS, Spackman M, Pearman A, Phillips LD (2009) Multi-criteria analysis: a manual. Department for Communities and Local Government, London, Available at http://eprints.lse.ac.uk/12761/1/Multi-criteria_Analysis.pdf
Donaldson C (2011) Willingness to pay and publicly funded health care: contradiction in terms? Briefing, OHE Seminar, Available at https://www.ohe.org/publications/willingness-pay-and-publicly-funded-health-care-contradiction-terms#sthash.2ffK4iYL.dpuf
Drummond MF, Sculpher MJ, Claxton K, Stoddart GL, Torrance GW (2015) Methods for the economic evaluation of health care programmes, 4th edn. Oxford Medical Publications, Oxford
EVIDEM (2015) Decision Criteria. Conceptual background, definitions, design & instructions. EVIDEM Collaboration. https://www.evidem.org/docs/2015/EVIDEM-v3-0-Decision-criteria-conceptual-background-definitions-and-instructions-June-2015.pdf
Garrido G, Rottingen B (2010) Developing health technology assessment to address health care system needs. Health Policy 94(3):196–202
Gilovich T, Griffin D, Kahneman D (2002) Heuristics and biases: the psychology of intuitive judgement. Cambridge University Press, New York
Golan O, Hansen P (2012) Which health technologies should be funded? A prioritization framework based explicitly on value for money. Isr J Health Policy Res 1:44
Golan O, Hansen P, Kaplan G, Tal O (2011) Health technology prioritization: which criteria for prioritizing new technologies and what are their relative weights? Health Policy 102(2–3):126–135
Hicks EP, Kluemper GT (2011) Heuristic reasoning and cognitive biases: are they hindrances to judgements and decision making in orthodontics? Am J Orthod Dentofacial Orthop 139(3):297–304
INAHTA. http://www.inahta.org/hta-tools-resources/
Kahneman D (2003) Maps of bounded rationality: psychology for behavioural economics. Am Econ Rev 93(5):1449–1475
Karlsberg Schaffer S, Sussex J, Devlin N, Walker A (2015) Local health care expenditure plans and their opportunity costs. Health Policy 119(9):1237–1244
Karlsberg Schaffer S, Sussex J, Hughes D, Devlin N (2016) Opportunity costs and local health service spending decisions: a qualitative study from Wales. BMC Health Serv Res 16:103
Kind P (2015) Cost-effectiveness analysis: a view into the abyss. Appl Health Econ Health Policy 13(3):269–271
Kitzhaber JA (1993) Prioritising health services in an era of limits: the Oregon experience. BMJ 307(6900):373–377
Marsh K et al (2014) Assessing the value of healthcare interventions using multi-criteria decision analysis: a review of the literature. Pharmacoeconomics 32:345–365. Value Health 19:125–137
Marsh K. et al. (2016) Multiple criteria decision analysis for health care decision making—Emerging good practices: report 2 of the ISPOR MCDA. Emerging GoodPracticesTaskForce
Mason H, Baker R, Donaldson C (2008) Willingness to pay for a QALY: past, present and future. Expert Rev Pharmacoecon Outcomes Res 8(6):575–582
Morris S, Devlin N, Parkin D (2007) Economic analysis in health care. Wiley, Chichester, p 236
National Institute for Health and Care Excellence – NICE (2013) Guide to the methods of technology appraisal 2013. NICE. Available at https://www.nice.org.uk/article/pmg9/resources/non-guidance-guide-to-the-methods-of-technology-appraisal-2013-pdf
Norheim OF, Baltussen R, Johri M et al (2014) Guidance on priority setting in health care (GPS-Health): the inclusion of equity criteria not captured by cost-effectiveness analysis. Cost Eff Res Alloc 12:18
Norman D, Sabin J (2008) Accountability for reasonableness: un updated. BMJ 337:a1850, Available at: http://www.bmj.com/content/337/bmj.a1850.full.print?
Paulden M, Stafinski T, Menon D, McCabe C (2015) Value-based reimbursement decisions for orphan drugs: a scoping review and decision framework. Pharmacoeconomics 33(3):255–269
Peacock S, Mitton C, Bate A, McCoy B, Donaldson C (2009) Overcoming barriers to priority setting using interdisciplinary methods. Health Policy 92(2):124–132

Phillips D (2007) Decision conferencing. In: Edwards W, Miles RF, von Winterfeldt D (eds) Advances in decision analysis: from foundations to applications. Cambridge University Press, Cambridge

Phillips LD, Fasolo B, Zafiropoulos N, Beyer A (2011) Is quantitative benefit-risk modelling of drugs desirable or possible? Drug Discov Today Technol 8(1):e3–e10

Sen AK (1977) Social choice theory: a re-examination. Econometrica 45:53–89

Shah KK, Praet C, Devlin NJ, Sussex JM, Appleby J, Parkin D (2012) Is the aim of the health care system to maximise QALYs? J Health Serv Res Policy 17(3):157–164

SMC (2015) PACE – patient and clinician engagement. Factsheet. https://www.scottishmedicines.org.uk/files/PACE/PACE_factsheet_FINAL.pdf

Sugden R (2008) Citizens, consumers and clients: Alan Williams and the political economy of cost–benefit analysis in The Ideas and Influence of Alan Williams. Ed. by Mason A, and Towse A. Available at https://www.ohe.org/publications/ideas-and-influence-alan-williams-be-reasonable-%E2%80%93-do-it-my-way

Sussex J, Rollet P, Garau M, Schmitt C, Kent A, Hutchings A (2013a) A pilot study of multicriteria decision analysis for valuing orphan medicines. Value Health 16(8):1163–1169

Sussex J, Towse A, Devlin N (2013b) Operationalising value based pricing of medicines: a taxonomy of approaches. Pharmacoeconomics 13(1):1–10

Thokala P, Duenas A (2012) Multiple criteria decision analysis for health technology assessment. Value Health 15(8):1172–1181

Thokala P, et al., for the ISPOR MCDA Task Force (2016) MCDA for Health care decision making – an introduction: report 1 of the ISPOR MCDA Emerging Good Practices Task Force. Value Health. 19(1):1–13

Towse A, Barnsley P (2013) Approaches to identifying, measuring, and aggregating elements of value. Int J Technol Assess Health Care 29(4):360–364

Towse A, Devlin N, Hawe E, Garrison L (2011) The evolution of HTA in emerging markets health care systems: analysis to support a policy response. OHE consulting report. Office of Health Economics, London

Van Til J, Groothius-Oudshoorn C, Lieferink M, Dolan J, Goetghebeur M (2014) Does techiques matter; a pilot study exploring weighting techniques for a multi-criteria decision support framework. Cost Eff Res Alloc 12:22

World Health Organization (WHO) (2010a) Health system financing. The path to universal coverage. Available at: http://www.who.int/whr/2010/en/

World Health Organization (WHO) (2010b) Media release on the Sixty-seventh World Health Assembly. Available at: http://www.who.int/mediacentre/news/releases/2014/WHA-20140524/en/

Youngkong S, Baltussen R, Tantivess S, Mohara A, Teerawattanon Y (2012) Multicriteria decision analysis for including health interventions in the Universal Health Coverage Benefit package in Thailand. Value Health 15:961–970

Chapter 15
Beyond Value Function Methods in MCDA for Health Care

Vakaramoko Diaby and Luis Dias

Abstract In health-care decision-making, the predominance of some value function multi-criteria decision analysis (MCDA) methods may obscure the existence and potential usefulness of alternative MCDA methods. The current chapter provides an introduction to alternative value function and non-value function methods. The alternative value function methods presented are approaches based on multi-attribute value theory (MAVT): measuring attractiveness by a categorical-based evaluation technique (MACBETH), Variable Interdependent Parameters (VIP) analysis, and stochastic multi-criteria acceptability analysis (SMAA). Non-value function methods described include goal programming models, dominance-based rough set approach, and outranking models. The chapter also reviews their use in health to date and ends with concluding remarks.

15.1 Introduction

MCDA, used as an umbrella term, is a decision-making framework that encompasses a large set of methods or approaches that simultaneously and explicitly take account of multiple and conflicting criteria (Baltussen and Niessen 2006). These methods can roughly be classified into five main families: elementary methods (Yoon and Hwang 1995), value function methods (Belton and Stewart 2002), goal and reference methods (Belton and Stewart 2002), outranking models, (Belton and Stewart 2002) and dominance-based approaches (Pawlak and Sowinski 1994; Greco et al. 2001; Moshkovich and Mechitov 2013). MCDA consists of three steps (Belton and Stewart 2002). The first step, referred to as problem identification and

V. Diaby (✉)
College of Pharmacy and Pharmaceutical Sciences, Florida A&M University, Tallahassee, FL, USA
e-mail: vakaramoko.diaby@famu.edu; diaby_v@yahoo.fr

L. Dias
INESCC, CeBER and Faculty of Economics, University of Coimbra, Coimbra, Portugal
e-mail: LMCDias@fe.uc.pt

© Springer International Publishing AG 2017
K. Marsh et al. (eds.), *Multi-Criteria Decision Analysis to Support Healthcare Decisions*, DOI 10.1007/978-3-319-47540-0_15

structuring, deals with identifying the decision-makers and setting their goals. At this step, the relevant competing options and their evaluation criteria are defined. The second step, called multi-criteria evaluation model development and use, requires the selection of the relevant aggregation model and the elicitation of the model's parameters, which defines the role played by each evaluation criterion when synthesizing the performance of the alternatives in multiple attributes. The last step, called the development of action plans, consists of making recommendations to decision-makers. Additionally, the presentation of sensitivity analyses informs the decision-makers regarding their level of confidence about the plans.

Even though analysts and researchers have access to a wide range of evaluation models in MCDA to respond to multifaceted problems in health care, the use has been confined to the application of only a few value function methods. Adunlin et al. conducted a systematic review to identify applications of MCDA in health care (Adunlin et al. 2015). The time horizon for the search spanned the years 1980–2013 and encompassed a wide range of bibliographic sources (electronic databases, gray literature). Of the 66 studies that met the inclusion criteria of the review, 91 % used a value function method, a method that computes a single value to summarize the performance of an alternative on multiple criteria (Adunlin et al. 2015).

Value function methods are techniques that compute an overall value for each competing alternative representing the global performance of each alternative on their attributes. As a result, these methods are referred to as full aggregation or compensatory methods. Other MCDA methods that do not compute an overall value and/or are not compensatory are available but have been applied less in health care.

The objective of this chapter is to highlight alternative MCDA methods that can be used to address health-care decision-making problems. The chapter is structured as follows. Sections 15.2 and 15.3 describe alternative value function methods and non-value function methods, respectively. Both sections review the use of these methods in health to date. The chapter ends with concluding remarks.

15.2 Alternative Value Function Methods

Multi-attribute utility theory (MAUT) and multi-attribute value theory (MAVT) (Keeney and Raiffa 1993) are well-known approaches in MCDA to obtain an overall score for an alternative being evaluated on multiple criteria. The main difference between these approaches is that MAUT makes use of utility functions that account for decision-makers' attitudes toward risk, utilizing the concept of lotteries, as opposed to MAVT where a global value function is constructed for each alternative to represent the global performance of the alternatives on the decision criteria, using the concept of preference intensity. This section briefly reviews how MAVT can be used to obtain an overall valuation for an alternative and suggests related approaches that can constitute an alternative to the traditional way of applying MAVT.

The implementation of the MAVT traditionally involves two main steps. The first step deals with the construction of a partial value function for each criterion.

A partial value function reflects how the value of an attribute varies along the measurement scale for the decision-maker. It can be an increasing function for an attribute such as quality of life or a decreasing function for an attribute such as cost. The second step aggregates the partial value functions to obtain a global value function. The most common aggregation model is the additive value function where the partial value of the alternative on each decision criterion is weighted by a scaling coefficient assigned to the respective value function, and these weighted values are then added yielding a global value. This requires the determination of scaling coefficients, which indicate the weight of each value function. Scaling coefficients can be elicited using a number of techniques including swing weighting (Diaby and Goeree 2014). The alternative with the highest global value is the preferred one. Construction of value functions needs to satisfy the transitivity of preference and indifference rule, while the additive aggregation model used in MAVT needs to satisfy the additive independence condition (namely, that trade-offs between two criteria do not depend on the level of the remaining criteria) (Belton and Stewart 2002).

There are only a few published applications of MAVT in health care. To our knowledge, there is only one study that applied the MAVT to patient-bed assignment in hospital admission management (Tsai and Lin 2014) in addition to a tutorial that illustrated the way to use MAVT to support reimbursement decision-making in health care (Diaby and Goeree 2014). Nevertheless, a recent project of the European Medicines Agency suggests using MAVT as the framework to support regulatory decisions about medicinal products (Phillips et al. 2012).

It is the authors' opinion that MAVT is an intuitive and easy-to-understand MCDA method, since it uses a way of aggregating scores that individuals are familiar with (e.g., computing GPA scores in academia, building composite indices such as United Nation's Human Development Index, etc.). It thus reflects the way data are aggregated in the above and many other examples. Like MAUT, MAVT defines an axiomatically based process for the construction of commensurable value scales and the definition of scaling coefficients.

A potential obstacle to using MAVT is the potential difficulty of eliciting precise values for the scaling coefficients that reflect the decision-maker's trade-offs (Dias and Clímaco 2000). However, to cope with this concern, it is possible to assess the robustness of conclusions through the use of software such as the Variable Interdependent Parameters (VIP) analysis (Dias and Clímaco 2000). VIP analysis suggests an alternative process to conduct an MAVT-based analysis consisting of eliciting only information that is easier to obtain, such as a ranking of the scaling coefficients, rather than precise numerical values. To the authors' best knowledge, there are no applications of VIP analysis in the health domain.

Another alternative approach to conduct an MAVT-based analysis is stochastic multi-criteria (or multiobjective) acceptability analysis (SMAA) (Lahdelma and Salminen 2001). Similar to the VIP analysis, this method does not require decision-makers to specify a vector of scaling coefficients. The space of all admissible scaling coefficients is sampled using Monte Carlo simulations in order to produce statistics about the ranking of each alternative. SMAA can also provide information about what scaling coefficients, if any, make each alternative a winner. The potential for SMAA has been advocated for health economic evaluation of medical interventions and was illustrated on a case of infertility treatment selection (Postmus et al. 2014).

A third alternative process to conduct an MAVT-based analysis is MACBETH (Ishizaka and Nemery 2013; Bana et al. 2012). MACBETH is distinguished from other MCDA methods by the fact that only qualitative judgments about the difference of attractiveness (desirability) between pairs of alternatives are needed. The decision-maker can state the difference of attractiveness between two alternatives using an ordinal qualitative scale composed of six levels, from "very weak" to "extreme." A consistency check is conducted to ensure the responses obtained from such pairwise comparisons do not conflict. The MACBETH procedure allows for the computation of numerical scores on an interval scale (0–100) for the alternatives on each criterion by the means of linear programming. A similar process is used to weight the criteria. A global score is estimated for each alternative using an additive aggregation, taking into account the scores of the alternative on the multiple criteria and the respective criteria weights. The alternative with the highest global score is considered the most attractive. The implementation of this method is supported by a software called M-MACBETH.

In health care, MACBETH has been applied to diagnosis and treat Alzheimer's and diabetes (de Castro et al. 2009a, b; de Moraes et al. 2010; Nunes et al. 2011). MACBETH shares similar features with the AHP. They both use pairwise comparisons to derive criteria and alternatives priorities, except that the MACBETH derives value functions based on linear programming, whereas AHP derives priorities using the eigenvalue method (Ishizaka and Nemery 2013; Dodgson et al. 2009). As a result, MACBETH may be of interest for decision-makers that would like to explore the use of other methods that convert verbal preferences into numerical scores. Recent works have demonstrated the feasibility of using MACBETH for group decision-making (Belton and Pictet 1997; Bana e Costa et al. 2014).

15.3 Non-value Function Methods for Health-Care Decision-Making

Using value function methods entails accepting that a very poor performance on one criterion can always be compensated by a very good performance on some other criterion. Therefore, these methods may not be the most appropriate when such compensatory effects are not considered to be adequate in the decision-making process. For instance, this type of compensability may be inadequate if criteria refer to impacts on different stakeholders (e.g., patients versus hospital managers or medical staff) or when criteria refer to rather different dimensions (economic, versus social or environmental risks, for instance) (Munda and Nardo 2005).

The following families of non-value function methods are presented in this section: (1) goal and reference point methods, (2) dominance-based approaches, and (3) outranking methods.

15.3.1 Goal and Reference Point Methods

There are several MCDA methods that evaluate alternatives by comparing them to some reference(s). The references can be internal (i.e., defined exclusively based on the set of alternatives) or can be external to the set of alternatives. The evaluation of each alternative does not depend only on its characteristics as in value-based approaches but also on the chosen references.

A popular MCDA method based on comparisons with internal references is TOPSIS (Yoon and Hwang 1995). In this case, there are two references defined with regard to the set of alternatives being evaluated. The first reference is the so-called ideal point, a fictitious alternative defined by selecting, for each criterion, the best observed performance in the set of the alternatives. The second reference is referred to as the anti-ideal point, a fictitious alternative defined by selecting, for each criterion, the worst observed performance in the set of the alternatives. The idea is to select an alternative that is near the ideal point and far from the anti-ideal point.

In TOPSIS, the evaluation score for an alternative is the distance to the anti-ideal solution divided by the sum of the same distance and the distance to the ideal solution. This yields a score between 0 and 1, like value function methods do. However, this value is not an evaluation of the alternative on its own merits but an evaluation of how the alternative compares to the chosen references. The chosen distance metric is the weighted euclidean distance, which allows placing different importances on different criteria. In order to make the distances comparable, a normalization operation is needed to transform the criteria scales into a common scale. The most common normalization in TOPSIS, performed separately for each criterion, consists of dividing each performance of an alternative by the square root of the sum of the squares of the performances of all alternatives on that criterion. An important concern about this method is that depending on the normalization method, the resulting scores can be different (Ishizaka and Nemery 2013). Another major concern is that introducing a poor and possibly irrelevant alternative that changes the anti-ideal point can reverse the relative positions of the remaining alternatives.

Upon reviewing the literature, one example framework was found using TOPSIS for health technology assessment (HTA) by Liang et al. (2014). This framework was built to appraise different medicines based on economic and health-related criteria. The method suggested by these authors was a variant of TOPSIS using judgment from different stakeholders, combined with the use of AHP to derive criteria weights. A similar combination of AHP, to derive weights, and TOPSIS, to rank alternatives, was used by Akdag et al. to evaluate the service quality of some hospitals in Turkey (Akdag et al. 2014). This study constitutes one of the several examples of TOPSIS applications to problems other than HTA in the health sector (Beheshtifar and Alimoahmmadi 2015; Sang et al. 2014; Bahadori et al. 2014).

There are many other methods based on distances to references (Ehrgott 2006), which include goal programming (Jones and Tamiz 2010). Such methods are used to set the value of decision variables subject to constraints, but the same principles can be used to rank a finite list of alternatives in order of their distance to a given reference point. Distances may or may not be weighted, attaching importance weights to the criteria. The reference alternative is usually an external reference indicating goals or aspiration levels.

In the health sector, goal programming has been mainly used for scheduling beds, staff, and/or patients (Thomas et al. 2013). No application of goal programming for HTA was identified in the literature, except for an illustration of how this approach could be used to support reimbursement decision-making in health care (Diaby and Goeree 2014).

Methods based on references may potentially be interesting for health-care decision-makers as they are often able to verbalize their aspirations by setting goals to be attained on each criterion. Then, a logical consequence is to seek which of the alternatives is closer to satisfying such goals, according to some metric, and possibly assigning a different weight to each goal. For instance, if a manager has a set of targets that he or she would like to attain (possibly including targets set by external entities), then it may be helpful to evaluate different decision alternatives considering their contribution to these targets. If the set of targets is very large and therefore they cannot all be met at the same time, then a reference-based approach will indicate which alternatives are most interesting with regard to those targets.

As a separate note, we might also mention data envelopment analysis (DEA) Cook and Seiford 2009; Thomas et al. 2013; Liu et al. 2013) as a close relative of MCDA (Ishizaka and Nemery 2013; Bouyssou 1999; Gouveia et al. 2008; Cooper 2005) that uses references. Indeed, DEA evaluates the performance of each alternative (decision-making unit in DEA terminology) considering the entire set of alternatives as potential references, rather than asking decision-makers to indicate aspiration levels. DEA could potentially be used to support decisions about whether or not to approve a new health technology, based on how it compares with the set of technologies already in operation.

15.3.2 Dominance-Based Approaches

A different way to perform a comparison of alternatives based on MCDA is to compare them directly, rather than computing an overall value (value-based approach) or comparing them with a reference. The simplest way to compare alternatives is to perform a pairwise comparison, i.e., a comparison of two alternatives, to check whether one of them is clearly superior to the other. An alternative x is said to dominate another alternative y if it is better on some criteria and is not worse in any other criterion. The resulting dominance relation does not require any subjective parameters such as criteria weights. If the purpose of the analysis is to identify a single best alternative, dominated alternatives can be discarded. However, the dominance relation typically applies to a few pairs of alternatives, and there are usually several non-dominated alternatives (especially if the number of criteria is large).

One of the most recent methods in MCDA, the dominance-based rough set approach (DRSA), is based on exploiting the idea of dominance using rough sets theory (RST) (Greco et al. 2005). This approach can be used in sorting problems (assigning alternatives to categories) or in problems where a ranking of the alternatives is sought. RST does not require setting any preference-related parameters (such as importance weights) but requires the decision-makers to provide examples of comparisons, e.g., stating that alternative x is better than alternative y. The method is able to extract *if-then* rules from such examples of preferences by an induction process. As an illustration, a rule might state "if alternative x is much better than alternative y on criterion 1 and it is not much worse on criterion 2, then x is better than y." Another approach that uses induction rules based on qualitative assessments is verbal decision analysis (VDA) (Moshkovich et al. 2002, 2005), which can also be used for sorting or ranking problems based on statements provided by a decision-maker.

In the health field, DRSA has been mainly used as a tool to discover knowledge from data, e.g., to identify metabolites involved in disease pathogenesis (Blasco et al. 2015) or to identify which factors predispose patients to return to intensive care units after cardiac surgery (Jarzabek et al. 2014). VDA has been mainly used as a diagnostic tool in the neuropsychology and neurologic disease domains (e.g., (Tamanini et al. 2011; Yevseyeva et al. 2008)).

Dominance-based approaches, particularly DRSA, are appealing for the modest information they require from decision-makers and for conveying results in the form of rules that are easy to understand. The method is particularly interesting when the set of alternatives is very large and when the decision-maker wishes to have a set of rules in natural language (*if… then…*) to sort alternatives. However, the requirement of comparing a few alternatives as examples can be difficult unless they differ only in a couple of criteria, and the resulting set of rules may be insufficient to provide a crisp sorting or a complete ranking of the alternatives as an output.

15.3.3 Outranking Approaches

As described in the previous section, the establishment of dominance relations does not require any subjective parameters such as criteria weights. That being said, the relation is usually poor, i.e., it applies to a few pairs of alternatives, not allowing to distinguish between alternatives which are not dominated. Outranking methods use additional inputs to enrich this relation such that even if an alternative x is not better than (or possibly equal to) an alternative y on every criterion, a decision-maker can conclude that x outranks y if a majority of the criteria support this assertion contingent upon the fact that there is no criterion on which x is too much worse than y (in which case this criterion might "veto" the outranking assertion). This is the basic principle of ELECTRE (Elimination Et Choix Traduisant la Réalité, in French or ELimination and Choice Expressing REality, when translated into English) methods, the first methods of this kind (Roy 1991; Greco et al. 2016).

In ELECTRE methods, each alternative is compared to every other alternative, one at a time (as in a round-robin tournament) to assert whether an alternative outranks (i.e., is as good as) another one. The outranking relations are established by taking into account the weights of the criteria in favor of the outranking relation (i.e., concordance) and also the possibility that an opposing criterion vetoes that outranking relation (i.e., discordance). These outranking relations obtained are then exploited using an appropriate method from the ELECTRE family. There are methods to select a winner (ELECTRE I and IS), to rank the alternatives (ELECTRE II, III, and IV), or to sort them into predefined categories (ELECTRE TRI). The outranking relation is not transitive (if x outranks y and y outranks z, then it does not necessarily hold that x outranks z), and it is not complete (it may happen that x does not outrank y and y does not outrank x, in which case they are said to be incomparable). In other words, the ELECTRE methods do not always yield a single winner or a complete ranking. This can be seen as a shortcoming of these methods (the method may not distinguish between some alternatives), or it can be seen as a plus in the sense that the method highlights situations where alternatives are incomparable and does not force a conclusion that is not supported by sufficiently strong arguments.

Another popular outranking method is PROMETHEE (Behzadian et al. 2010; Brans et al. 1986). Contrary to ELECTRE, PROMETHEE does not require a majority threshold and does include the possibility of one criterion vetoing an outranking assertion. PROMETHEE is able to provide a partial or a complete ranking of the alternatives by considering, on average, how much an alternative outranks or is outranked by its competitors. Other outranking methods that deserve consideration, but less known, are NAIADE (Munda 1995) and methods that use qualitative information such as ORESTE, QUALIFLEX, and REGIME (Martel and Matarazzo 2005).

There are numerous examples of application of outranking methods to support health-care decision-making. ELECTRE IS has been used in France to select strategies for screening hemoglobinopathies taking into account cost-effectiveness and five other qualitative criteria (Gales and Moatti 1990). More recently, Diaby and Goeree illustrated how ELECTRE IS could be used for a hypothetical HTA problem. ELECTRE TRI has been used in several applications (Diaby and Goeree 2014). Figueira et al. (2011) used this method to assign couples seeking assisted reproduction to embryo transfer categories defining the number of embryos to be implanted (Figueira et al. 2011). The use of PROMETHEE for health-care decision-making includes, but is not limited to, the ranking of alternative strategies to deal with an overcrowded emergency room in Brazil (Amaral and Costa 2014) and the ranking of regional hospitals assessing their degree of specialization (D'Avignon and Mareschal 1989). Chen et al. used a variant of QUALIFLEX to select the best treatment to a patient with a diagnosis of acute inflammatory demyelinating disease, evaluating three therapies against eight health-related criteria and a cost criterion (Chen et al. 2013).

Outranking methods were devised to avoid one of the main characteristics of value function models, full compensation. As a result, it is the authors' opinion that outranking methods may be appealing to decision-makers who wish to avoid making trade-offs or those who deem that an alternative's poor performances on some decision criteria should not be compensated by its high performances on other criteria.

15.4 Concluding Remarks

MCDA was developed outside health care but has been increasingly applied in this field. It provides a unique opportunity to align decision-makers' preferences with their choices and provide a systematic and transparent way of making health-care decisions. Even though value functions are largely used in health care, MCDA users should be aware of the existence of alternative families of MCDA methods. Within value function methods, which synthesize the merits of each alternative into a global value figure, there are methods that have been applied less in health care, such as MACBETH, which were presented in this chapter. However, value function methods have certain key characteristics. First, these methods allow compensation, i.e., an alternative can make up for its poor performance on some criteria by compensating with higher performance on other criteria. Second, the weights represent the trade-offs between criteria, which need to satisfy conditions such as the preferential independence of criteria. Third, there is a requirement to elicit precise numerical weights for all criteria and scores for each alternative on all criteria. These characteristics may be too restrictive for some decision problems, where alternative methods to function methods may be more appropriate.

This chapter reviewed these other methods besides value function methods. A different way of evaluating alternatives is to compare these with given references, which can be based on the best observations (e.g., TOPSIS) or be externally provided. This type of approach may best suit situations in which decision-makers have a clear idea of the goals they wish to achieve. However, if the reference is derived from the actual performances of the alternatives, adding or removing an alternative may alter the conclusions pertaining the remaining alternatives.

Dominance-based approaches may be particularly interesting if the decision-makers prefer to reason in terms of examples rather than weights. DRSA, in particular, only requires modest information from end users (parsimonious models). This allows decision-makers to avoid dealing with the parameters of a mathematical model, provided that they have a set of exemplary decisions (e.g., from past experience) that can be provided as an input to the method. Although decision-makers may be quite unfamiliar with RST (hindering transparency), the results it produces are in the form of decision rules that can be easily understood.

Finally, outranking methods are particularly suited to decision-makers that are not willing to define substitution trade-offs between criteria. Outranking methods may also be useful if the goal is to identify a small subset of alternatives that fulfill a minimum requirement from a large set of alternatives as developing a total value score for each alternative using value function methods might be impractical. However, outranking methods do not always provide a clear-cut result, i.e., these approaches might lead to incomparability between two alternatives; that being said, one could argue that this is appropriate as further deliberation might be needed to choose between them.

By offering this large set of methods, MCDA proves to be flexible enough to accommodate the needs of decision-makers. However, as presented in this chapter, there are a diverse set of MCDA techniques each with different features and advantages/disadvantages. There is a long way to go before the potential of MCDA is used to its fullest extent. To that end, we call for further research with the decision-makers to identify which of these alternative methods in health care are suitable in different decision contexts.

Acknowledgement The authors are grateful to Praveen Thokala, Kevin Marsh, and Ellen Campbell for their insightful comments on earlier versions of this book chapter.

References

Adunlin G, Diaby V, Xiao H (2015) Application of multicriteria decision analysis in health care: a systematic review and bibliometric analysis. Health Expect 18:1894–1905

Akdag H, Kalaycı T, Karagöz S, Zülfikar H, Giz D (2014) The evaluation of hospital service quality by fuzzy MCDM. Appl Soft Comput 23:239–248

Amaral TM, Costa AP (2014) Improving decision-making and management of hospital resources: an application of the PROMETHEE II method in an Emergency Department. Oper Res Health Care 3(1):1–6

Bahadori M, Izadi M, Karamali M, Teymourzadeh E, Yaghoubi M (2014) Research priorities in a military health organization using multi criteria decision making techniques. J Mil Med 16(1):37–44

Baltussen R, Niessen L (2006) Priority setting of health interventions: the need for multi-criteria decision analysis. Cost Eff Resour Alloc 4:14

Bana e Costa CA, Lourenço JC, Oliveira MD, Bana e Costa JC (2014) A socio-technical approach for group decision support in public strategic planning: the pernambuco PPA case. Group Decis Negot 23(1):5–29

Bana e Costa CA, De Corte JM, Vansnick J (2012) Macbeth. Int J Info Tech Dec Mak 11(02):359–387

Beheshtifar S, Alimoahmmadi A (2015) A multiobjective optimization approach for location-allocation of clinics. Int Trans Oper Res. 22(2):313–28.

Behzadian M, Kazemzadeh RB, Albadvi A, Aghdasi M (2010) PROMETHEE: a comprehensive literature review on methodologies and applications. Eur J Oper Res 200(1):198–215

Belton V, Pictet J (1997) A framework for group decision using a MCDA model: sharing, aggregating or comparing individual information? J Decis Sys 6(3):283–303

Belton V, Stewart T (2002) Multiple criteria decision analysis: an integrated approach. Springer Science & Business Media. Norwell, Massachussets, US and Dordrecht, The Netherlands
Blasco H, Błaszczyński J, Billaut J et al (2015) Comparative analysis of targeted metabolomics: dominance-based rough set approach versus orthogonal partial least square-discriminant analysis. J Biomed Inform 53:291–299
Bouyssou D (1999) Using DEA, as a tool for MCDM: some remarks. J Oper Res Soc 50(9):974–978
Brans J, Vincke P, Mareschal B (1986) How to select and how to rank projects: the PROMETHEE method. Eur J Oper Res 24(2) 228–238
Chen T, Chang C, Lu JR (2013) The extended QUALIFLEX method for multiple criteria decision analysis based on interval type-2 fuzzy sets and applications to medical decision making. Eur J Oper Res 226(3):615–625
Cook WD, Seiford LM (2009) Data envelopment analysis (DEA)–thirty years on. Eur J Oper Res 192(1):1–17
Cooper W (2005) Origins, uses of, and relations between goal programming and data envelopment analysis. J Multi-Criteria Decis Anal 13(1):3–11
D'Avignon G, Mareschal B (1989) Specialization of hospital services in Québec: an application of the PROMETHEE and GAIA methods. Math Comput Model 12(10):1393–1400
de Castro AKA, Pinheiro PR, Pinheiro MCD (2009a) An approach for the neuropsychological diagnosis of Alzheimer's disease: a hybrid model in decision making. In: Rough sets and knowledge technology. Springer, Berlin, pp 216–223
de Castro AKA, Pinheiro PR, Pinheiro MCD (2009b) Towards the neuropsychological diagnosis of Alzheimer's disease: a hybrid model in decision making. In: Best practices for the knowledge society. Knowledge, learning, development and technology for all. Springer, Berlin, pp 522–531
de Moraes L, Garcia R, Ensslin L, da Conceição MJ, de Carvalho SM (2010) The multicriteria analysis for construction of benchmarkers to support the Clinical Engineering in the Healthcare Technology Management. Eur J Oper Res 200(2):607–615
Diaby V, Goeree R (2014) How to use multi-criteria decision analysis methods for reimbursement decision-making in healthcare: a step-by-step guide. Expert Rev Pharmacoecon Outcomes Res 14(1):81–99
Dias L, Clímaco J (2000) Additive aggregation with variable interdependent parameters: the VIP analysis software. J Oper Res Soc 51(9):1070–1082
Dodgson J, Spackman M, Pearman A, Phillips L (2009) Multi-criteria analysis: a manual. Department for Communities and Local Government, London
Ehrgott M (2006) Multicriteria optimization. Springer Science & Business Media. New York (original version)
Figueira JR, Almeida-Dias J, Matias S, Roy B, Carvalho MJ, Plancha CE (2011) Electre Tri-C, a multiple criteria decision aiding sorting model applied to assisted reproduction. Int J Med Inform 80(4):262–273
Gales CL, Moatti J (1990) Searching for consensus through multicriteria decision analysis. Int J Technol Assess Health Care 6(03):430–449
Gouveia M, Dias L, Antunes C (2008) Additive DEA based on MCDA with imprecise information. J Oper Res Soc 59(1):54–63
Greco S, Matarazzo B, Slowinski R (2001) Rough sets theory for multicriteria decision analysis. Eur J Oper Res 129(1):1–47
Greco S, Matarazzo B, Słowiński R (2005) Rough membership and bayesian confirmation measures for parameterized rough sets. In: Rough sets, fuzzy sets, data mining, and granular computing. Springer, Berlin, pp 314–324
Greco S, Ehrgott M, Figueira J (2016) Multiple criteria decision analysis: state of the art surveys, 2nd edn. Springer, New York
Ishizaka A, Nemery P (2013) Multi-criteria decision analysis: methods and software. John Wiley & Sons, Chichester

Jarzabek R, Bugajski P, Greberski K, Blaszczynski J, Slowinska-Jarzabek B, Kalawski R (2014) Readmission to an intensive care unit after cardiac surgery: reasons and outcomes. Kardiol Pol 72(8):740–747

Jones D, Tamiz M (2010) History and philosophy of goal programming. In: Practical goal programming. Springer, New York, pp 1–9

Keeney R, Raiffa H (1993) Decisions with multiple objectives: preferences and value trade-offs. Cambridge University Press

Lahdelma R, Salminen P (2001) SMAA-2: stochastic multicriteria acceptability analysis for group decision making. Oper Res 49:444–454

Liang L, Liu Z, Wang H (2014) Appling the EVIDEM framework with fuzzy multicriteria group decision making method to medicines appraisal⋆. J Comput Inf Syst 10(4):1659–1667

Liu JS, Lu LY, Lu W, Lin BJ (2013) A survey of DEA applications. Omega 41(5):893–902

Martel J, Matarazzo B (2005) Other outranking approaches. In: Multiple criteria decision analysis: state of the art surveys. Springer, New York, pp 197–259

Moshkovich HM, Mechitov AI (2013) Verbal decision analysis: foundations and trends. Adv Decis Sci 2013:9

Moshkovich HM, Mechitov AI, Olson DL (2002) Ordinal judgments in multiattribute decision analysis. Eur J Oper Res 137(3):625–641

Moshkovich H, Mechitov A, Olson D (2005) Verbal decision analysis. In: Multiple criteria decision analysis: state of the art surveys. Springer, New York, pp 609–633

Munda G (1995) Multicriteria evaluation in a fuzzy environment: theory and applications in ecological economics. Physica-Verlag, Heidelberg

Munda G, Nardo M (2005) Constructing consistent composite indicators: the issue of weights. European Commission – Joint Research Center, Office for Official Publications of the European Communities, Luxembourg [EUR 21834 EN]

Nunes LC, Pinheiro PR, Pequeno TC, Pinheiro MCD (2011) Toward an application to psychological disorders diagnosis. In: Software tools and algorithms for biological systems. Springer, New York, pp 573–580

Pawlak Z, Sowinski R (1994) Rough set approach to multi-attribute decision analysis. Eur J Oper Res 72(3):443–459

Phillips LD, et al (2012) Benefit-risk methodology project: work package 4 report: benefit-risk tools and processes. European Medicines Agency, London. Available at: http://www.ema.europa.eu/docs/en_GB/document_library/Report/2012/03/WC500123819.pdf

Postmus D, Tervonen T, van Valkenhoef G, Hillege HL, Buskens E (2014) A multi-criteria decision analysis perspective on the health economic evaluation of medical interventions. Eur J Health Econ 15(7):709–716

Roy B (1991) The outranking approach and the foundations of ELECTRE methods. Theor Decis 31(1):49–73

Sang S, Wang Z, Yu C (2014) Evaluation of health care system reform in Hubei Province, China. Int J Environ Res Public Health 11(2):2262–2277

Tamanini I, de Castro AK, Pinheiro PR, Pinheiro MCD (2011) Verbal decision analysis applied on the optimization of alzheimer's disease diagnosis: a case study based on neuroimaging. In: Software tools and algorithms for biological systems. Springer, New York, pp 555–564

Thomas BG, Bollapragada S, Akbay K et al (2013) Automated bed assignments in a complex and dynamic hospital environment. Interfaces 43(5):435–448

Tsai P, Lin F (2014) An application of multi-attribute value theory to patient-bed assignment in hospital admission management: an empirical study. J Healthc Eng 5(4):439–456

Yevseyeva I, Miettinen K, Räsänen P (2008) Verbal ordinal classification with multicriteria decision aiding. Eur J Oper Res 185(3):964–983

Yoon KP, Hwang C (1995) Multiple attribute decision making: an introduction, vol 104. Sage Publications, Thousand Oaks

Chapter 16
Best Practice for MCDA in Healthcare

Lawrence D. Phillips

Abstract This chapter begins with a short overview of decision theory—four self-evident characteristics of coherent preference that lead logically to the three considerations for ensuring the consistency of decisions: (1) the utility of decision consequences, (2) the probabilities those consequences will occur and (3) the expected utility rule for combining utilities and probabilities as a guide to action. Extending the theory to accommodate multiple criteria for evaluating the values of the alternatives provides the simple weighted average rule for combining values across the criteria, preserving the goal of coherence in decisions. This simple rule provides the basis for multi-criteria decision analysis (MCDA). As applied to healthcare, MCDA takes account of both measurable data and subjective judgements about the data, with the latter often representing clinical judgement or patient preferences.

An eight-step framework for constructing an MCDA model is described and used to formulate 16 best practice principles, with a focus on creating a model in a facilitated group workshop. Working collectively enables a group to identify a requisite set of criteria and provides the expertise to evaluate the alternatives against the criteria. The overall goal is to create a model that best reflects the current state of knowledge and judgement, which enables uncertainty and different perspectives to be explored, thus supporting but not automating any final decision.

16.1 Introduction

MCDA means different things to different people, but whatever the interpretation, all approaches are intended to improve decisions when conflicting objectives mean that no single decision can be best for all of its possible consequences. However, the deeper value of MCDA is that when the modelling is carried out in a facilitated

L.D. Phillips
London School of Economics and Political Science, London, UK
e-mail: larry_phillips@msn.com

© Springer International Publishing AG 2017

K. Marsh et al. (eds.), *Multi-Criteria Decision Analysis to Support Healthcare Decisions*, DOI 10.1007/978-3-319-47540-0_16

workshop attended by a diverse group of knowledgeable key players, the process allows participants to develop a shared understanding of the issues, generate a sense of common purpose and agree recommendations for the way forwards (Phillips 2007; Franco and Montibeller 2010). In short, the process aligns participants so everyone is pulling in the same direction while preserving the important differences in paths.

Two social scientists, Charles Kepner and Benjamin Tregoe, reported these advantages for problem-solving and group decision-making when managers in organisations applied the structured process described in their 1965 book *The Rational Manager* (Kepner and Tregoe 1965). Chapter 6 listed the steps of the process they called 'decision analysis', the term they used to describe their approach to problem-solving and decision-making:

1. Set objectives against which to choose.
2. Classify objectives as to importance.
3. Develop alternatives from which to choose.
4. Evaluate alternatives against the objectives to make a choice.
5. Choose the best alternative as a tentative decision.
6. Assess adverse consequences from the choice.
7. Control effects of the final decision.

Fast forward 35 years, and here is MCDA described in the UK Government's *Multi-Criteria Analysis: A Manual* (Dodgson et al. 2000):

1. Establish the decision context.
2. Identify options to be appraised.
3. Identify objectives and criteria.
4. Score each option against the criteria.
5. Assign weights for each criterion to reflect their relative importance.
6. Combine weights and scores.
7. Examine the results.
8. Conduct sensitivity analyses.

Some differences, but both are concerned with multiple objectives and both engage in scoring options on criteria, incorporating uncertainty in the scoring process and weighting the criteria, so it would appear that not much changed over those 35 years. But in fact, a great deal happened, with applications for healthcare arising only recently. However, as Marsh et al. point out in their recent review, '… [MCDA] approaches and methods are very diverse, with limited correspondence between approaches employed and the type of healthcare decision or product evaluated (Marsh et al. 2014)'.

Perhaps this chapter can begin to provide some focus. Let's start with a brief history of the theory on which MCDA is based, which will illuminate the best practice section of this chapter. Along the way, we will discover the three key principles of decision analysis that are as important to decision-making as Newton's three laws of motion are to an understanding of the universe.

16.2 Decision Theory

It was Frank Ramsey, a brilliant Cambridge mathematician, philosopher and economist and younger brother of the former Archbishop of Canterbury, Michael, who introduced in 1926 the concept of consistency as logically implying probabilities that represent an individual's degrees of belief (Ramsey 1926). John von Neumann and Oskar Morgenstern (1947) extended the consistency argument by further developing Ramsey's axioms sufficiently to introduce utilities. Jimmie Savage took the additional step of starting with an axiom system that assumed neither probabilities nor utilities, only coherent preferences, which he showed leads logically to the existence of probabilities and utilities and to the expected utility rule as a guide to coherent decisions (Savage 1954). But what is meant by 'coherent preference', and what is its importance to MCDA?

Savage's axioms of coherent preferences are simple and elegant. The four most important are ordering, transitivity, dominance and the sure-thing principle. Without doing too much damage to his complete exposition, here are my descriptions of a hypothetical person whose preferences obey these axioms.

Ordering Either you prefer A to B or B to A, or you are indifferent between them. This requires only knowing your order of preferences, even if you don't know your actual preferences.

Transitivity If you prefer A to B and B to C, then you should prefer A to C. This is a requirement for any form of measurement.

Dominance If all the possible consequences of action A are at least as good as all the consequences of action B, and in one or more ways, A's consequences are better than B's, then you should prefer A to B.

Sure-thing If A and B are characterised by one or more consequences that are identical, then your preference should not take these consequences into consideration, for whether you choose A or B, you are certain to obtain the consequence that is identical.

A few technical axioms are included, like the list of alternatives must be finite, but nobody seems to worry too much about these as they are unobjectionable within Savage's 'small world' of practical applications, whose decisions contingent on anticipated future events can be reasonably defined, in contrast to the 'grand world' he recognised as constituting many linked decisions and possible future events that cannot sensibly be foreseen. As yet, nobody, Savage included, has developed a wholly satisfactory 'grand world' approach to coherent decision-making.

It's not difficult to find instances in which real people violate these axioms, but that's not the point. Here we are considering a real person who on a particular occasion wishes to make choices that are not in conflict with his or her objectives. You wouldn't, for example, place bets on the outcome of a single horse race such that no matter which horse wins, you are certain to lose money (with apologies to

Dutch colleagues, that sort of gamble is called a 'Dutch book' in the English-speaking world; I understand you call it an 'English book'). It seems reasonable to enquire if there are any principles that a person could apply so that a Dutch book wouldn't be accepted, because the axioms aren't very helpful. For example, sometimes people are unsure of their preferences and as a result might well violate the first axiom.

What would be helpful? The answer is 'the theorems': they make clear we should consider (1) utilities of consequences, (2) the probabilities of realising those consequences and (3) the expected utility rule—choosing the course of action with the highest 'expected' (weighted average) utility. Those three principles are as important to decision-making as Newton's laws are to understanding bodies in motion. But, some would say, the three theorems at the heart of decision-making are not the same as Newton's laws, which apply to the real world. In answer, Newton's laws apply to ideal bodies, with mass concentrated at a point and moving in a vacuum, yet they can be applied in the real world to very complex physical systems. Similarly, the theorems of coherent preference can be applied to construct 'small world' models that will enable effective decisions, but the calculus of probabilities and the mathematics of utilities restrict our freedom in applying them, just as the relationship between force, mass and acceleration restrict the movement of physical bodies.

Savage's theorems are implied by the axioms, but the implication works in the other direction, too: the theorems imply the axioms (though not uniquely—other, similar axioms of coherent preference also lead to the same theorems). Thus, it is perfectly acceptable to work with people whose preferences may not be coherent and to engage them in building a decision theory model, which will in the process help them to construct coherent preferences that ensure their decisions are consistent with their objectives.

16.3 Decision Analysis

Those restrictions became more evident as decision theory morphed into an applied technology in the 1960s and 1970s, following the 1961 exposition by Raiffa and Schlaifer (1961), *Applied Statistical Decision Theory*. Ron Howard developed a systems analysis approach to decision theory, which he called 'decision analysis'(Howard 1966), apparently unaware that Kepner and Tregoe had first contributed the term a year earlier. Raiffa's 1968 book, *Decision Analysis* (Raiffa 1968), and Schlaifer's 1969 book, *Analysis of Decisions Under Uncertainty* (Schlaifer 1969) (accompanied by an informative Instructor's Manual, book of computer programmes and case studies developed by the Harvard team, an astonishing intellectual achievement), explained in great detail how this new technology could be applied as an aid to decision-making.

In 1976, the focus on modelling uncertainty expanded to include decisions with multiple objectives, as Howard Raiffa's then student, Ralph Keeney, turned Raiffa's 1969 RAND Corporation report, *Preferences for Multi-Attributed Alternatives* (Raiffa 1969), into a full exposition of what we now know as Keeney-Raiffa MCDA.

By extending the axioms of coherent preference, they showed how multiple, conflicting objectives could be included in the analysis, along with uncertainty and risk, which establishes the best practice principles (Keeney and Raiffa 1976). Methods such as MACBETH, PAPRIKA, discrete choice experiments, conjoint analysis and the analytic hierarchy process all use ranking or rating measurement procedures, whereas unique interval or ratio scales are required for the expected utility or value calculations that link MCDA to decision-making in the face of uncertainty. My choice of MCDA for defining best practice is based on its generality, completeness and theoretically sound foundation in the Savage axioms. That's not to deny the usefulness of other methods that might be easier to use and produce useful results, but like all models, they are limited in validity, scope and applicability.

An MCDA model is often created in a facilitated workshop attended by key players who represent the various perspectives on the issues. One form of facilitated workshop is decision conferencing (Phillips 2007), in which the impartial facilitator guides the process of creating a model, while the leader and participants contribute the content. This separation of responsibility for process from content makes possible the rapid development and exploration of the model, which usually is completed in 1–3 days, though refinements may well take place subsequently for complex problems, often between a series of workshops. A workshop setting will be assumed throughout this presentation of best practice principles.

Most multi-criteria approaches are characterised by a process of scoring options (projects, programmes, policies, strategies, systems, etc.) on criteria, weighting the criteria to accommodate the different metrics used by the criteria and then combining the weighted scores to provide an overall ordering of the options. The various forms of multi-criteria analysis are briefly reviewed in Dodgson et al. (2000) and explained in detail by Belton and Stewart (2002). Dodgson et al. felt that the most appropriate approach for policy development in the UK was Keeney-Raiffa MCDA. The eight-step process at the start of this chapter is further defined and elaborated by the 16 best practice principles that follow. Throughout, the objective is to create a 'requisite' decision model, which is just sufficient in form and content to resolve the issues at hand (Phillips 1984).

16.4 Principles for Establishing the Decision Context

Principle 1: Define the Bounds of the Problem

Savage (1954) argued that coherence of preference is always bounded; we can only manage coherence within a defined 'small world'. In other words, coherence is always conditional on our assumptions about the limits of a decision's context. For example, a utility function for a department's budget in an organisation often shows more risk aversion than the corporate utility function. This inconsistency arises in part because the department's portion of the total budget is so much smaller that its utility functions appear to be almost linear over the same range on the corporate utility function. A related reason appears in the 'commons dilemma' (Hardin 1968): choosing actions that maximise expected utility in each of several departments may not collectively maximise expected utility for the whole organisation. What is best for the 'grand world', to use Savage's terminology, is not the sum of what is best in a collection of 'small worlds'. This problem is caused by the failure to consider trade-offs, which would consider opportunity costs, between departments than it is to the incompatibilities of risk attitudes between small and grand worlds. This is a serious problem for health technology assessment organisations because there is no universal, fungible measure of health outcomes that is acceptable across different small worlds.

Principle 2: Identify the Purpose and Key Players

A further aspect of the context involves identifying the stakeholders and key players who will be consulted or engaged in a workshop. Key players include experts and others who can make a useful contribution to the analysis; they are not necessarily stakeholders, who are those affected by the consequences of the decisions. It is also important to consider people who could reject the recommendations of the workshop. Ministers and others may not be available to participate in the appraisal study, but their perspectives could be contributed by representatives. Also, before a workshop it would be wise for the facilitator to engage with the problem owners to identify the key players, establish the objectives of the workshop, outline the main tasks that will constitute the work of the workshop and indicate the preparation expected of invited participants. These features sent to participants before the workshop in a 'calling note' will establish their expectations for the event and ensure a high degree of motivation and engagement. For most healthcare applications, it is particularly important to include clinicians in the workshops, whose experience with patients is critically important in assessing the clinical value of measured data.

Principle 3: Explore Context and Issues with the Group

At the start of the workshop, after introductions and a restatement of the objectives for the meeting, the facilitator asks the group to discuss the issues that are important to consider for achieving the objectives. Depending on participants' responses, prompting by the facilitator could establish relevant internal and external influences; the political, economic, social, technological, environmental and legal (PESTEL) factors; or the organisation's mission (why are we here?) or core values (what we care deeply about), any of which will affect the MCDA model. In particular, the context will provide meaning to subsequent value judgements.

16.5 *Principles for Identifying Options*

The second and third steps are interchangeable, identify the options and identify the objectives and criteria. If options are given, ask questions of the group about objectives. If objectives are given, ask questions about options. When neither has been clearly identified, discussing objectives and options becomes, appropriately, a reflexive process; each informs the other. Let's start with the options.

Principle 4: Establish a Requisite Set of Clearly Defined Options
When options are already on the table or easily identified from the start, the facilitator might ask if there could be other uses of the available resources, i.e. other decision opportunities. Budget constraints often inhibit thinking about new options, so the facilitator could encourage 'blue-sky' thinking without considering the budget. This can be an important step in finding alternatives that are more promising uses of the available resource, which might not emerge from the MCDA model until a later stage. Encouraging the group to create 'win-win' options helps to prevent 'win-lose' arguments that are often raised by anxious participants, which prevents real progress. Including the 'status quo' or 'do nothing' as options, even if they aren't realistic, can serve as a reference point for assessing added value at later stages. Each option should be defined clearly. In MCDA, unlike a decision tree, the options do not have to be mutually exclusive. They could be decisions, strategies, policies, subsystems, projects, programmes or anything that could lead to achievement of objectives.

16.6 Principles for Identifying Objectives and Criteria

Objectives are desirable end states at some time in the future, made operational by identifying and defining criteria (or attributes), which are measurable goals. For example, 'alleviating suffering' is an objective, while 'reducing disease severity' is a measurable criterion. Both are characterised by a verb and a noun.

Principle 5: Establish a Requisite Set of Clearly Defined, Operational Criteria
Recent research by Bond et al. (2010) showed that individuals were limited in the number of objectives they were able to bring to mind, and those they did make explicit were limited in range and in depth of thinking. They found that

providing category-based prompts at the start of the elicitation process was less successful than giving the prompts *after* asking the individual to extend their list. For example, the chair of the Advisory Council on the Misuse of Drugs suggested to members discussing the meaning of 'harm' that they consider physical, psychological and social harms separately and that they distinguish between harms to the user and to others. Those categories served as prompts, which helped to structure the discussion of harm criteria and resulted in 16 criteria altogether (Advisory Council on the Misuse of Drugs 2010).

A criterion's definition should be operational in the sense that each alternative's effects can be judged or measured for the criterion on a scale that is monotonic in preference (either larger or smaller effects are preferred to intermediate effects).

Principle 6: Ensure the Criteria Are Nonredundant

Eliminate unnecessary or duplicate criteria. For example, regulators generally ignore minor side effects that won't affect the decision about a new drug, so they are eliminated from consideration. Also, a physician's global assessment (PGA) of a patient's psoriasis might be repeated in a scoring system that included PGA in an application for a new drug; the regulator should consider only one or the other of these duplicates.

Principle 7: Ensure There Is No Double Counting Within and Across Criteria

Make sure that a single data point appears once and only once across several criteria and for a given criterion. For example, mean months of survival, median months of survival and mean progression-free months double count the same data points across those three criteria. But as they may reveal somewhat different effects, they can all be included in an MCDA model, but only one should be operational—by giving the other two criteria zero weights—in each of three different runs of the model.

Double counting of patients is another example. Patients surviving at 12 months, 18 months and 24 months, as separate criteria, are double-counting patients: anyone surviving to the longer periods has survived to the shorter ones. Either only one criterion at a time should be given non-zero weight, or the three criteria should be represented as a proper frequency distribution: 12–17 months, 18–23 months and 24 months or greater.

Principle 8: Ensure the Criteria Are Mutually Preference Independent
The preference order of options on any one criterion is unaffected by the preference order on any other criterion and vice versa. This condition is weaker than statistical independence. Scores on criteria are typically statistically correlated across the criteria, but a high correlation might imply violation of preference independence. If participants ask to see the scores on criterion Y while scoring options on criterion X, that suggests a violation of this principle. Lacking such requests suggests, but does not guarantee, mutual preference independence. This requirement must be met if weighted scores are to be interpreted unambiguously, for *any* weighted average model. Statistical correlation doesn't matter if criteria are preference independent, which is a weaker requirement.

Principle 9: Iterate Between Options and Objectives to Create a Requisite Set of Each
More typically, moving back and forth between this and the previous step is helpful because neither options nor objectives may at the start be well established. Engage in value-focused thinking (Keeney 1992): be clear about your values (what you care about), imagine desirable and undesirable health outcomes, develop your objectives (verb and noun), and separate ends (your fundamental objectives) from means, all in the service of creating desirable alternatives.

16.7 Principles for Scoring the Options

The purpose of scoring is to convert input performance measures into preference values, the first step for establishing a single, common metric that will legitimise comparisons of all the options across all the criteria. At this stage, the consequences of the options are expressed as performance measures; these are usually real-world measurements, though they may also be direct preference judgements. A value function over the performance measures is determined next, where value is defined as the extent to which the outcome achieves the objective. The value function may be linear, but sometimes in healthcare it is not. Are 20 life-years gained twice as desirable as 10? Possibly not—and perhaps the value function also depends on how old the person is now. Note that scoring the options requires data or judgements about the performance of each separate option on a given criterion. It is not differences between options that are inputs for MCDA; weighted differences between options emerge as outputs, whereas for other approaches, like cost-benefit analysis, they are inputs. Sometimes data may be absent or in qualitative form, in which case preference values are assessed directly, preferably by group consensus to minimise bias of individually assessed preferences. Published data all too frequently report odds or risk ratios, without sufficient information to recover the numerator and denominator of the ratio. Unless one or the other is identical for all options, it isn't possible to form preferences for these ratios. Separate measures are required for each option in MCDA.

Principle 10: Ensure That Assessors Understand the Type and Meaning of the Preference Scale
In healthcare, options are typically interventions, and the consequences of the interventions are expected to provide added value in the form of favourable effects, at a possible loss of value for unfavourable effects. Three types of scales are used in MCDA: absolute, ratio and interval, which differ in their scale's origin and unit of measure. In measurement theory (Krantz et al. 1971), counting is an absolute scale; the origin, zero, means an absence of the property in whatever is being counted, and the counts are one integer at a time, representing, for example, the number of patients exhibiting the favourable or unfavourable effect, often reported as a percentage of the total number of patients. For a ratio scale, the origin is also zero, with the same meaning, for example, in measuring speed of onset for noticeable pain relief in which no pain relief at all, following a treatment, would be scored zero. The unit is a matter of choice, as in measuring time in minutes or hours. For an interval scale, both the origin and unit are matters of choice, as in measuring temperature on scales in which the boiling and freezing points of water at sea level provide two reference points, 212 and 32 for Fahrenheit or 100 and 0 for Celsius. Value scales in MCDA are often defined as interval scales, with reference points chosen to encompass a range of realisable data, as a thermometer for an inhabitable room would show a plausible range. It's useful to draw a value scale on a flipchart so participants understand that the numbers represent strength of preference and what 100 and 0 mean, as shown in Fig. 16.1 for an interval scale (some modellers use a value scale from 0 to 1.0, but the 0–100 scale avoids decimals and possible confusion with probabilities).

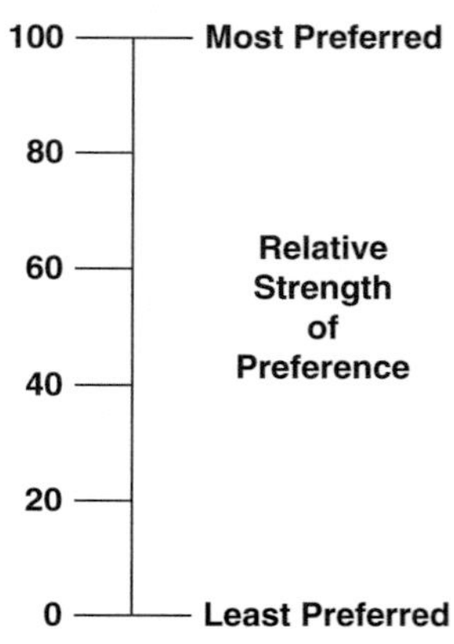

Fig. 16.1 Interval preference scale

The reason the choice of scale type matters is that it provides guidance for defining the reference points on the scales, for interpreting the preference values while they are being assessed and determining the type of consistency checks that are consistent with the scale type (see Principle 11). It also enables the weighted preference values to be properly interpreted, as is noted below in the principles for interpreting results. For example, in modelling the harm of psychoactive drugs, Nutt et al. used ratio scales, with zero representing 'no harm' and 100 as the most harmful drug uniquely for each criterion (Nutt et al. 2010). For modelling prescription drugs, most of the PROTECT Benefit-Risk project teams (2015) used interval scales, with predefined levels of the effects chosen to include the observed data about the effects, plus or minus realistic amounts that might arise if more data were available. Ranges that are too large will make it difficult or impossible to assess trade-off weights because unrealistic upper and lower limits are not within the experience of the assessors. More generally, 100 might represent the maximum realisable performance and zero the lowest acceptable performance on a given criterion, instead of the best and worst actually realised. When the 0–100 scale is defined by specific levels of the input performance measure, it is referred to as a 'global' scale by Belton and Stewart (2002) and in the V.I.S.A MCDA software or a 'fixed' scale in the Hiview software (LSE/Catalyze 2011).

Defining two points on a criterion scale by assigning 0 and 100 to the least and most preferred options is an understandable and convenient way to establish an interval scale, as contrasted to pre-establishing ranges. It has the advantage of focusing the judgements of experts on only the options under consideration and the data actually observed. These scales are called 'local' by Belton and Stewart and 'relative' in the Hiview software. Whether performance measures are positive or negative, it is important to establish the direction of preference: are smaller numbers or larger numbers more preferred? Lesser pain is more preferred, and more fever is less preferred. Chapter 4 gives additional information on scoring.

Principle 11: Carry Out Consistency Checks During and After Scoring the Options

Consistency checks are easiest when assessments employ a ratio scale. For example, if option A is given a preference value of 100 and option B a 50, then the facilitator might ask the group if A is really twice as desirable as B for its effect on the criterion under consideration or twice as good or twice the value (provided that the facilitator has made clear that 'value' is meant in its nonmonetary sense).

For interval scales, differences in preference values are the basis for consistency checks. For example, if option A scores 100, B is 80 and C is 20, then assessors might note that the 60-point difference in preference between B and C is three times that of A compared to B. Because the zero point was arbitrarily chosen, it would be incorrect to say that B is four times better than C.

16.8 Principles for Weighting the Criteria

Weights are scale constants that represent trade-offs in preference values; they equate the units of preference value across all criteria within the small world of the MCDA. To equate units of preference value across many small worlds, such as healthcare decisions at system level, requires judging trade-offs among key criteria across the small worlds, which is well established in MCDA, e.g. resource al location across all departments in a hospital (Kleinmuntz 2007). The weights are relative measures that show how a fixed difference in preference on one value scale corresponds to a fixed difference in preference on another value scale. Both Fahrenheit and Celsius scales, for instance, include 0–100 portions, but the Celsius increment represents a larger increment of temperature than the 0–100 increment on the Fahrenheit scale, so it takes 9 Fahrenheit degrees to equal 5 Celsius degrees.

Principle 12: Ensure That Ranges of Comparisons Are Taken into Account in Assessing Value Trade-Offs

A common misinterpretation of weights is that they represent the importance of the criteria; that's only half true. The range from least to most preferred points on a scale is also a consideration, with weights representing the importance of the range. In purchasing a car, most people consider cost to be an important criterion. However, if the difference between the most and least costly car being considered is small, then cost isn't so important. And a big difference would be given more weight, unless the purchaser is very wealthy, in which case cost might not be important. The operative question for assessing weights is this: 'how big is the difference between least and most preferred positions on this criterion, and how much do you care about that difference'? The first part of the question is often about hard data; the second might be a clinical judgement about the added value to the patient, and that depends on the healthcare context. That's why it is important at the start to understand the context.

Here's a simple example. Imagine you are suffering pain from a strained muscle and decide to take either aspirin, ibuprofen or paracetamol. Which of the following three criteria would you rate as most and least important to you: the speed of the first noticeable reduction in your pain, the extent of pain relief (percent of patients who report at least a 50 % reduction in pain within 2 h) or the duration of action (the time to re-medication for 50 % of patients). (Note the application of Principle 10.) Make your choice before reading on. (For the purpose of illustration, ignore side effects.)

The data, based on the findings of two workshops attended by UK experts on pain, including the swing weights they assigned to the three criteria, are shown in Table 16.1.

Table 16.1 Data: linear conversion of the data to preference values (in parentheses) and weights on three criteria for three painkiller drugs

	Speed of onset Minutes	Pain relief % of patients	Duration of action Hours	Weighted preference value
Aspirin	50 (20)	20 (0)	5.0 (67)	16
Ibuprofen	55 (0)	48 (100)	5.5 (100)	47
Paracetamol	30 (100)	33 (46)	4.0 (0)	71
Swing weights	*100*	*75*	*15*	
Normalised wts	*0.53*	*0.39*	*0.08*	

Overall, paracetamol obtains the highest weighted preference value largely because of its speed of onset, the most heavily weighted criterion. The swing on that criterion is from 30 to 55 min; ibuprofen, which gives better pain relief, is 25 min slower. And the low weight on duration of action arises from the modest range of data, a difference of only 1.5 h. You may not agree with these weights, but the example provides a salient reason for attending to ranges in assessing weights. In general, larger differences that matter receive higher weights.

Principle 13: Keep It Simple!

Deploying the operative question can vary; what works for some groups does not work so well for others. Sometimes asking assessors to imagine a hypothetical option that scores zero on all criteria and then inviting the group to decide which criterion would add the most value if moving from least to most preferred positions on only one criterion could be achieved; which would it be? That establishes a standard for comparing the ranges on each of the other criteria, one at a time, always compared to the one large change. This is an example of the paired comparison method, which is based on the law of comparative judgement, first developed in 1927 by Thurstone (1959) and still widely applied in psychology because it is the simplest way of obtaining reliable and valid judgements.

Another useful paired comparison approach is to ask which of the following combinations of positions on speed of onset and pain relief is better:

Option A : speed of onset 30 min and pain relief for 20% of patients

OR

Option B : speed of onset 55 min and pain relief for 48% of patients

If A is chosen, the speed of onset range has been judged as more preferred; otherwise B's range is larger. Next, successively compare the range on the larger criterion with the ranges on the remaining criteria, until the longest range that matters is identified. Assign a weight of 100 to the criterion with the longest range that matters, and then engage in paired comparisons to establish weights on the remaining criteria. The similarity to conjoint analysis (Johnson 2006) should be evident. The best-worst/worst-best process doesn't work very well when the preference scales are statistically correlated, which is often the case in healthcare. Respondents are likely to say that an option is a combination they can't imagine because it never occurs in the real world. More is said about this approach in Chapter 4.

Since weights are ratios, you can ask consistency check questions, e.g. a weight of 60 adds twice the preference value over the range as compared to a 30. It's wise to make those comparisons during the assessment process, for a reduction of the weights compared to 100 is almost always the result, largely because assessors start off thinking that everything is important until the concept of added value over ranges is introduced. A simple consistency check on the weights assigned in Table 16.1 is to note that the added preference values on pain relief and on duration of action (75 plus 15) were judged to be 90 % of the added value of the range in pain relief. Finally, since subjective judgement is the source of the weights, it can be informative to involve stakeholders in those judgements as well. This is another reason to be clear at the start about the purpose of the model. Chapter 4 gives other approaches to weighting.

16.9 Principles for Calculating Weighted Scores

Whatever the inputs to an MCDA, scores and weights or ratings of pairs of differences, it is algorithms, or mathematical formulae, that combine the inputs. With scoring and weighting completed, isn't the result obvious? Why can't aggregation be done intuitively? The answer has been known for 60 years, since the publication of clinical psychologist Paul Meehl's 1954 book, *Clinical versus Statistical Prediction* (Meehl 1996), which dropped a bombshell on clinical psychology. Meehl found that simple, linear, additive models consistently outperformed clinical predictions of behaviour in the 20 studies he could find reported in the literature. He identified integration of multiple pieces of data as the problem, not the judgements about the pieces. Among many subsequent studies, Phillips et al. (1966) compared various ways of judging and aggregating uncertain data, and their findings agreed with Meehl's conclusions. Today, with over 200 studies now published, the conclusion still stands. Indeed, Kahneman devoted an entire chapter to the topic in *Thinking, Fast and Slow* (Kahneman 2011). So, the best practice principle is simple.

Principle 14: Use an Algorithm to Aggregate the Evidence and Judgements
For most MCDA models, the algorithm simply multiplies each preference value by the criterion weight and sums across all criteria. That simple weighted additive model applies when the criteria are judged to be mutually preference independent. Keeney and Raiffa (1976) provide the mathematics for situations in which mutual preference independence does not apply. The mathematics are still simple, but the additional assessments are often more difficult, so most decision analysts will suggest rephrasing the criteria so that the independence requirement is met. Others will ignore it, arguing that little is usually gained by moving to the more complex model.

Application of the analytic hierarchy process (AHP) doesn't require separate preference values and weights. Rather, its inputs are matrices of paired comparisons using a 9-point scale representing differences. The mathematics applied to the matrices is based on matrix algebra, not the expected utility or weighted value model, so it can lead to violations of the axioms of coherent preference (Belton and Gear 1983) and has led to Dyer's criticism (Dyer 1990) that the output weights from the AHP are 'arbitrary'. Conjoint analysis and discrete choice experiments also conflate preference values and weights, which might be sufficient in some situations. The added capability to separate them in MCDA enables experts about the data to do the scoring, with decision-makers who may have a better understanding of trade-offs assessing the weights.

16.10 Principles for Examining Results

Examining the results begins with the overall ordering of options (as in the rightmost column of the table for painkillers). Next, overall benefits might be compared to overall costs, or to risks, or one cluster of benefits to another cluster. Each of these can be represented by a two-dimensional graph that gives a clear pictorial representation for establishing the dominance relationships among the options by showing the efficient frontier. Paired comparisons of options show the relative advantages and disadvantages of each member of the pair. A detailed survey of graphs for displaying inputs and results can be found in two major reports of the IMI-PROTECT project (Mt-Isa et al. 2013a, b).

Principle 15: Rely on Software to Provide the Graphs and Tables to Display Results
As for best practice, here are some guidelines:

1. Interval-scale input data are best shown in thermometer displays (which make differences more visually salient; ratios are not interpretable), while ratio-scale data are more usefully shown with horizontal bar graphs (which make ratios of scores more obvious).
2. Vertical (or horizontal) stacked bar graphs are also good for displaying overall weighted scores at any node in the value tree, with the sectors of each bar giving the weighted contributions of the lower-level constituents.
3. X-Y scatterplots for MCDA option-evaluation models show the efficient frontier for any two criteria. The efficient frontier for MCDA models of prioritisation and resource allocation, showing the investment options in order of their benefit-to-cost ratio, can help decision-makers 'steer' a feasible solution onto or close to the efficient frontier (Phillips and Bana e Costa 2007).
4. Difference displays and waterfall charts are good for comparing one option against another on each of the criteria.

16.11 Principles for Sensitivity Analyses and Scenario Analyses

Sensitivity analyses provide ways to explore the effects on final results of imprecision in the data and differences of opinion about input scores, value functions and weights. MCDA displays remarkable insensitivity to precision in the inputs, a topic so important that it constitutes all of Chapter 11 in von Winterfeldt and Edwards (1986). Because of this insensitivity, it is possible for key players to agree about the best option without agreeing about the precise values of the inputs. Scenario analyses provide 'what if' analyses: combinations of scores and weights that might be more appropriate as more data are obtained or the context changes. This can be a useful way of testing whether or not to collect additional data—there is no point in collecting data if it won't change the overall result. Sensitivity analyses are displayed as line graphs, one line for each option.

Principle 16: Explore the Robustness of Conclusions Using Sensitivity Analyses and Scenario Analyses
These methods are commonly used in MCDA modelling to explore uncertainty about outcomes. As mentioned at the start of the chapter, MCDA can also accommodate probabilities, which provide another way to deal with uncertainty: through application of the expected value or utility rule. More information about this approach is given in Chapter 5.

It is important to recognise that the overall purpose of an MCDA is to provide a guide to action, not to give 'the right answer'. An MCDA model helps to stimulate creative thinking, deepens insight and lends structure to clarify thinking. Often an initial, rough model is constructed, mainly relying on the judgements of experts, with participants role-playing alternative points of view to identify those areas needing more work. This focuses subsequent efforts on only those aspects that are crucial to obtaining an agreed result and guides the data collection process.

Applying these principles for creating an MCDA model can result in a model that truly represents the collective expertise of a group of experts and that could be replicated with another group of competent experts. This was demonstrated by a replication in 2013 for the European Union of the 2010 UK drug harms study (van Amsterdam et al. 2015). The correlation between the final weighted preference values in the two studies was 0.993, quite unexpected from two different groups of experts using the same criteria after changing about 10 % of the scores and reassessing all the weights. Future research should look for opportunities to confirm this capability of 'best practice' MCDA modelling in other settings.

16.12 Conclusion

Some critics have objected that MCDA is just a process of collecting opinions and personal judgements, disqualifying it from being considered a proper scientific approach. As we have seen, MCDA is based on an axiomatic theory that derives expected utility and weighted utility as consequences of the assumption that decision-makers are concerned to make decisions that are not self-contradictory. The result is a theory whose elements for healthcare are usually measureable data and subjective judgements, with the latter representing clinical judgement. Expressing those judgements in the explicit, quantified form of value functions and criterion weights is at first difficult for many experts, but I have found that gentle assistance is usually welcomed and after a brief period becomes almost second nature, with those quick to adapt, challenging others to 'stop waffling and give us a number'. It takes time to learn how to express one's intuition about clinical value as a preference score or clinical relevance as a numerical weight or uncertainty as a probability.

When data are sparse, as in the case of drug harms, care is taken to enquire on what basis the scores are assigned. For example, in the original decision conference for the six painkiller drugs, the experts provided data for the three favourable effects and one unfavourable effect (adverse skin reactions). But they were unable to locate good studies for any of the remaining seven unfavourable effects (an astonishing fact in itself given how many billions of tablets have been consumed over many years worldwide), so they made direct assessments of the options on 0–100 preference scales. To do this, they relied on their extensive experience with the drugs, their knowledge of the mechanisms of action of the drugs, theories about pain and other considerations, all of which were openly discussed to consensus. It is informed judgements that form the inputs to an MCDA model, not opinions.

When data are available, they are used. If data are absent, then judgements are made, but on predefined scales with two points on the scale clearly defined. This enables experts to assess meaningful relative values and weights, with consistency checks made to ensure that the relative scores of several options and the criteria weights are defensible. Impartial facilitation helps to legitimise information, whatever the source, and to ensure that all experts have their say. Participants are chosen to represent the diversity of opinion about the topic, and peer review is most vigorous at the stage of scoring and weighting, as participants express their judgements in numerical form. It is common for experts to disagree, but assigning numbers often reveals differences in perspective that reflect each person's past experience. Sharing that experience in a workshop setting provides a degree of learning that enables a model to be constructed. The point is to create a model that represents the current state of knowledge and judgement of a collection of experts, which contributes to the validity and reliability of the final results.

Acknowledgements I am indebted to Kevin Marsh, Mireille Goetghebeur, Praveen Thokala and Rob Baltussen for their comments on the original draft, as well as suggestions from colleagues at the June 2015 meeting of all authors of this book's chapters. These have improved the text by helping me to broaden, sharpen and illustrate the discussion to apply across the many methods that deal with multiple criteria.

References

Advisory Council on the Misuse of Drugs (2010) Consideration of the use of multi-criteria decision analysis in drug harm decision making. Home Office, London

Belton V, Gear AE (1983) On a short-coming of Saaty's method of analytic hierarchies. Omega 11(3):228–230

Belton V, Stewart TJ (2002) Multiple criteria decision analysis: an integrated approach. Kluwer Academic Publishers, Boston/Dordrecht/London

Bond SD, Carlson KA, Keeney R (2010) Improving the generation of decision objectives. Decis Anal 7(3):238–255

Dodgson J, Spackman M, Pearman A, Phillips L (2000) Multi-criteria analysis: a manual. London: Department of the Environment, Transport and the Regions, republished 2009 by the Department for Communities and Local Government

Dyer JS (1990) Remarks on the analytic hierarchy process. Manage Sci 36(3):249–258

Franco LA, Montibeller G (2010) Facilitated modelling in operational research. Eur J Oper Res 205(3):489–500

Hardin G (1968) The tragedy of the commons. Science 162:1243–1248

Howard RA (1966) Decision analysis: applied decision theory. In: Hertz DB, Melese J (eds) Proceedings of the fourth international conference on operational research. Wiley-Interscience, New York, pp 55–71

Johnson FR (2006) Measuring conjoint stated preferences for pharmaceuticals: a brief introduction. RTI Health Solutions, Research Triangle Park

Kahneman D (2011) Thinking, fast and slow. Allen Lane, London

Keeney RL (1992) Value-focused thinking: a path to creative decisionmaking. Harvard University Press, Cambridge

Keeney RL, Raiffa H (1976) Decisions with multiple objectives: preferences and value tradeoffs. John Wiley, New York

Kepner CH, Tregoe BB (1965) The rational manager. Kepner-Tregoe, Princeton

Kleinmuntz DN (2007) Resource allocation decisions. In: Edwards W, Miles RF Jr, Von Winterfeldt D (eds) Advances in decision analysis: from foundations to applications. Cambridge University Press, Cambridge, pp 400–418

Krantz DH, Luce RD, Suppes P, Tveresky A (1971) Foundations of measurement. Academic, San Diego/London

LSE/Catalyze (2011) Hiview3 starter guide. Catalyze Ltd, Winchester

Marsh K, Lanitis T, Neasham D, Orfanos P, Caro J (2014) Assessing the value of healthcare interventions using multi-criteria decision analysis: a review of the literature. Pharmacoeconomics 32(4):345–365

Meehl PE (1996) Clinical versus statistical prediction: a theoretical analysis and a review of the evidence. Jason Aronson; Original 1954 edition, University of Minnesota Press, Northvale

Mt-Isa S, Peters R, Phillips LD, Chan K, Hockley KS, Wang N et al (2013a) Review of visualisation methods for the representation of benefit-risk assessment of medication: stage 1 of 2. PROTECT Consortium, London

Mt-Isa S, Hallgreen CE, Asiimwe A, Downey G, Genov G, Hermann R et al (2013b) Review of visualisation methods for the representation of benefit-risk assessment of medication: stage 2 of 2. PROTECT Consortium, London

Nutt DJ, King LA, Phillips LD, on behalf of the Independent Scientific Committee on Drugs (2010) Drug harms in the UK: a multicriteria decision analysis. Lancet 376:1558–1565

Phillips LD (1984) A theory of requisite decision models. Acta Psychol (Amst) 56:29–48

Phillips LD (2007) Decision conferencing. In: Edwards W, Miles RF, von Winterfeldt D (eds) Advances in decision analysis: from foundations to applications. Cambridge University Press, Cambridge

Phillips LD, Bana e Costa CA (2007) Transparent prioritisation, budgeting and resource allocation with multi-criteria decision analysis and decision conferencing. Ann Oper Res 154(1):51–68

Phillips LD, Hays WL, Edwards W (1966) Conservatism in complex probabilistic inference. IEEE Trans Hum Factors Electron HFE-7:7–18

PROTECT Benefit-Risk Project. PROTECT Benefit-Risk website. 2015. Cited; Available from: PROTECTBenefitRisk.eu

Raiffa H (1968) Decision analysis. Addison-Wesley, Reading

Raiffa H (1969) Preferences for multi-attributed alternatives. Santa Monica: The RAND Corporation. Report No.: RM-5868-DOT/RC

Raiffa H, Schlaifer R (1961) Applied statistical decision theory. Harvard University Press, Cambridge

Ramsey FP (1926) Truth and probability. Published 1931 in. The foundations of mathematics and other logical essays, Ch VII: edited by R.B. Braithwaite, Kegan, Paul, Trench, Trubner & Co., London/Harcourt, Brace and Company, New York. 1999 electronic edition. pp 156–198

Savage LJ (1954) The foundations of statistics. 2nd edn, 1972. Dover ed. Wiley, New York

Schlaifer R (1969) Analysis of decisions under uncertainty. McGraw-Hill, New York

Thurstone LL (1959) The measurement of values. University of Chicago Press, Chicago

van Amsterdam J, Nutt D, Phillips L, van den Brink W (2015) European rating of drug harms. J Psychopharmacol 29(6):655–660

von Neumann J, Morgenstern O (1947) Theory of games and economic behavior, 2nd edn. Princeton University Press, Princeton

von Winterfeldt D, Edwards W (1986) Decision analysis and behavioral research. Cambridge University Press, Cambridge

MIX
Papier aus verantwortungsvollen Quellen
Paper from responsible sources
FSC® C105338

If you have any concerns about our products,
you can contact us on
ProductSafety@springernature.com

In case Publisher is established outside the EU,
the EU authorized representative is:
Springer Nature Customer Service Center GmbH
Europaplatz 3, 69115 Heidelberg, Germany

Printed by Libri Plureos GmbH
in Hamburg, Germany